Diagnosis in color

Neurology

Malcolm Parsons
MA, FRCP

Lately Consultant Neurologist
The General Infirmary at Leeds

**Senior Clinical Lecturer
in Neurology**
University of Leeds

Michael Johnson
DM, FRCP

Consultant Neurologist
St James's University Hospital, Leeds

**Senior Clinical Lecturer
in Neurology**
University of Leeds

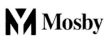 Mosby

EDINBURGH LONDON NEW YORK PHILADELPHIA SYDNEY TORONTO 2001

MOSBY

An imprint of Harcourt Publishers Limited

© Mosby International Ltd 2001

M is a registered trademark of Harcourt Publishers Limited

The rights of Malcolm Parsons and Michael Johnson to be identified as authors of this work have been asserted by them in accordance with the Copyright, Designs and Patents Act 1988.

First published 2001

ISBN 0 7234 3179 5

British Library Cataloguing in Publication Data
A catalogue record for this book is available from the British Library

Library of Congress Cataloging in Publication Data
A catalog record for this book is available from the Library of Congress

Note
Medical knowledge is constantly changing. As new information becomes available, changes in treatment, procedures, equipment and the use of drugs become necessary. The authors and the publishers have taken care to ensure that the information given in this text is accurate and up-to-date. However, readers are strongly advised to confirm that the information, especially with regard to drug usage, complies with the latest legislation and standards of practice.

Printed in China

The publisher's policy is to use **paper manufactured from sustainable forests**

Commissioning Editor: Richard Furn
Project Development Manager: Siân Jarman
Design Direction: Judith Wright
Project Manager: Frances Affleck

Contents

'Many cases conform to no recognisable type with which we are familiar. This is especially true of cases of diseases of the nervous system. The only way to deal with them is to perceive what the symptoms mean, individually or combined, and to treat each case as if it were a new problem'. (WR Gowers)

Preface

Neurological demonstrations have always been popular because of their wealth of visible signs. The apparent complexity of these signs has, however, earned the subject an (undeserved) reputation of being difficult. It is therefore surprising that among the innumerable textbooks of neurology there is virtually none which attempts to illustrate them and to explain their anatomical basis and significance. This we have tried to do.

The book is in essence a third, more affordable edition of the *Wolfe Colour Atlas of Clinical Neurology*. It covers the same ground as the earlier book and contains approximately the same number of illustrations, although the text has been shortened and only essential references have been retained. It gives examples of virtually all the abnormalities likely to be seen on a neurological ward and uses simple anatomical diagrams to explain their origin. It shows, in the context of brief case histories, how these signs should be interpreted and investigated and demonstrates the causative lesions radiologically and, in many instances, with surgical photographs or pathological specimens. The material is arranged in a conventional manner and each section, which is complete in itself, starts from a basic level. We have, however, worked our way through to some difficult and unusual cases, partly to give them publicity but mainly to show how, with a logical approach, the site and the nature of the lesion can still be elucidated. In this way we hope that a student, in addition to seeing and understanding all the major signs, will be able to learn how the 'neurological mind' works.

This is not another textbook of neurology, of which there are already far too many. Rather it is an attempt to bridge the gap between a theoretical knowledge of the subject and the practicalities of examining patients and interpreting and investigating their signs. As such, we hope that it will be of value to students at every level of training.

Leeds   M.P.
2000   M.J.

Acknowledgements

First and foremost we would like to thank the patients whose histories are discussed for their generous cooperation. At a time when conflicts between the public and the profession receive so much publicity it is perhaps worth mentioning that in over 30 years there have only been two occasions on which a request for clinical photographs for teaching purposes met with anything other than enthusiastic cooperation.

We would also like to thank the many colleagues in various parts of the country who have invited us to see their patients, Miss Rennee Bailey and Mr H. Grayshon Lumby for the illustrations and the many photographers, pathologists, radiologists, radiographers and technicians whose work is illustrated. In particular we would like to thank Mr Miles Gibson and Mr P. van Hille who provided many of the surgical illustrations and Dr Graham Bonsor who loaned some additional scans and advised on the radiological reports. We would also like to express our gratitude for permission to reproduce the following illustrations:

13.16	Dr D. A. Burns
7.15	Dr D. G. F. Harriman
3.78	Mr A. and Dr M. Jefferson and the *British Journal of Surgery*
3.58, 6.9	Mr A. and Dr M. Jefferson and the *Proceedings of the Royal Society of Medicine*
3.24	Dr R. E. Laidlaw and the *St Louis Mosby Year Book*
3.7–3.9	Mrs J. MacKarell and the *National Society for Education in Art and Design*
9.31	Dr S. Nurick and the *British Journal of Hospital Medicine*
6.44	Prof. M. A. Smith
7.84	The *British Medical Journal*.

1.

Higher functions

Assessment of the 'higher functions' of the brain – the most difficult and neglected part of the neurological examination – tests the integrity of the 'silent areas' of the hemispheres. Focal lesions may produce impairment of mood, aphasia, apraxia or agnosia. Diffuse lesions (which can of course produce similar symptoms) may also cause dementia and impairment of consciousness. The manifestations of these lesions, which are sometimes bizarre, often occur in isolation. It is therefore important not only that they should be recognised as organic in origin but also that they should be recognised as a sign (and often a localising sign) of damage to the hemispheres.

Cooperation and mood

The accuracy of a history can be impaired by a patient's mood. Some, having been asked to repeat their story several times, have simply become uncooperative. In others the problem is one of apathy due to depression or of inattention due to euphoria. Euphoria can be an important sign in patients with multiple sclerosis or lesions in the frontal lobes.

Aphasia

Aphasia is defined as an inability to exchange spoken or written ideas when the mechanisms of speech and writing are intact and the patient is not demented, blind or deaf. In some instances this disability is so mild that it can only be demonstrated when the patient is deliberately flustered and to detect it speech, writing and the ability to comprehend the spoken and written word have to be scrutinised individually. In others the loss of expression or comprehension is so profound that the conscious but uncommunicative patient is thought to be 'confused'. But the majority show, through expletives or interjections ('goodbye!') or the ability to chant or sing that the 'mechanism of speech' is intact. The importance of the sign is that it shows that there is a lesion in a cerebral hemisphere, usually on the dominant side.

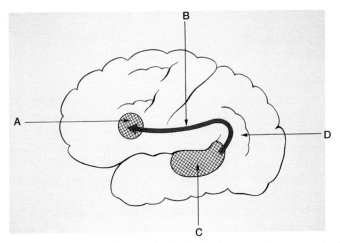

1.1 The anatomy of speech. Textbook diagrams give an oversimplified impression of the organisation of speech. Broadly speaking, however, lesions in the inferior frontal gyrus (Broca's area) produce a non-fluent, expressive aphasia (A). Those with lesions in the arcuate fasciculus (B) have normal comprehension but are unable to repeat what they hear. More posteriorly placed lesions in the superior temporal gyrus (Wernicke's area, C) produce jargon aphasia in a patient who cannot understand speech or writing. Lesions in the angular gyrus (D) produce alexia and agraphia.

1.2 Expressive aphasia. A patient who complained that when trying to write a message her 'hand had gone funny – I just couldn't spell'. The non-fluent nature of the text, her inability to find words and her awareness of the many errors are evident.

1.3 Fluent aphasia. In marked contrast to the previous example the flow of words is uninterrupted, although a patient with normal comprehension would have been dissatisfied with the repetition of the same simple message (perseveration).

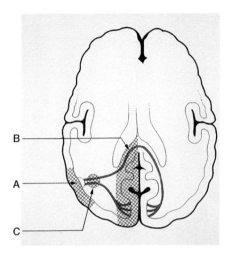

1.4 Word blindness. Lesions in the region of the dominant angular gyrus (A) produce alexia, agraphia, acalculia, left/right disorientation and finger agnosia (inability to identify individual digits) – Gerstmann's syndrome. Occlusion of the posterior cerebral artery may however produce alexia without agraphia by destroying the left visual cortex and severing the association fibres from the intact cortex on the right (B). Subcortical lesions (C) have a similar effect without producing a hemianopia.

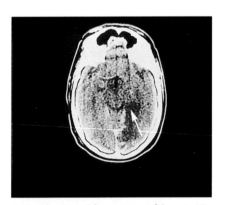

1.5 Alexia without agraphia. A 57-year-old man who complained of bumping into things on the right and of impairment of memory. These symptoms were due to infarction in the territory of the left posterior cerebral artery (arrow) which had destroyed the visual cortex and extended into the medial aspect of the temporal lobe and hippocampus. The angular gyrus was intact, so he could still write. He was however unable to read his own writing because the visual cortex on the left and the association fibres from the right had been destroyed (1.4B). As is often the case with such lesions he also had colour and object agnosia. He could match colours but could not name them and mistook an electric razor for a camera until it was switched on and he recognised the sound. Note that here and elsewhere we have followed the convention of showing the left side of the body on the right side of the scan.

Apraxia

Apraxia is defined as an inability to make movements to order when the nature of the request is understood and there is no significant impairment of power, sensation or coordination. Thus in apraxia of gait – one of the most common forms – a patient who cannot put one foot in front of the other when walking is yet able to lie on his back and 'pedal' with his feet in the air. Apraxia and aphasia are closely linked anatomically, for the lesion usually lies in the supramarginal gyrus of the dominant hemisphere (1.6). It is therefore important to ensure that the failure to respond is due to apraxia and not to receptive aphasia (i.e. incomprehension). As with aphasia the manifestations range from trivia evident only on close scrutiny (e.g. the use of the fist as a hammer or the palm as a saw blade when miming the use of tools) to the gross misuse of everyday objects. Constructional and dressing apraxia, which are based on a faulty conception of space, are usually due to lesions in the non-dominant hemisphere.

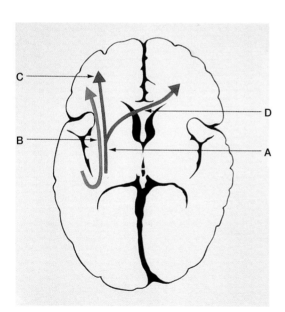

1.6 Apraxia. Lesions in the left supramarginal gyrus (A) produce bilateral apraxia which is often associated with aphasia due to involvement of the arcuate fasciculus and adjacent parts of the speech mechanism (B). Lesions in the left frontal lobe (C) produce apraxia in the limbs on the right while damage to fibres to or in the right frontal lobe (D) produces apraxia on the left.

Agnosia

An alert patient with normal sensation who is unable to recognise familiar objects, colours, sounds etc. is said to have agnosia. This disorder, which tends to affect one modality of sensation, can often be bypassed if another is used. Thus a patient with tactile agnosia may describe the size, shape and texture of the object in his hand, but is unable to recognise it as an orange until it is seen, smelt or tasted. Patients who can see but cannot recognise common objects are said to have *visual associative agnosia*. Those who only identify certain fragments or features of the object presented but fail to grasp the whole are said to have *apperceptive agnosia* – a condition which may in fact be due to a complex disorder of visual exploration rather than true agnosia.

Agnosia may loosely be regarded as the sensory counterpart and mirror image of apraxia as the causative lesion usually lies in the non-dominant parietal lobe. This, however, is not an absolute rule, for object and colour agnosia are sometimes found with lesions in the dominant occipital lobe and *prosopagnosia* – an inability to recognise individual faces, buildings etc. – is usually associated with bilateral occipital lesions.

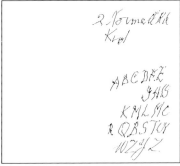

1.7

1.7–1.9 Neglect. Patients with lesions in the non-dominant hemisphere may also display defects of body image. Those with *tactile agnosia*, who appear to have normal sensation, ignore stimuli on the left when both sides are stimulated simultaneously. Those with *left–right disorientation* confuse the two sides of the body while those with *autotopagnosia* ignore the left side of the body and surrounding space. As a result they may fail to write on one side of a page (1.7), to copy the left side of a diagram (1.8) or to wash or even to recognise the left side of their bodies. The effects of this disorder can be bewildering. Thus one patient, a skilled amateur photographer, began to produce batches of films which were all clearly 'off centre' (1.9). As with the other two patients illustrated this was the only obvious sign of cerebral damage.

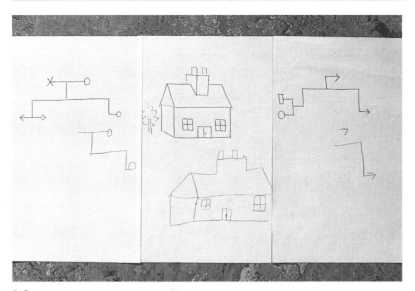

1.8

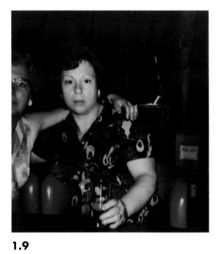

1.9

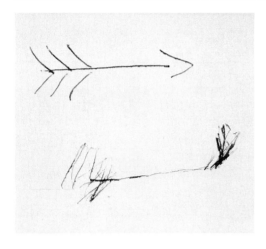

1.10 Constructional apraxia. Lesions in the non-dominant parietal lobe can also produce *topographical agnosia* in which a patient is unable to learn the layout of a strange ward or house and *constructional apraxia* in which he is unable to place one object correctly in relationship to another (e.g. when laying a table or drawing a diagram). This young patient, who appeared to have recovered from a cardiac arrest, was unable to copy the arrow. Constructional apraxia may also be seen with lesions of the angular gyrus.

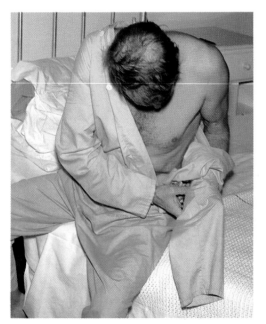

1.11 Dressing apraxia. Agnosia and spatial disorientation produced by injury to the non-dominant parietal lobe may account for dressing apraxia – a sign which is often concealed by well-meaning 'helpers'. Patients should therefore be left to dress themselves after examination (see also 6.30).

Dementia

Aphasia, apraxia and agnosia can all be caused by focal damage to the hemispheres. Dementia, with which all three can be associated, implies the presence of a more extensive, acquired and progressive lesion that cannot be attributed to any other cerebral disorder. Global deterioration is no longer required but in addition to increasingly severe impairment of memory the patient shows at least one other cognitive defect (aphasia, apraxia, agnosia or a disorder of executive function). Dementia must not be confused with depression or with delirium – an acute disturbance of cerebral function usually caused by (extrinsic and possibly reversible) factors such as infection, metabolic disorders, drugs or toxins.

The assessment of intelligence is a complicated process which involves comparing the patient's performance not only with the norm but also with what would be expected in the light of academic and occupational attainments. When testing for dementia the patient's account is rarely of value. Information from the family or from colleagues at work may however establish that there has been a clearcut deterioration in performance or behaviour. For comprehensive testing in borderline cases it is usually necessary to enlist the aid of a psychologist. In more straightforward cases the mini-mental state examination may suffice (see Folstein MF et al, *Journal of Psychiatric Research* 1975; 12: 189–198 or Harrison MJG, *Neurological Skills*, Butterworth, 1987, p 6).

Consciousness

As detailed assessment of consciousness requires a knowledge of the integration of the cranial nerves, which is discussed in Chapter 3, this topic is considered in Chapter 4.

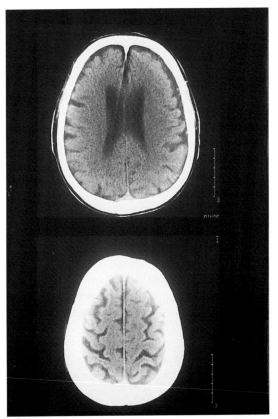

1.12 Investigation of dementia. Enquiries must be made about a family history of dementia or Huntington's chorea and a past history of alcoholism, trauma, anoxia, meningitis or encephalitis. Tests for syphilis, AIDS, hypothyroidism and B12 deficiency will be required. A CT scan will exclude a tumour and hydrocephalus (especially normal pressure hydrocephalus with enlarged ventricles but normal sulci in those with a history of subarachnoid haemorrhage, head injury or meningitis). In the majority, however, the scan will be normal or (as in the illustration) will show widening of the sulci and exposure of the falx by cerebral atrophy.

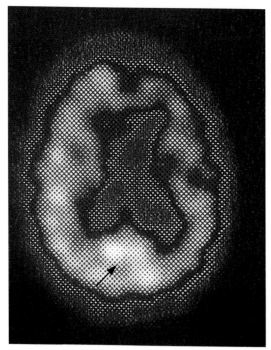

1.13 Investigation of dementia. Different forms of dementia produce lesions at different sites and by using MR and Single Photon Emission Computed Tomography (SPECT scanning) it is possible to study the regional anatomy and physiology. In this instance the normal, bright appearance of the cortex is only found in the posterior part of the brain (arrow). The darker image elsewhere – particularly on the right of the picture – is abnormal.

2.

Involuntary movements

Involuntary movements, unlike the majority of neurological disorders, do not lend themselves to precise analysis. Apart from doubts about the anatomical and biochemical basis of these conditions there may even be uncertainty about the nature of the movement under consideration, for in some instances different movements co-exist or merge into one another. Detailed discussion of this topic, which is not one which lends itself to illustration by still photography, is beyond the scope of this book, but examples of the main disorders are given below.

Tremor
Tremor, a rapid, repetitive, rhythmic movement, is classified as follows:

Resting tremor – present when the limb is at rest (e.g. Parkinson's disease).

Action tremor – present throughout movement (e.g. essential tremor).

Intention tremor – worse towards the end of a movement (cerebellar tremor).

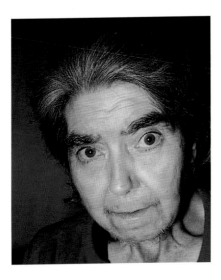

2.1 Parkinson's disease. The three components of this condition are tremor, plastic or cogwheel rigidity and akinesia. The 'pill-rolling' resting tremor characteristically disappears when the limb is in use, but does not always do so. Tremor of the head is uncommon. Tremor may indeed be absent and the insidious development of unilateral 'weakness' is often attributed to a cerebral tumour because the nature of the rigidity responsible and the patient's expressionless face have not been observed.

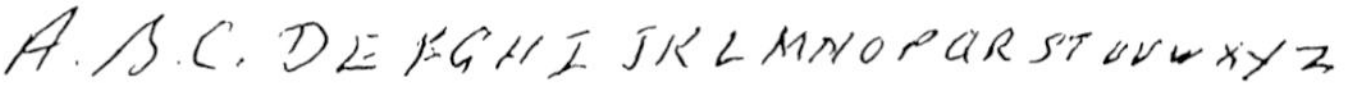

A·B·C·DEFGHIJKLMNOPQRSTUVWXYZ

2.2

Pinderfields   General Hospital   Wakefield

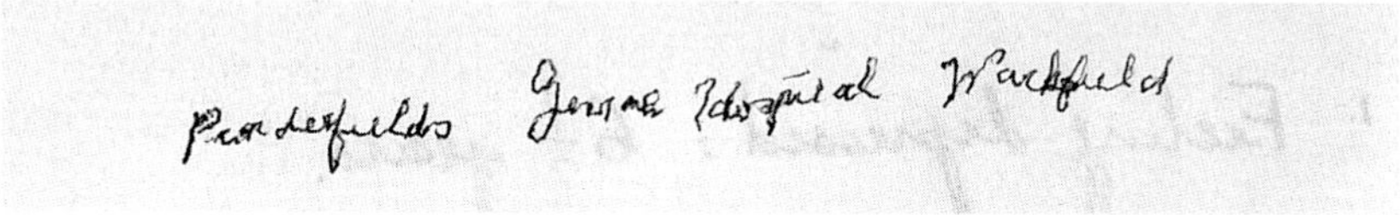

2.3A

Sample of her writing on discharge:

J.G.T. /

Pinderfields   General   Hospital

is a   good   hospital

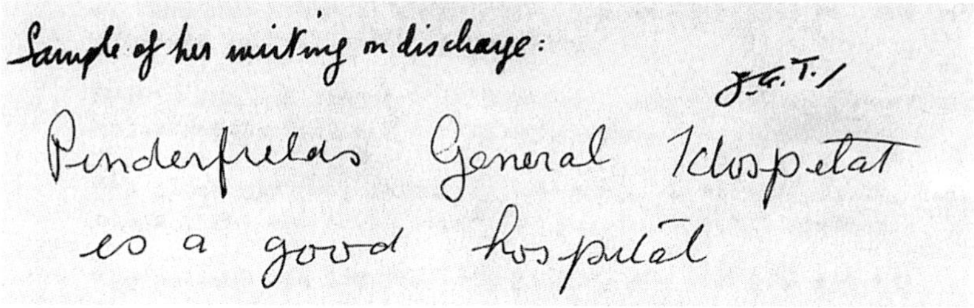

2.3B

2.2, 2.3A,B Writing in Parkinson's disease. The striking feature of Parkinsonian writing is not the tremor but a gradual diminution in size (micrographia 2.2). The severity of this problem is most evident when, with the withdrawal of phenothiazines, the condition is 'cured' (2.3A,B).

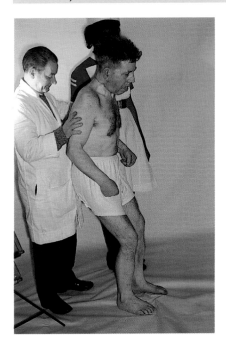

2.4 Posture in Parkinson's disease. Much of the disability in Parkinson's disease is caused by difficulty in initiating movements due to akinesia. This is often associated with a devastating tendency to fall without making any attempt to regain balance. Note the posture of the hands.

WASHING (AND ROUTINE TASKS   THE CUT OFF POINT IS QUITE

SUDDEN AND OFTEN LEAVES ONE IN AN EMBARESSING POSITION

WITH AMOUTH FULL OF UNCHEWED FOOD ETC.   ASSUMING THE

PRESENT LOW LEVELS OF ENERGY TO BE CONSUMED A PRACTICAL

DOSE WOULD BE ABOUT 16 TABLETS A DAY

2.5 Intellect in Parkinson's disease. Parkinson's statement that 'the senses and intellects are uninjured' is not, unfortunately, correct, for in the later stages of the disease dementia can occur. It is, however, far more likely that an expressionless, drooling, mute patient will be wrongly assumed to be demented. This patient was seen because he was thought to be incapable of making a will. Closer examination showed that he was in full possession of his faculties and, given a printing device, he produced this perceptive and well-phrased commentary on his treatment.

14.5.84.   *NORAH   MADDEN*   UNTREATED

14.6.84.   *NORAH MADDEN*   PROPRANOLOL
40 mgs. t.d.s.

2.6 Essential tremor. Unlike a Parkinsonian (resting) tremor an essential (action) tremor is present throughout movement. Patients therefore complain that they spill tea and soup and that their writing is illegible. The size of the letters, however, remains unchanged. The condition is inherited as a Mendelian dominant and often responds to alcohol or (as in this instance) to propranolol. Other causes of action tremor include thyrotoxicosis and a variety of toxic and metabolic disorders.

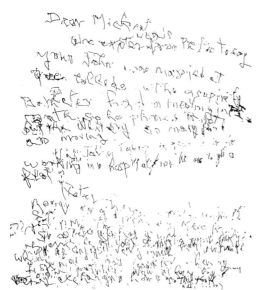

2.7 Cerebellar tremor. Cerebellar or intention tremor can be caused by a wide variety of toxic, demyelinating, infective, vascular and neoplastic disorders. It ranges in severity from a minor lack of precision at the extremes of the finger–nose test to a gross and disabling incoordination that makes the handwriting illegible.

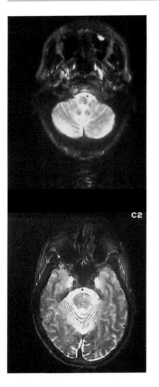

2.8 Shy–Drager syndrome. Progressive and often hereditary degeneration of the cerebellum is seen in a variety of disorders. It may appear in childhood (Friedreich's ataxia) or develop in middle life as a multi-system disorder (e.g. olivo-ponto-cerebellar atrophy), Parkinsonism (striato-nigral degeneration), axial stiffness and defective ocular movements (progressive supranuclear palsy) or – as here – with bladder dysfunction, impotence and postural hypotension (Shy–Drager syndrome). The MR scan, on which the CSF appears white, shows widening of the cerebellar sulci.

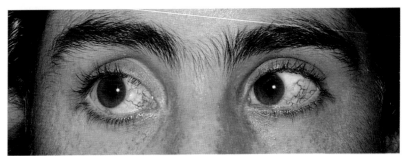

2.9 Ataxia telangiectasia. This autosomal recessive disorder may cause mild mental retardation but usually presents in childhood with ataxia and disorders of ocular movement. Telangiectasia of the conjunctiva, nose, ears and joint creases appears after the age of 5 and most patients die in their teens of a lymphoma or of an infection precipitated by a globulin deficiency.

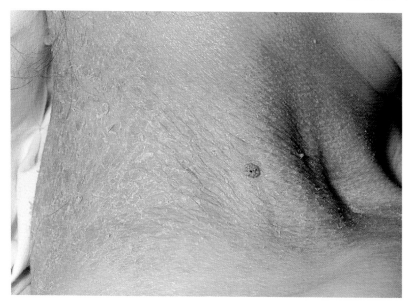

2.10 Refsum's syndrome. Icthyosis of the neck in a 40-year-old patient who presented with a 9-year history of difficulty with walking. A high serum phytanic acid level showed that she had Refsum's syndrome. Other manifestations include retinal pigmentation, deafness, hypertrophic polyneuritis, cerebellar ataxia, skeletal abnormalities and a high CSF protein. The condition improves if the chlorophyll derivative phytanic acid is excluded from the diet.

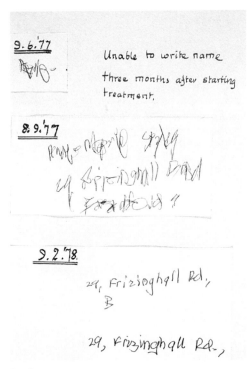

2.11

2.11, 2.12 Wilson's disease.

Therapeutic as well as eugenic considerations are also implicated in Wilson's disease. This 23-year-old student became tremulous, clumsy, apathetic, forgetful and depressed. Variable cerebellar and extrapyramidal signs were found and tests confirmed that she had Wilson's disease. Entries in her address book (2.11) show the gradual deterioration in her writing which improved (2.12) after treatment with penicillamine.

9.6.77

Unable to write name three months after starting treatment.

8.9.77

9.2.78.

29, Frizioghall Rd,
B

29, Frizinghall Rd,

2.12

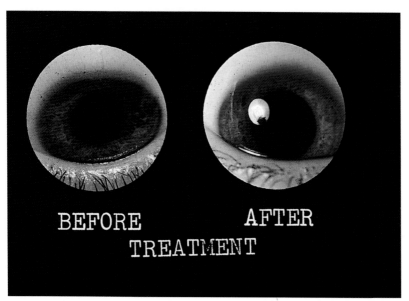

BEFORE   **AFTER**
TREATMENT

2.13 Kayser–Fleischer ring. The diagnosis of Wilson's disease can be confirmed by the observation of a Kayser–Fleischer ring – an area of golden-brown pigmentation at the periphery of the cornea. In most patients this lesion can only be seen on slit lamp examination, but here its presence and resolution during treatment are visible to the naked eye.

Other metabolic disorders associated with ataxia include type C Niemann–Pick disease, vitamin E deficiency and cholestanolosis.

Dystonia

The term dystonia is used to describe athetoid writhing movements or abnormal postures which are maintained for longer periods. *Primary dystonias* – which are often inherited – are rarely associated with other neurological abnormalities. In children the movement commonly starts in one foot and spreads to produce a devastating generalised abnormality known as dystonia musculorum deformans. Generalised dystonia may also be paroxysmal. Adults are more likely to have a segmental dystonia such as torticollis, blepharospasm or writer's cramp. *Secondary dystonias* are often associated with fits, spasticity or low IQ as in athetoid cerebral palsy due to anoxia or kernicterus and the unilateral dystonia that sometimes follows a stroke or surgery. The most common cause of secondary dystonia however is drugs such as phenothiazines, butyrophenones and metoclopramide. Rare but important causes include juvenile Huntington's chorea (which is hereditary) and Wilson's disease and the juvenile hereditary dystonic parkinsonian syndrome which are amenable to treatment.

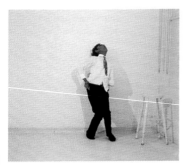 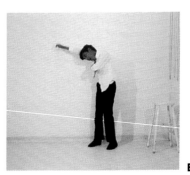

a   B

2.14A,B Paroxysmal dystonia. Pictures, taken over the course of a few seconds, of a child with kinesigenic dystonia. This disorder produces severe but transient athetoid movements when the patient is startled or moves suddenly as at the start of a race. It can be prevented if, when action is anticipated, the patient makes gentle jogging movements. A second form, induced by fatigue, tension, coffee and alcohol, causes bouts of athetosis that last for hours. A third form develops as the day progresses and responds to L-DOPA. All are inherited, usually as a dominant.

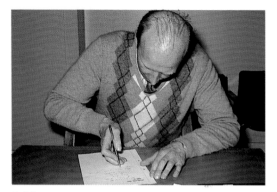

2.15

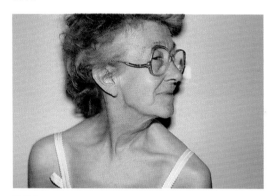

2.16

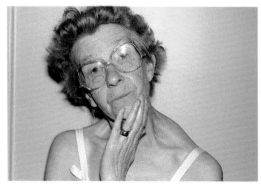

2.17

2.15 Writer's cramp. In this condition a patient's hand, which for other purposes is normal, assumes an increasingly abnormal posture as he tries to overcome diffi-culties with writing. This is one of a wide variety of occupational cramps that impede the main activity of musicians, watchmakers, golfers, painters, tellers etc. An occasional association with torticollis and the subsequent development of Parkinsonism or torsion dystonia in a few patients suggests an organic as opposed to a psychiatric cause. The condition is now being treated with botulinum toxin.

2.16,2.17 Spasmodic torticollis. The head may be rotated to one side (torticollis), backwards (retrocollis) or forwards (antecollis). Initially the movement is paroxysmal, is most evident when the patient is tense and can be controlled by a light touch on the side of the face (the geste antagonistique). In many the position of the head later becomes fixed and the patient develops cervical spondylosis. Although no pathological cause has been demonstrated, this is now regarded as a segmental dystonia which can be treated with botulinum toxin.

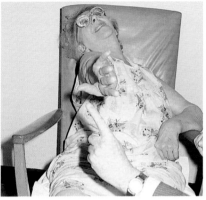 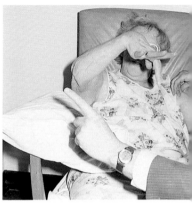

2.18   **2.19**

2.18,2.19 Secondary dystonia. Dystonic movements in a 70-year-old woman recovering from hemiballismus. The arm is characteristically extended and hyperpronated with flexion at the wrist and extension of the fingers. The foot was inverted and plantar-flexed with extension of the great toe. The head is turned to one side or backwards and there is an excessive lordosis and/or scoliosis.

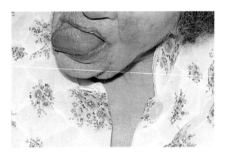

2.20 Orofacial dyskinesia. Involuntary chewing and grimacing movements with protrusion of the tongue (flycatcher tongue), restlessness (akathisia) and sometimes swaying of the trunk are common in patients treated for long periods with phenothiazines. No clearcut pathological cause has been demonstrated.

Chorea

Patients with chorea display a succession of irregular, unpredictable, jerky movements affecting all parts of the body. They range from twitches of a finger or eyebrow to more violent movements that may impair the use of a limb. Many look almost deliberate, and patients may try to conceal them by incorporating them in other movements, giving a general appearance of restlessness. Rheumatic or Sydenham's chorea is now rare but hereditary chorea and chorea due to L-DOPA are common. The movement may also be seen in thyrotoxicosis, disseminated lupus, polycythaemia, encephalitis, anoxia and after vascular accidents.

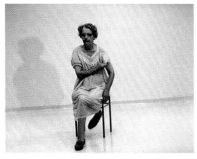 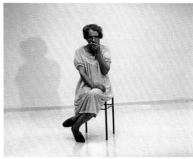

A   **B**

2.21A,B Chorea. Two pictures taken over a brief period with the patient 'sitting still'. In isolation, the way in which she pushes her handkerchief into her sleeve could pass as normal. However, seen in the context of a succession of other actions (entwining the legs, kicking the heel, wiping the mouth, pursing the lips etc.) it becomes evident that it was a 'camouflaged' choreiform movement.

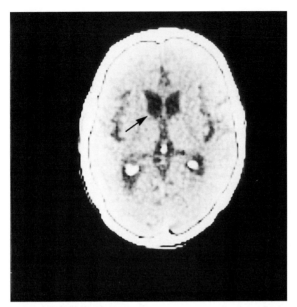

2.22 Huntington's chorea. Huntington's chorea, which is inherited as a dominant, usually presents in middle life with a combination of chorea and dementia. Some authorities believe that senile chorea without dementia is a variation of the same disorder. The juvenile (Westphal) form which presents with dementia, rigidity and epilepsy must not be confused with the benign hereditary chorea of childhood that does not affect the intellect or shorten life. The scan, from an adult patient, shows generalised atrophy and atrophy of the caudate nucleus which normally indents the lower lateral part of the lateral ventricle. This gives the ventricle a 'square' appearance (arrow – cf. 3.82)

Myoclonus

Myoclonic jerks are irregular, brief, shock-like movements that may be focal or diffuse. They may occur *in isolation* as in benign nocturnal myoclonus or *in association with epilepsy*, including salaam attacks and the sudden muscular inhibition (negative myoclonus) that causes the falls sometimes seen with absences. They may be associated *with progressive ataxia and epilepsy* – the condition once known as the Ramsay Hunt syndrome but now usually attributed to a mitochondrial cytopathy – or *with dementia* as in subacute sclerosing panencephalitis and spongiform encephalopathy. They may also be seen *with anoxia, uraemia, liver failure and after the withdrawal of alcohol and certain drugs.*

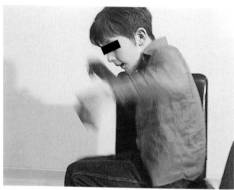

2.23

2.23, 2.24 Myoclonus. A 9-year-old child whose academic deterioration was attributed to 'late nights' until, some months later, he began to wet the bed and developed violent myoclonic jerks. He had had an attack of measles 3 years earlier, but the antibody level was still abnormally high and periodic discharges typical of sclerosing panencephalitis were found on the EEG (2.24 arrows). The diagnosis was confirmed by brain biopsy.

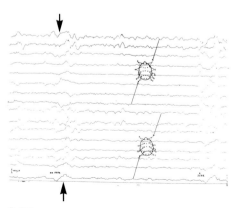

2.24

Involuntary movements of the face

The head may be the site of a senile or cerebellar tremor, and a tremor of the lips or tongue is sometimes seen in Parkinson's disease. Dystonic movements such as torticollis, orofacial dyskinesia and blepharospasm can occur, and facial tics (which occur in up to 25% of children) have to be distinguished from chorea by the fact that they are stereotyped and can, for a time at least, be suppressed. Partial seizures sometimes present with twitching around the angle of the mouth and patients with multiple sclerosis may develop a peculiar squirming of the muscles known as facial myokymia. Other involuntary movements are discussed below.

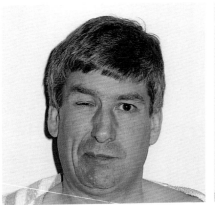 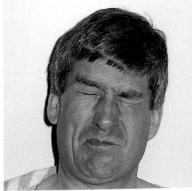

2.25　　　　　**2.26**

2.25,2.26 Hemifacial spasm. A visible twitching of one eyelid – benign myokymia – is a commonplace symptom. Some patients, however, develop paroxysmal involuntary closure of one eye that later spreads to involve the whole of one side of the face (2.25). In time this is associated with mild weakness of the affected side as shown by the inability to bury the eyelashes on screwing up the eyes (2.26). The condition has been attributed to compression of the facial nerve by an aberrant blood vessel, but treatment by decompression has been replaced with injections of botulinum toxin.

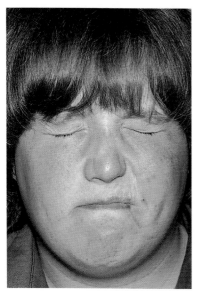 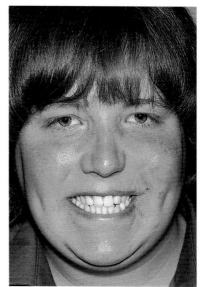

2.27   **2.28**

2.27,2.28 Aberrant regeneration of the facial nerve. When closing the eyes the patient seems to have weakness of the right side of the face (2.27). The appearance, however, is caused by involuntary contraction on the left due to aberrant regeneration of the facial nerve (note the facial scar). As shown on (2.28) movements of the right side of the face are in fact unimpaired.

3.

Cranial nerves

Visual acuity

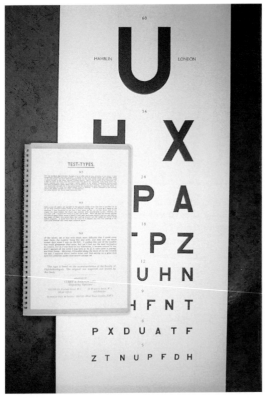

3.1 Visual acuity. When doing a neurological examination the visual acuity should be recorded. Near vision is tested with the patient holding a Faculty of Ophthalmologists' chart. Distant vision is tested with a Snellen wall chart at 6 metres. Patients who use glasses should wear them and the eyes should be tested individually. Note the smallest print which is legible (e.g. right N5, left N6) adding the word 'aided' if glasses were used. Distant vision is scored 6/6 if the patient can read 6-metre print at 6 metres, 6/9 if he can only read 9-metre print etc. This is a more sensitive test.

The fundus – papilloedema

Florid papilloedema can be recognised at a glance, but in early cases the components (3.2) have to be considered individually. The main causes are:

1. Intracranial hypertension – bilateral, with the emphasis on disc swelling.
2. Hypertension – bilateral, but with haemorrhages, exudates and vascular changes.
3. Retinal vein thrombosis – unilateral with distended veins and massive haemorrhages.
4. Retrobulbar neuritis at nerve head (papillitis) – unilateral with severe loss of vision.
5. Acute ischaemic neuropathy – unilateral, with severe loss of vision and often with contralateral optic atrophy.

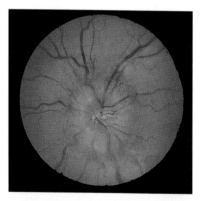

3.2 Papilloedema in a patient with benign intracranial hypertension. The disc is pink, the cup is obliterated and the veins are distended. The disc margin is ill-defined and it is impossible to trace the course of some vessels as they arch upwards over its swollen border.

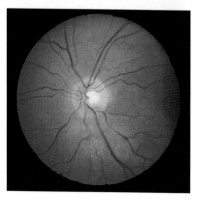

3.3 Normal fundus. Case 3.2 after recovery. The fundus is now virtually normal. The disc is paler, the cup is visible and the veins are no longer distended. The disc margin is sharp and crossing vessels are clearly visible.

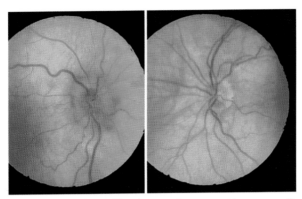

3.4 Unilateral papilloedema. A patient with gross swelling on the right but a relatively normal disc on the left. This not uncommon finding may be due to a variation in the structure of the optic nerve sheath which protects one eye from the effects of intracranial hypertension. A subfrontal tumour may have a similar effect, producing ipsilateral optic atrophy – sometimes with anosmia – and contralateral papilloedema (the Foster Kennedy syndrome – see 6.15).

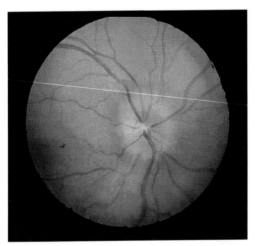

3.5 Papillitis (demyelination at the tip of the optic nerve). The appearance is that of papilloedema. In papilloedema, however, vision is usually normal, except perhaps during exertion when transient blurring occurs because venous stasis exposes the retina to the effect of hypotension. In papillitis, by contrast, vision is severely impaired.

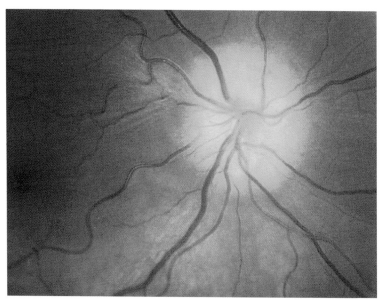

3.6 Pseudopapilloedema. Some healthy patients have discs which look abnormal. This man had symptoms suggestive of raised intracranial pressure. The disc and cup are ill defined and the vessels appear to arch upwards over the disc margin. The scan and the CSF pressure were, however, normal and fluorescin angiography confirmed that the patient had not got papilloedema.

The fundus – retrobulbar neuritis

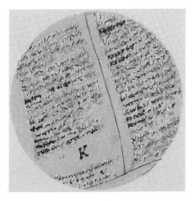

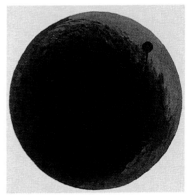

3.7

3.8

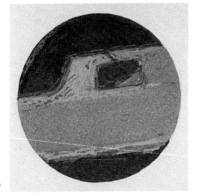

3.9

3.7–3.9 Retrobulbar neuritis is the most common neurological cause of monocular impairment of vision. Symptoms range from 'mistiness' to total blindness, but the characteristic defect is a central scotoma. As illustrated by the artist Peter MacKarell, this produces 'an infuriating bouncing grey dot' in the centre of the visual field which, in this 'patient's eye view', obscured an entry in a dictionary (3.7). He subsequently became completely blind on that side but a few weeks later, when 'looking at the examiner's voice' with his defective eye, he became aware of the (colourless) head of a medical pin beyond the edge of a central scotoma (3.8). Later still, when being driven home, he could see the shape of the car mirror and sun visor, although 'the outside world in the spring sunshine was enveloped in fog' (3.9). (From *Depictions of an Odyssey*, reproduced by kind permission of his widow and the National Society for Education in Art and Design.) Seventy per cent of patients with 'idiopathic' retrobulbar neuritis go on to develop multiple sclerosis.

The fundus – optic atrophy

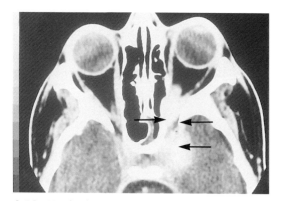

3.10 Meningioma compressing optic nerve. Compression of the optic nerve can also produce a central scotoma because the papillo-macular bundle is particularly susceptible to pressure. Like demyelination, this results in optic atrophy. In contrast to demyelination, however, the patient is often unaware of the defect until the 'good' eye is covered. Moreover, whereas patients with demyelination often have normal vision despite a very pale disc, patients with severe loss of vision due to compression of the optic nerve may (as in this instance) have a disc that looks normal. Here a meningioma has widened and eroded the optic canal (arrows) and extended backwards into the parasellar region (arrow).

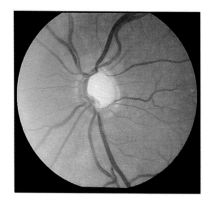

3.11 Optic atrophy. In optic atrophy the disc is pale, the response to light is impaired and the visual evoked response is abnormal. The pallor may be generalised, or may be confined to the temporal border where the papillo-macular fibres lie. Unless severe or asymmetrical it can be difficult to recognise, as the temporal border of the disc is always a little paler. Pigmentation around the disc, the pallor of the cup and a myopic disc can also cause confusion. In *primary* optic atrophy (due to demyelination, compression, ischaemia, trauma, toxins such as alcohol and tobacco, vitamin B12 deficiency, syphilis, hereditary and retinal disorders) the disc margin is sharp. In optic atrophy *secondary* to papilloedema the margin – at least initially – is blurred.

Visual fields

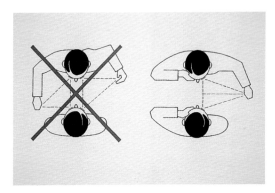

3.12 Examination of the visual fields. The visual fields must always be tested because patients are sometimes unaware that a defect is present. The arms should be fully extended and the hands must be kept midway between the examiner and the patient so that neither is working at an advantage. The ability to detect movements or count fingers is tested in each quadrant of each eye individually. When an abnormality is suspected (as in the case of a pituitary tumour) the ability to see the colour of a red hatpin provides an even more rigorous test.

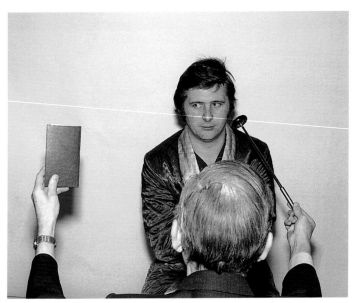

3.13 Testing fields in an uncooperative patient. A field defect may also be detected by showing that an object can be 'infiltrated' into one quadrant or half-field without attracting the patient's attention.

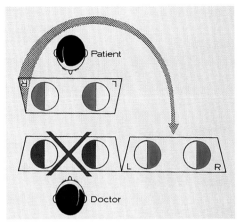

3.14 Charting the visual fields. It is customary to chart the fields as seen by the patient – a practice which produces a mirror image of the diagram most people draw instinctively. To avoid confusion the sides should be labelled.

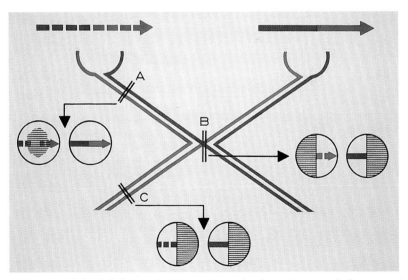

3.15 Visual field defects. Lesions anterior to the chiasm (e.g. retrobulbar neuritis) produce a defect in one eye (A). Lesions of the chiasm interrupt decussating fibres from the nasal half of each retina and produce a bitemporal field defect (B). Lesions behind the chiasm produce an homonymous hemianopia (C). Lesions in the occipital lobes produce generalised impairment of vision.

Visual fields – bitemporal hemianopia

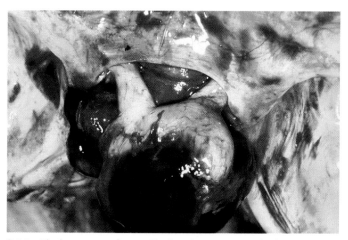

3.16 Pituitary apoplexy. The best known cause of a bitemporal hemianopia is compression of the decussating fibres in the chiasm by a pituitary tumour. In this instance a lethal haemorrhage (pituitary apoplexy, which presents with meningism, visual failure and/or ophthalmoplegia) has left the chiasm stretched tightly over the gland. Other causes of compression from below include aneurysms and meningiomas.

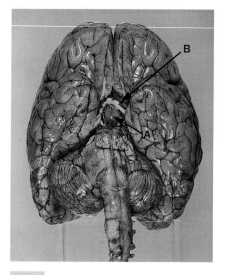

3.17 Enlargement of the third ventricle. In severe hydrocephalus enlargement of the third ventricle (A) can compress the chiasm (B) from above. Unlike pituitary tumours, which mainly affect the fibres from the lower part of the retina, such lesions (like craniopharyngiomas) affect fibres from the upper part, producing a predominantly inferior quadrantic bitemporal hemianopia (see 8.2–8.4).

Visual fields – homonymous hemianopia

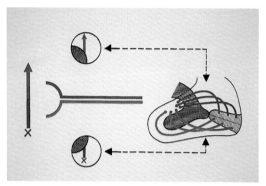

3.18 Homonymous hemianopia. Lesions behind the chiasm produce an homonymous hemianopia. Those in the geniculate body and radiation cause a defect of which the patient is aware because they 'split' the macula, making reading difficult. With vascular lesions in the calcarine cortex the macula, which is represented in the occipital pole and has a separate blood supply from the middle cerebral artery, is spared. Patients may therefore be unaware of the field defect, and this is a potent cause of road accidents. Lesions in the temporal lobes, which impinge on fibres from the lower part of the retina, produce a predominantly upper quadrantic defect. The converse applies to lesions in the parietal lobes.

Visual fields – occipital lobe lesions

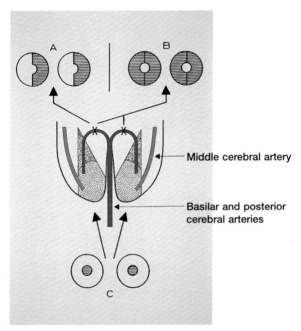

Middle cerebral artery

Basilar and posterior cerebral arteries

3.19 Occipital lobe lesions. Bilateral ischaemia of the occipital lobes, as in basilar migraine, produces an almost complete loss of vision. Patients with occlusion of one posterior cerebral artery have an homonymous hemianopia with macular sparing because the macula, represented in the occipital pole, has a separate supply from the middle cerebral artery (A). If subsequently the other posterior cerebral artery is occluded they are reduced to macular vision (B). Watershed infarcts (see 7.73) have a similar effect. Such patients – who cannot see large objects, but can see small ones which fit into their 'gunbarrel fields' – are often thought to be hysterics. By contrast, injury to the occipital poles produces a bilateral macular (central) field defect (C).

Proptosis

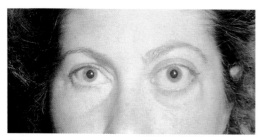

3.20

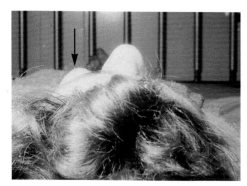

3.21

3.20, 3.21 Meningioma of optic nerve sheath.

A patient is said to have proptosis when, with the head erect and the gaze directed forwards, sclera is visible between the iris and the lower lid. The presence of unilateral proptosis can be confirmed by looking down onto the head and moving backwards until the 'eyes disappear over the horizon' (3.21 arrow). The situation of the lesion can often be determined from the position of the pupil which, in this instance, has been displaced upwards and outwards. Benign tumours – in this case a meningioma of the optic nerve sheath – progress slowly and cause pain but do not impair vision.

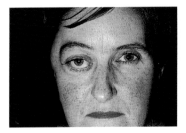

3.22

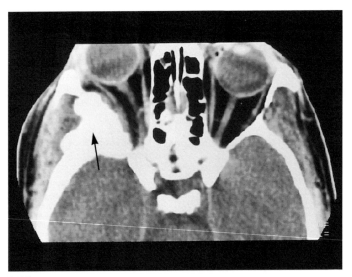

3.23

3.22,3.23 Sphenoid wing meningioma. A middle-aged woman with slowly developing right-sided proptosis and downward displacement of the globe. She also has a mass over the right temple. This (along with a tendency to train the hair forwards so as to conceal the mass) is the characteristic picture of a meningioma on the lateral third of the sphenoid wing, which produces the massive hyperostosis seen on the scan (arrow).

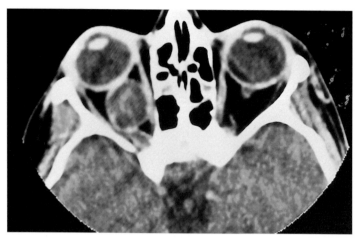

3.24 MR scan of orbital tumour. The investigation of proptosis is an area in which the technique of MR scanning has been of enormous value. In this film a cavernous haemangioma in the right orbit can be seen displacing the recti, indenting the globe and causing proptosis. (Reproduced by kind permission from *MR and CT Imaging of the Head, Neck and Spine*, RE Laidlaw (ed), Mosby-Year Book, St Louis, 1985.)

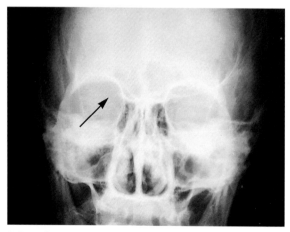

3.25 The 'empty orbit'. Proptosis due to a malignant tumour develops more rapidly and is associated with loss of vision. In this instance a secondary deposit from a bronchial carcinoma has eroded the lesser wing of the sphenoid on the right (arrow) producing the appearance of an 'empty orbit'.

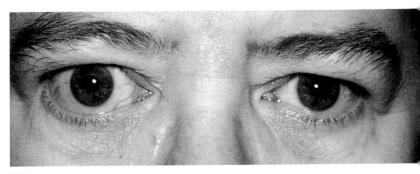

3.26

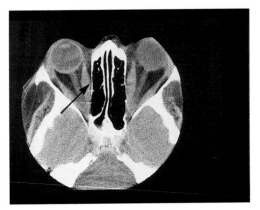

3.27

3.26,3.27 Endocrine exophthalmos. Patients with hyperthyroidism usually have bilateral proptosis and have, or have had, a goitre and thyrotoxicosis. The condition known as endocrine exophthalmos or ophthalmic Graves' disease is of more interest to neurologists as 50% of these patients – who have no history of thyrotoxicosis, no evidence of hyperthyroidism on basic tests and often no goitre – have proptosis which is confined to or worse on one side. Careful examination usually reveals unilateral or (as in this case) bilateral lid retraction, lid lag and/or impairment of upward gaze. A CT scan shows swelling of the extraocular muscles – especially the medial recti (arrow) – and more sophisticated tests of thyroid function are usually abnormal.

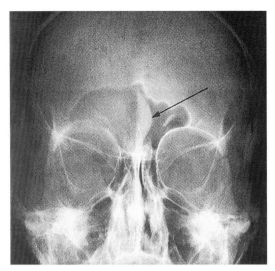

3.28 Mucocele. This defect is due to obstruction of the exit from the right frontal sinus. The sinus is opaque and distended, causing proptosis and displacement of the medial septum to the left (arrow).

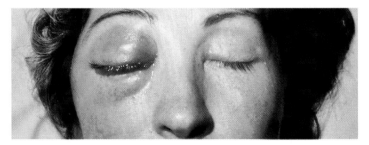

3.29 Carotico-cavernous fistula. Head injury or rupture of an atherosclerotic aneurysm in the cavernous sinus can result in a carotico-cavernous fistula. The patient develops proptosis which tends to be worse on bending and to be relieved by compression of the carotid artery. A bruit – of which the patient may be aware – is audible over the globe. Such lesions are best treated by balloon occlusion.

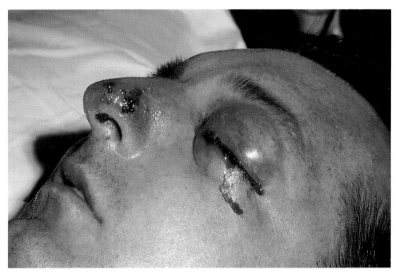

3.30 Cavernous sinus thrombosis. A patient who developed a boil on his nose followed, 24 hours later, by left-sided proptosis. He lost the eye and had a pulmonary embolus but survived after intensive treatment. Infections of the face, the sinuses, the teeth and the ear can travel via the veins to the cavernous sinus. They spread rapidly from one side to the other, producing unilateral and then bilateral proptosis and ophthalmoplegia. Unless controlled, they then extend backwards into the meninges or the brain. This is a lethal condition which requires intensive and prolonged antibiotic treatment. The use of heparin is also advised, particularly if haemorrhage can be excluded.

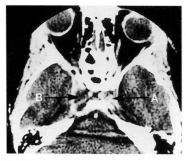

3.31

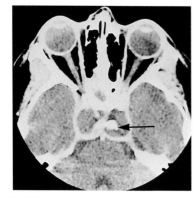

3.32

3.31–3.33 Cavernous sinus thrombosis.

This teenage child presented with a 3-week history of nasal obstruction followed by fever, headache and swelling of the right eye. She was found to have pansinusitis and 'orbital cellulitis', was treated with antibiotics and a sinus washout and was discharged in 5 days. She returned 3 weeks later with a right internal and external ophthalmoplegia. A CT scan showed that the left cavernous sinus was normal (3.31A) but that the right cavernous sinus was occluded by clot (3.31B). She had an ethmoidectomy and a further course of antibiotics, and 2 weeks later was said to be 'nearly normal'. Two weeks later still she was admitted for a third time with fever, left frontal headache, a left third nerve palsy and a right hemiplegia. A second scan showed that the left cavernous sinus was now also occluded (3.32 arrow) and that a large infarct was visible in the left hemisphere (3.33 arrow). This illustrates the danger of inadequate treatment with antibiotics and the aggressive nature of the infection (*see also 3.73–3.75*).

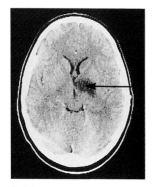

3.33

The pupil – reflex reactions

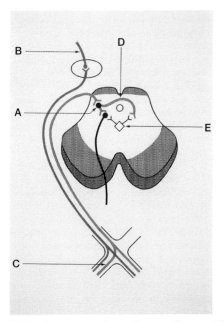

3.34 Anatomy of pupillary reflexes. The normal pupil contracts when exposed to light and when the eyes focus on a nearby object. When testing the light response it is important to use a powerful beam and to ensure that the patient does not produce a bogus reaction by fixing on the torch.

The light reflex is a midbrain reflex mediated via parasympathetic fibres from the Edinger Westphal component of the third nerve nucleus. As each nucleus receives afferent fibres from both eyes (A) the pupil of a blind eye will contract when the sound eye is illuminated. Likewise, because this is a brainstem reflex, the pupils of a patient with cortical blindness react to light (B).

With lesions in the afferent fibres – and especially with those in the optic nerve (C) – the response to light is slower, weaker and less well sustained. This is demonstrated with the 'swinging light test' in which the eyes are illuminated alternately for a few seconds at a time. As the beam falls on the defective eye the pupil appears to dilate – a Marcus Gunn pupil.

Pineal tumours and other lesions of the tectum (D) may damage the decussating afferent fibres as a result of which the pupils are fixed and dilated. The reaction of accommodation is, however, preserved because the nucleus of Perlia is intact (E).

Dilation of the pupil

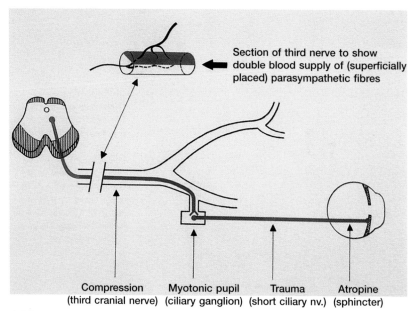

Section of third nerve to show double blood supply of (superficially placed) parasympathetic fibres

Compression	Myotonic pupil	Trauma	Atropine
(third cranial nerve)	(ciliary ganglion)	(short ciliary nv.)	(sphincter)

3.35

Anatomy of the parasympathetic pupilloconstrictor fibres. The size of the pupil is determined by the balance of parasympathetic pupilloconstrictor and sympathetic pupillodilator activity. The commonest cause of a dilated pupil is compression of the third cranial nerve to which the pupillo-constrictor fibres – which run superficially – are particularly susceptible. Such compression may be due to a tentorial pressure cone (3.36–3.37), a berry aneurysm (3.54–3.59) or to an aneurysm in the cavernous sinus (3.60–3.63). With ischaemic lesions, by contrast, the parasympathetic fibres are usually spared because they have a supply both from the core and the surface of the nerve. After leaving the third nerve the parasympathetic fibres may be damaged in the ciliary ganglion producing a myotonic pupil (3.38A,B), by trauma to the ciliary nerves or by atropine eye drops.

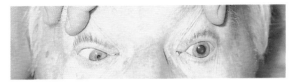

3.36

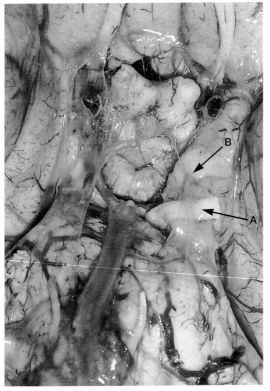

3.37

3.36, 3.37
Hutchinson's pupil.
The fixed dilated pupil of a patient with raised intracranial pressure (3.36) is due to a tentorial pressure cone. The third nerve (3.37A) is compressed by the temporal lobe (B) as it is forced between the midbrain and the tentorium.

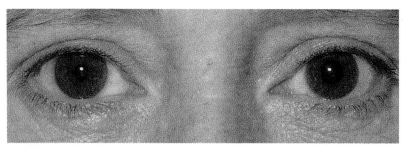

3.38A

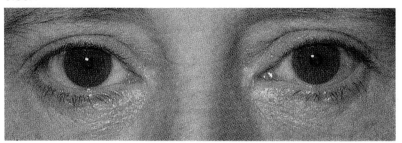

3.38B

3.38A,B Holmes Adie (myotonic) pupil. Young female patients occasionally
present with a dilated, regular pupil which has been noticed by chance or because the
patient complained of being dazzled by oncoming headlights (3.38A). The pupil does
not react to light but does constrict slowly on accommodation. The abnormality is due
to degeneration of the ciliary ganglion, and the residual response is due to inhibition
of the sympathetic fibres. As might be expected with a denervated muscle, the pupil
constricts with pilocarpine at a dilution (0.05%) that would not affect a normal eye
(3.38B). Loss of the light reaction and an associated loss of tendon reflexes in the legs
may raise the possibility of an Argyll Robertson pupil. The youth of the patient and the
size and regularity of the pupil make this improbable, although in later years (when
the pupil constricts) differentiation can be more difficult.

Constriction of the pupil

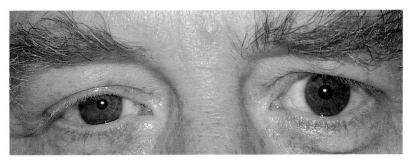

3.39 Horner's syndrome. Constriction of the pupil is seen in Horner's syndrome, in syphilis and with drugs such as pilocarpine and opium. Loss of sympathetic control allows the parasympathetic pupillo-constrictor fibres to act unopposed. It also causes ptosis, for the sympathetic shares with the third nerve the innervation of the levator palpebrae superioris, supplying the smooth muscle component. This lesion (Horner's syndrome) is easily overlooked, for the small pupil will not be evident in a bright light and the ptosis, which is slight and variable, is easily overcome by the third nerve.

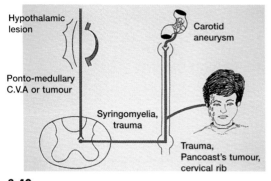

3.40

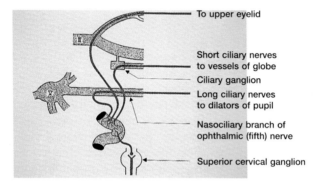

3.41

3.40,3.41 Anatomy of the cervical sympathetic. In isolation, Horner's syndrome is of little diagnostic value. It may be idiopathic or may occur with a variety of migraine-like syndromes such as cluster headache and Raeder's syndrome. It may also be a feature of lesions at various points along the long course of the sympathetic fibres. These arise in the hypothalamus and run ipsilaterally in the brainstem and cord to the first thoracic root (3.40). Here they leave the cord and ascend through the sympathetic chain to the superior cervical ganglion. From there they pass to the carotid artery and divide (3.41), fibres to the upper lid and conjunctival vessels running with the third nerve while those that control the pupil join the nasociliary branch of the ophthalmic. Horner's syndrome may therefore be a feature of pontine haemorrhage, of a lateral medullary syndrome (see 7.75–7.77), of syringomyelia (see 8.23–8.30), of Pancoast's tumour (see 11.24,11.25) or of injury to the brachial plexus (see 11.22,11.23). It is noteworthy that sweating is controlled by fibres which leave below the superior cervical ganglion. Facial anhydrosis therefore implies a lesion below that point (see 11.24).

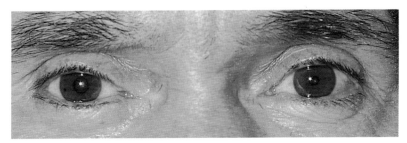

3.42 Argyll Robertson pupils are small, irregular and unequal. They do not react to light but react briskly on accommodation. The abnormality may be due to a tectal lesion of the type described in 3.34 which also involves the sympathetic tracts. Traditionally associated with tabes dorsalis and general paralysis of the insane it is now most commonly seen in diabetes.

Ptosis

Asymmetry or drooping of the lids over the pupil when the head is erect and for which there is no local cause is known as ptosis. Mild unilateral ptosis with a constricted pupil (Horner's syndrome) and total unilateral ptosis with a dilated pupil (third nerve palsy) are discussed elsewhere (3.39–3.41,3.54–3.56). Diseases of muscle, the myo-neural junction and the peripheral nerves can also cause ptosis. Here the disorder tends to be bilateral but not necessarily symmetrical. The furrowing of the brow seen with a third nerve palsy may be absent because the facial muscles are also affected.

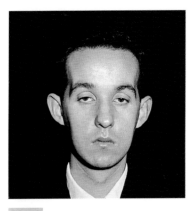

3.43 Dystrophia myotonica. In addition to bilateral ptosis the patient has a receding hairline, wasting of the temporalis muscles and an expressionless face. The facial weakness accounts for the absence of frontalis overactivity.

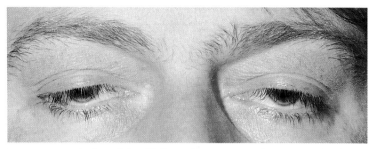

3.44 Congenital and familial ptosis. Ptosis may be congenital or familial. Ocular myopathy – often a mitochondrial myopathy known as the Kearns–Sayre syndrome – presents in early adult life with bilateral ptosis followed by external ophthalmoplegia and possibly facial palsy.

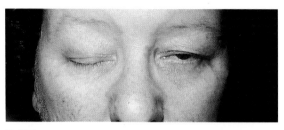

3.45A

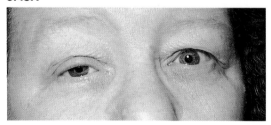

3.45B

3.45A,B Myasthenia gravis. Complete unilateral ptosis suggestive of a third nerve palsy which draws attention away from the fact that the other lid is also abnormal (3.45A). In fact the patient had myasthenia gravis with asymmetrical ptosis and responded to edrophonium (3.45B).

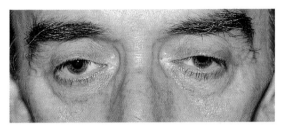

3.46 Miller Fisher syndrome. A 53-year-old man who had developed a nasal voice and diplopia. He had mild bilateral ptosis which he did not attempt to correct because of weakness of the facial muscles. He went on to develop a bilateral internal and external ophthalmoplegia and a bulbar palsy. Apart from areflexia his limbs were normal. He recovered spontaneously. The syndrome of cranial polyneuritis, ataxia and areflexia is known as the Miller Fisher variant of inflammatory demyelinating polyneuritis.

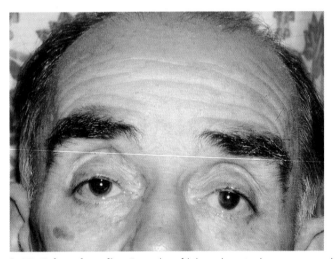

3.47 Tabes dorsalis. Examples of bilateral ptosis due to a myopathy, myasthenia and polyneuritis have already been given. The bilateral ptosis of tabes dorsalis, like the Argyll Robertson pupils with which it is associated, can also for convenience be thought of as attributable to destruction of sympathetic fibres in the midbrain. Note the compensatory contraction in the intact frontalis muscles.

The third and fourth cranial nerves

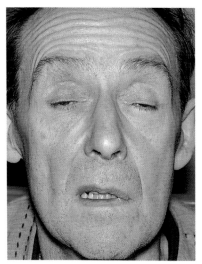

3.48

3.48–3.52 Ptosis due to infarction of the third nerve nucleus. This 56-year-old man, who had a strong history of vascular disease, had an ophthalmic examination in March and was normal. In April he had two fits during a bout of ventricular fibrillation. On recovery, despite overactivity of the frontalis, he was unable to open his eyes (3.48). Facial movements (3.49), convergence and the pupillary responses were normal but the eyes did not adduct on lateral gaze (3.50A,B) and initially he was unable to look upwards or downwards (3.51,3.52).

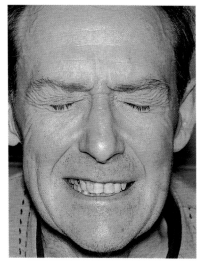

3.49

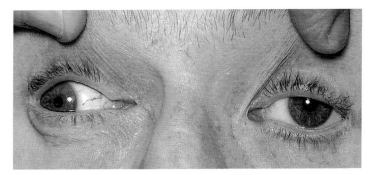

3.50A

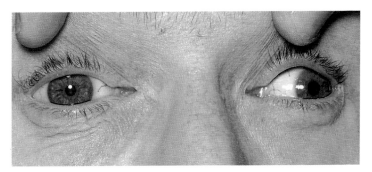

3.50B

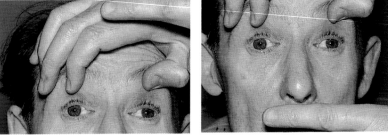

3.51

3.52

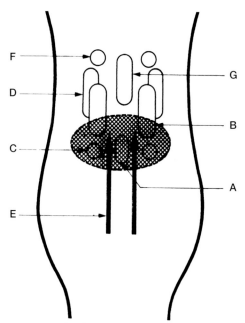

3.53 Ptosis due to infarction of third nerve nucleus (cont.). These findings are readily explained on the basis of an infarct in the shaded area of the third nerve nucleus. This structure is a series of parallel cylinders arranged in a rostro-caudal direction. In this instance the central caudal nucleus (A) which controls the levator palpebrae superioris, the ventrimedial nucleus (B) and the adjacent fourth nerve nucleus (C) which control downward gaze and the dorsilateral nuclei (D) which control upward gaze have been damaged. So too have the terminal parts of the medial longitudinal bundles (E) producing an internuclear ophthalmoplegia (see 3.93–3.95). The reaction to light controlled by the Edinger Westphal nuclei (F) and convergence controlled by the nucleus of Perlia (G) have been spared (Growdon et al, *Archives of Neurology* 1974; 30: 179). Because of the proximity of the two nuclei nuclear lesions are usually bilateral. They are also characteristically partial because a lesion at this site large enough to obliterate the nucleus would be lethal.

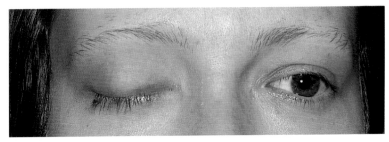

3.54A

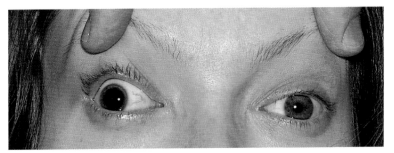

3.54B

3.54A,B–3.56 Third nerve palsy. A 23-year-old woman with a 4-week history of right retro-orbital pain leading, shortly before admission, to diplopia followed by closure of the right eye. She had a complete right ptosis (3.54A). The right eye was externally deviated by the intact sixth nerve and the pupil was dilated and fixed (3.54B). Lateral gaze to the right was normal (3.55A). On looking to the left the right eye moved inwards (due to inhibition of the sixth nerve) but did not adduct (3.55B). Note how on looking downwards the scleral vessels medial to the iris move downwards due to clockwise rotation of the globe (compare 3.55B and 3.56).

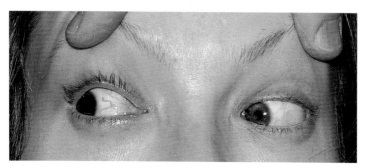

3.55A

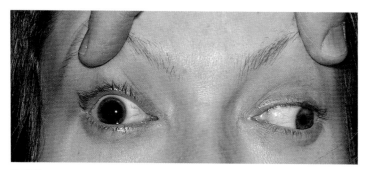

3.55B

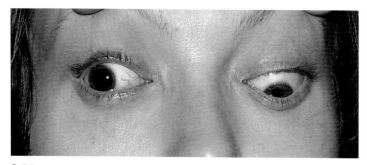

3.56

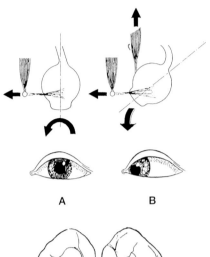

A   B

3.57A,B Testing the fourth cranial nerve. The rotatory movement of the eye described above indicates that the fourth nerve is intact, for it innervates the superior oblique muscle which is inserted across the top of the globe and induces such a movement when the eye is in a neutral position (3.57A). It is only when the eye is adducted by the medial rectus, bringing the line of pull of the superior oblique along the axis of the globe, that depression is produced (3.57B).

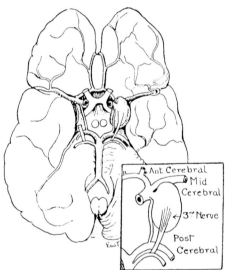

Ant Cerebral
Mid Cerebral
3ʳᵈ Nerve
Post Cerebral

3.58 Aneurysm of the posterior communicating artery. An isolated but complete third nerve palsy with dilation of the pupil suggests that the nerve has been compressed by an aneurysm on the posterior communicating artery. After emerging from the midbrain it passes between the posterior cerebral and the superior cerebellar arteries and runs alongside this vessel. The problem is well illustrated in Geoffrey Jefferson's paper (*Proceedings of the Royal Society of Medicine* 1947; 40: 419–431) from which this picture is reproduced.

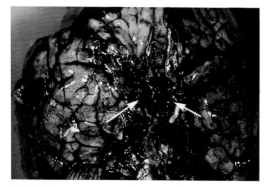

3.59 Aneurysms on the posterior communicating arteries. The brain of a patient who died after a subarachnoid haemorrhage. The glistening third nerves lie just external to the threadlike posterior communicating arteries on each of which there is an aneurysm (arrows) (see 7.21).

Lesions in the cavernous sinus

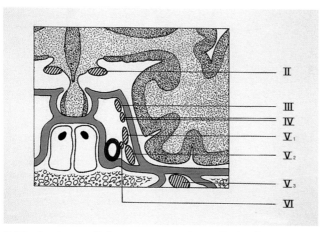

3.60 Anatomy of the cavernous sinus. Within the cavernous sinus the third nerve is near the carotid artery and the fourth, the first two divisions of the fifth and the sixth cranial nerves. The third division of the fifth leaves via the foramen ovale without entering the sinus.

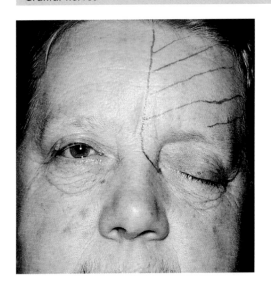

3.61 Atherosclerotic aneurysm in the cavernous sinus. A
67-year-old woman who suddenly developed severe pain over the left temple, followed soon after by a complete left ptosis, complete external ophthalmoplegia, a fixed dilated pupil and numbness over the brow. This combination of signs indicates a lesion in the cavernous sinus and the sudden onset of symptoms and the discovery of a bruit over the orbit suggested that it was probably an atherosclerotic aneurysm.

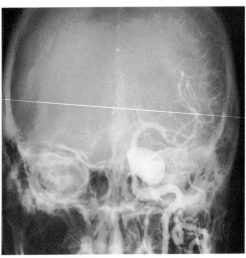

3.62 Angiogram of cavernous sinus aneurysm (cont.).
Angiography confirmed that there was a large swelling on the trunk of the internal carotid artery. Such lesions (which can also be seen on a scan (see 3.111)) usually present with pressure symptoms, although they occasionally rupture to produce a carotico-cavernous fistula (see 3.29). By contrast berry aneurysms, with the exception of aneurysms on the posterior communicating artery, usually present when they rupture.

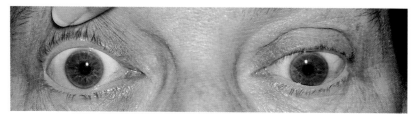

3.63 Atherosclerotic aneurysm of cavernous sinus. The fixed dilated pupil commonly seen with these lesions implies that the parasympathetic supply to the pupil has been destroyed but that the sympathetic supply is intact. Sympathetic fibres, however, traverse the nasociliary branch of the ophthalmic nerve before entering the long ciliary nerves so they too are sometimes damaged. This patient, who gave the customary story of right retro-orbital pain, facial numbness, diplopia and ptosis had a complete internal and external ophthalmoplegia with a *constricted* pupil.

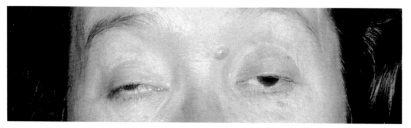

3.64

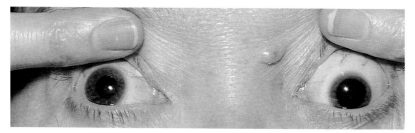

3.65

3.64,3.65 Bilateral third nerve palsies due to midline carcinoma. A 47-year-old woman who complained of right frontal headache and, over 3 years, developed numbness of the right and then of the left side of the face. Over the same period she developed severe bilateral ptosis, virtually complete external ophthalmoplegia and fixed dilated pupils. She therefore appeared to have lesions in the cavernous sinus on both sides.

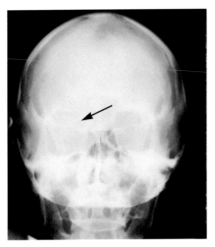

3.66

3.66,3.67 Bilateral third nerve palsies due to midline carcinoma (cont.). An X-ray done in 1966 showed destruction of the wall of the right orbit (3.66 arrow). Three years later this was more evident (3.67A) and an opacity had appeared in the nasal sinuses (3.67B). A biopsy of the ethmoid sinus showed that the patient had an adenocarcinoma.

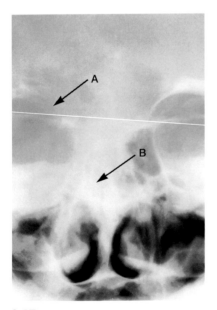

3.67

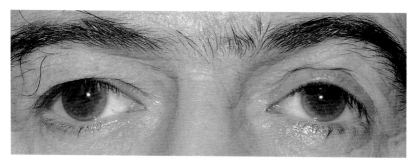

3.68

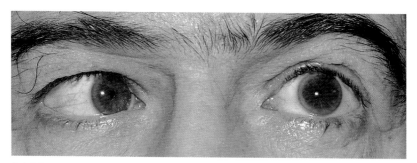

3.69A

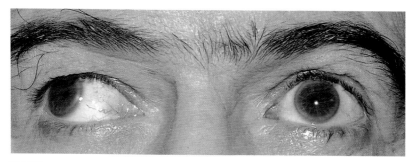

3.69B

3.68–3.70A,B Ischaemic lesion simulating cavernous sinus aneurysm.
Seven days before admission this 57-year-old patient, a heavy smoker with a history of coronary artery disease, developed intense pain over the left eyebrow and along the side of the nose. The following day he developed diplopia and a complete left ptosis. When seen the ptosis had diminished, but it was evident that all movements of the left eye were impaired. The pupil was normal.

65

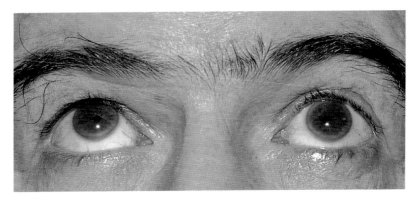

3.70A

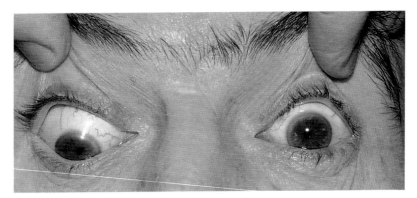

3.70B

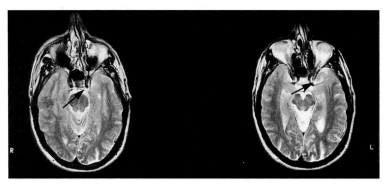

3.71

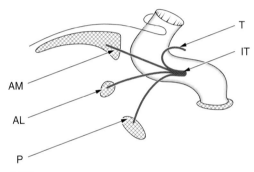

3.72

3.71,3.72 Ischaemic lesion simulating cavernous sinus aneurysm (cont.)
The sudden onset of left-sided symptoms, the involvement of all the extra-ocular muscles and the distribution of the pain in the territory of the first division of the trigeminus suggested once more that the patient had an aneurysm in the cavernous sinus. An MR scan showed, however, that the diameter of the carotid artery was normal (3.71 arrow). In fact this is a good example of the effects of occlusion of the inferolateral trunk (IT) which arises from the intracavernous part of the carotid artery and divides into four branches. The tentorial branch (T) supplies the third and fourth cranial nerves and the anteromedial branch (AM) enters the superior orbital fissure to supply the third, fourth, sixth and the ophthalmic division of the fifth cranial nerves. The anterolateral (AL) and posterior (P) branches enter the foramina rotundum and ovale to supply the maxillary and mandibular nerves. These two vessels anastomose with and may indeed arise from another source (3.72). Ischaemic neuritis due to occlusion of one of the three arteries which supply the cranial nerves (see also 3.118,3.147–3.150) was originally associated with diabetes and zoster, but has come into prominence as a result of complications of interventional radiology (J Lapresle and P Lasjaunias, *Brain* 1986; 109: 207). Note how, in an ischaemic lesion, the pupil is spared.

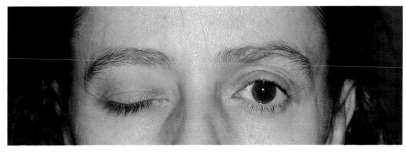

3.73

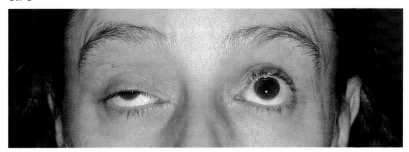

3.74

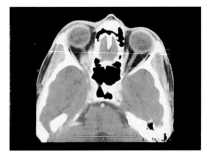

3.75

3.73–3.75 Tolosa Hunt syndrome. Lesions in the region of the superior orbital fissure also present with paralysis of the third, fourth and sixth nerves and pain or impairment of sensation in the territory of the first (but not the second) division of the trigeminus. Because of their situation they also cause proptosis. In addition to tumours, which clearly have to be excluded, this syndrome can be caused by a steroid-responsive inflammatory disorder known as the Tolosa Hunt syndrome. Over the course of 5 years this 40-year-old patient had had recurrent episodes of right- or left-sided orbital pain with proptosis, ptosis and diplopia. A CT scan showed a mass at the apex of the right orbit (3.75 arrow). There was a rapid response to treatment with steroids.

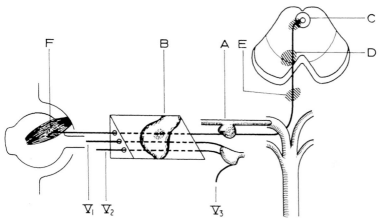

3.76 Other causes of a third nerve palsy. Palsies caused by berry aneurysms on the posterior communicating artery (A), by atherosclerotic aneurysms in the cavernous sinus (B), by adjacent lesions in the superior orbital fissure and by lesions in the nucleus (C) have been discussed above. Injury to the nerve as it leaves the midbrain anteriorly close to the pyramidal tract produces a complete palsy with a contralateral hemiparesis (Weber's syndrome, D). The third nerve, along with others, can be damaged by meningitis, neoplastic infiltration, sarcoidosis and basal fractures (E). The extra-ocular muscles may be affected by a variety of neuromuscular disorders including myasthenia (F). Aneurysms and (?ischaemic) neuropathy, e.g. due to diabetes account for nearly 50% of cases.

The sixth cranial nerve

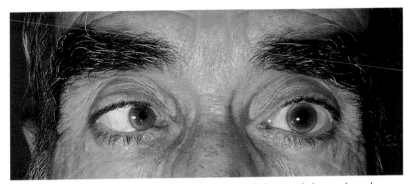

3.77 Left sixth nerve palsy. The only defect is failure to abduct on lateral gaze to the left. This provides a good model on which to test the rules for analysis of diplopia which are:

1. Muscles work in pairs whose names are 'as opposite as possible' – e.g. left superior rectus/right inferior oblique.
2. Separation of images is greatest along the line of pull of the defective muscle.
3. The outer (fainter) image comes from the defective eye.

Vision is tested by looking laterally, and upwards and downwards to left and right to determine the point at which the diplopia is most marked. The eyes are then covered in turn to find which one is defective. In this instance the images were most widely separated on looking to the left. The affected muscle must therefore be the right medial or the left lateral rectus. The outer image went when the left eye was covered, thereby showing that it was the left lateral rectus which was defective.

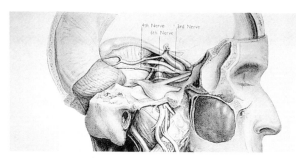

3.78 Causes of a sixth nerve palsy. By contrast with the third nerve an isolated sixth nerve palsy is rarely due to aneurysmal compression for, as the illustration from Geoffrey Jefferson's paper (*British Journal of Surgery* 1938; 26: 267–302) shows, the sixth nerve (unlike the third) is well away from the posterior communicating artery.

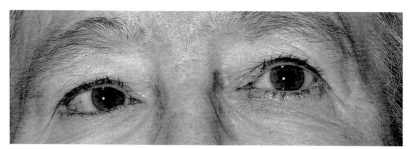

3.79A

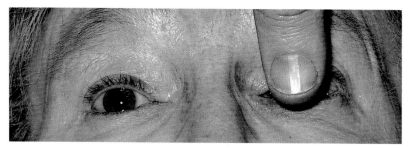

3.79B

3.79A,B Concomitant strabismus. A sixth nerve palsy is sometimes confused with a concomitant squint. This condition usually occurs in a defective eye and rarely causes diplopia. If the fixating eye is covered the defective one (which is capable of a full range of movement) comes into line.

Brainstem control of ocular movements – convergence and vertical gaze

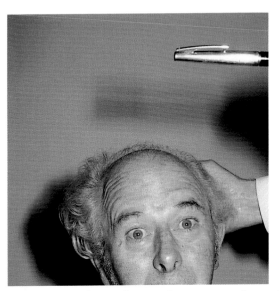

3.80 Parinaud's syndrome. Convergence and vertical gaze are controlled by centres in the roof of the midbrain. Patients with destructive lesions in this area lose the ability to look upwards and may develop lid retraction (Collier's sign) when trying so to do. Convergence and the response to light may be impaired and there is often an uncontrollable tendency to topple backwards. (Overactivity, as seen in postencephalitic parkinsonism or after treatment with phenothiazines, butyrophenones or metoclopramide, results in oculogyric crises.)

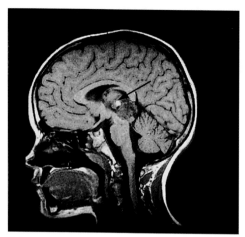

3.81

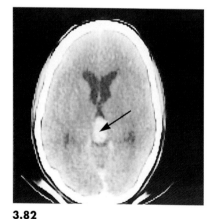

3.82

3.81,3.82 Pinealoma. The centre for vertical gaze may be damaged by vascular accidents, demyelination, encephalitis and vitamin deficiency but Parinaud's syndrome is particularly associated with tumours (especially pinealomas) in the region of the quadrigeminal plate (3.81 arrow). Because the aqueduct is also compressed, interfering with the flow of CSF, a complaint of headache is common.

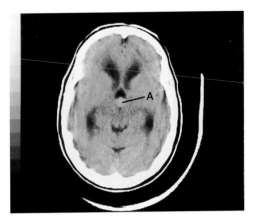

3.83

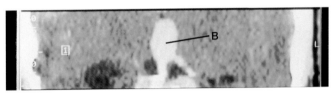

3.84

3.83,3.84 Basilar tip aneurysm. 'Tumours' indenting the posterior end of the third ventricle (cf. 3.82,3.83) are not always pinealomas. The frontal reconstruction of this scan shows that this lesion (A) is in fact an aneurysm at the bifurcation at the tip of the basilar artery (B).

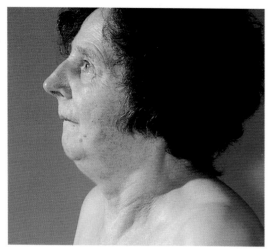

3.85 Progressive supranuclear palsy. This condition is most often caused by the Steele–Richardson–Olszewski syndrome, a progressive multi-system degeneration which presents in or after middle life with a tendency to fall backwards, dysarthria, dysphagia, frontal lobe signs and a peculiar disorder of ocular movement. In particular there is a defect of voluntary downward gaze which, coupled with a tendency to hold the head in an extended position, makes walking even more difficult. Although often mistaken for parkinsonism, the limbs do not necessarily show the signs of that condition.

Brainstem control of ocular movements – lateral gaze

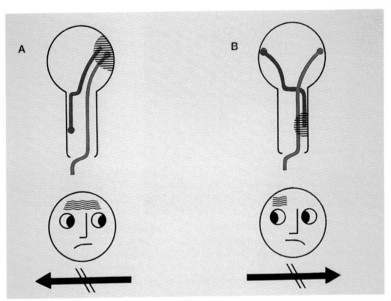

3.86 The pontine centre for lateral gaze. Centres in the hemisphere control conjugate gaze to the opposite side. Lesions in the left hemisphere therefore impair conjugate gaze to the right as a result of which the eyes 'look towards the (hemisphere) lesion' because conjugate gaze to the left is intact (A). The tracts concerned decussate at the top of the midbrain and travel to pontine centres for conjugate lateral gaze. These lie close to the abducens nuclei and are surrounded by the seventh nerves. A lesion on the left side of the brainstem therefore impairs conjugate gaze to the *left* and is often associated with a facial palsy (B). In both instances, pyramidal tract damage will be to (as yet uncrossed) fibres from the left hemisphere. Patients with brainstem lesions, unlike those with hemisphere lesions, therefore look *towards* their paralysed side.

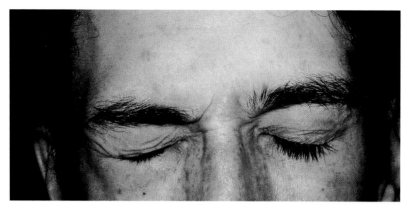

3.87

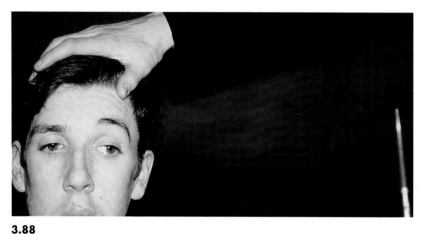

3.88

3.87,3.88 Brainstem lesion with lateral gaze palsy to left. A patient with multiple sclerosis and a mild left facial palsy (note inability to bury eyelashes). He was unable to look or to follow to the left because the left pontine centre for conjugate lateral gaze was damaged.

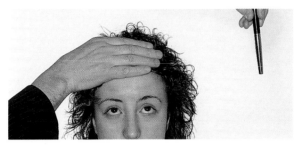

3.89

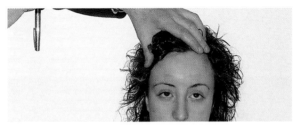

3.90

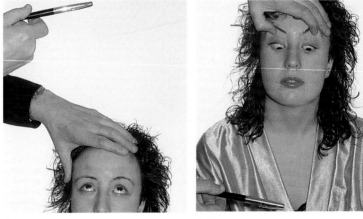

3.91   **3.92**

3.89–3.92 Brainstem lesion with bilateral lateral gaze palsy. Another patient with demyelination who presented with diplopia and ataxia and was found to have bilateral facial nerve palsies. She was unable to look to left or right because the adjacent pontine centres had been damaged. Vertical gaze, controlled from a separate centre in the midbrain, was intact.

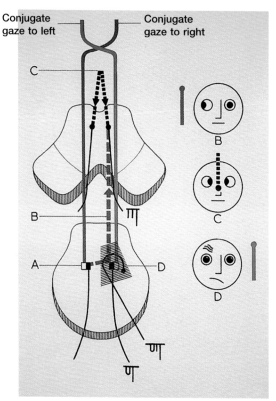

Conjugate
gaze to left

Conjugate
gaze to right

3.93 Internuclear ophthalmoplegia and the 'one-and-a-half' syndrome.
The pontine centre for conjugate gaze to the right (A) is controlled by fibres from the
left hemisphere (continuous red line). It in turn controls the adjacent sixth nerve and
part of the contralateral third nerve nucleus. The latter function is effected via the
medial longitudinal bundle (broken red line) which crosses the midline at once and
ascends on the opposite side of the brainstem. A lesion in the medial longitudinal
bundle will produce an internuclear ophthalmoplegia (B) wherein on lateral gaze
abduction is normal but adduction is defective. The left medial rectus and the
third nerve are however intact so convergence (which is controlled from above) is
normal (C).

The patient shown on 3.87 and 3.88 had a lesion which had destroyed the centre for
conjugate gaze to the left and the adjacent facial nerve (D). Such a lesion, as the
diagram shows, can also damage the medial longitudinal bundle from the opposite
side with the result that in addition to loss of conjugate gaze to the left there is also
loss of adduction on looking to the right – the 'one-and-a-half' syndrome.

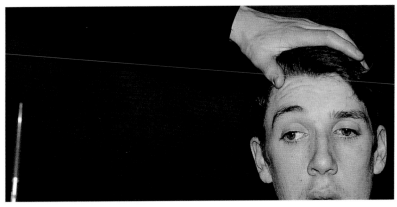

3.94

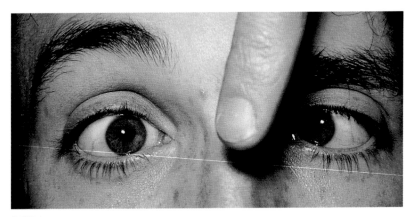

3.95

3.94,3.95 Internuclear ophthalmoplegia. This in fact proved to be the case for the left eye did not adduct on lateral gaze although it worked normally on convergence. A unilateral internuclear ophthalmoplegia is commonly due to a vascular accident whereas a bilateral lesion is more likely to be due to demyelination. In multiple sclerosis the sign is often associated with *ataxic nystagmus* in which the jerking movements in the abducting eye are of greater amplitude.

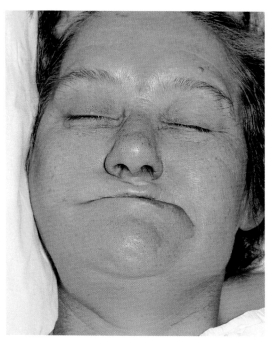

3.96 Combined pontine and midbrain lesion. The lesions described above do not always occur in isolation. This 57-year-old woman, a heavy smoker, suddenly complained of headache and developed right-sided tinnitus and a left hemiplegia. She had weakness of the right masseter and temporalis muscles, a profound right lower motor neurone facial palsy (shown by the way in which the right cheek 'billows' during respiration while asleep) and although she could abduct the left eye all other horizontal eye movements were absent. She therefore had a lesion on the right side of the brainstem affecting the fifth, seventh and eighth nerves, the pontine centre for lateral gaze, the medial longitudinal bundle and the pyramidal tract from the right hemisphere.

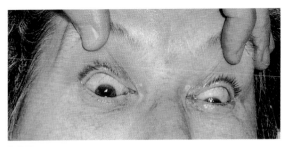

3.97

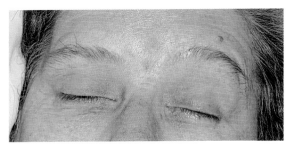

3.98

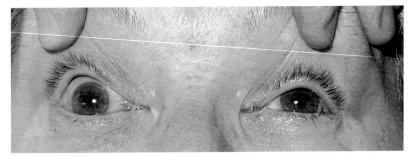

3.99

3.97–3.99 Combined pontine and midbrain lesion (cont.). Vertical gaze was normal, showing that the upper part of the third nerve nucleus was intact (3.97). There was, however, severe bilateral ptosis which, despite vigorous use of the intact left frontalis muscle (note position of left eyebrow) the patient could not overcome (3.98) and the pupils were greatly constricted (3.99). The lesion was therefore also affecting the caudal part of the third nerve nucleus and the sympathetic fibres in the midbrain (cf. 3.48–3.53).

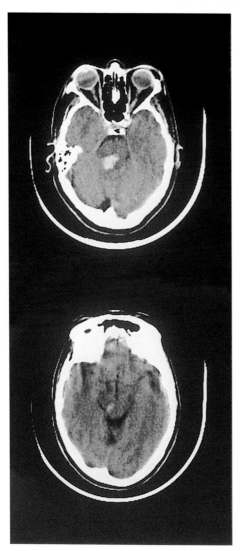

3.100 Combined pontine and midbrain lesion (cont.). The sudden onset of symptoms suggested a vascular accident and the CT scan showed an extensive but predominantly right-sided haemorrhage in the midbrain and pons. The introduction of scanning has shown that non-fatal lesions of this sort are not, in fact, uncommon.

Cortical control of ocular movements

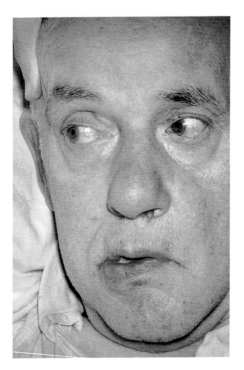

3.101 Unilateral lesions. Centres in each hemisphere control conjugate gaze to the opposite side. If, as in this instance, the centres in the right hemisphere are damaged those on the left are unopposed and the eyes 'look towards the (hemisphere) lesion'. If, on the other hand, the hemisphere lesion is the focus of an epileptic discharge the head and eyes will turn away from the damaged side in an adversive attack.

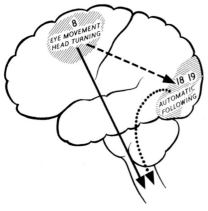

3.102 Bilateral lesions. There are in fact two centres which control conjugate gaze to the opposite side in each hemisphere. The function of those in the occipital lobe is to hold a target in focus once it has been brought into view regardless of movements made by it or by the patient. This subconscious action is done with great precision, and if both occipital centres are damaged a patient whose eyes appear to move perfectly well will complain of blurring of vision. Coupled with severe difficulty in judging the position and distance of objects this condition (*Balint's syndrome*) poses a greater disability than straightforward blindness.

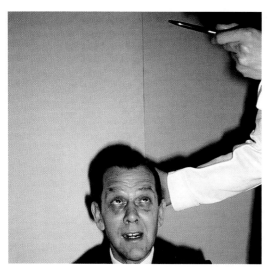

3.103

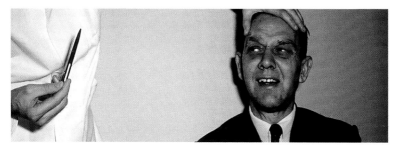

3.104

3.103–3.106 Bilateral lesions (cont.). The functions of the frontal centres for conjugate gaze (3.102) are to suppress the fixation/following reflex and to direct the eyes onto a new target. Bilateral damage produces a condition known as *ocular motor apraxia*. Using the occipital centres for fixation and following the patient can track a moving target with ease (3.103,3.104) but when asked to turn his eyes to the side or upwards he is unable so to do, although he struggles to turn his head in the appropriate direction (3.105,3.106). Children with a congenital disorder of this sort learn to overcome the reflex by blinking or with sudden violent turning movements (often mistaken for a tic) that drag the eyes from the existing target onto a new one.

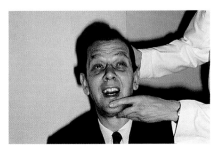

3.105

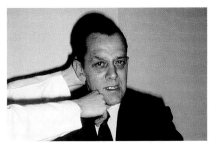

3.106

The trigeminal nerve

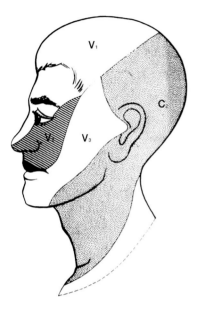

3.107 Cutaneous distribution of the trigeminal nerve.
The precise distribution of the branches of the trigeminal nerve is important. Note that the territory of the first division extends well towards the back of the head and onto the outside of the nose, and that the third division does not innervate the angle of the jaw or much of the ear.

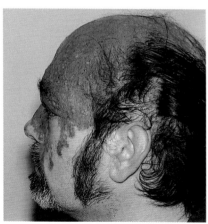

3.108 Sturge–Weber syndrome.
The area supplied by the trigeminus is often well outlined in this condition. The posterior extent of the territory of the first division is clearly visible, as is the extension of the nasociliary branch onto the side of the nose. The latter is important in zoster, for the risk of corneal damage is said to be diminished if this area is unaffected.

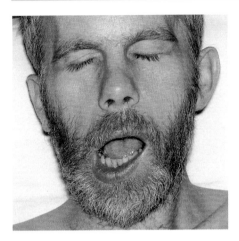

3.109 Motor root of the trigeminal. Damage to the motor root produces weakness and wasting of the masseter and temporalis muscles. It also damages the pterygoids, as a result of which the jaw swings to the affected side on opening the mouth.

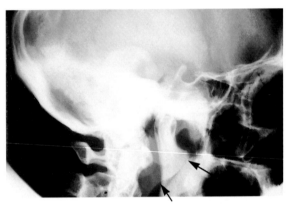

3.110 Trigeminal neuropathy. Facial numbness may be caused by tumours, aneurysms, vascular accidents, sarcoidosis, syphilis, collagen diseases and a variety of iatrogenic dental disorders. 'Idiopathic' facial numbness is sometimes associated with extensive destruction of the nose. In recent years the importance of Sjögren's syndrome has become apparent and nasopharyngeal carcinomas (arrows) are a well known trap. This patient presented with nasal obstruction, headache and deafness. He had had sinus washouts and insufflation of the Eustachian tube before, 4 months later, epistaxis and a squint revealed the true diagnosis.

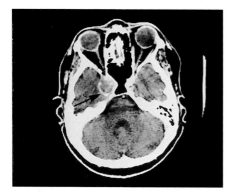

3.111 Facial pain. The diagnosis of dangerous disorders such as cranial arteritis, glaucoma and sphenoid sinusitis and of treatable disorders such as cluster headache and trigeminal neuralgia depends on awareness and appropriate questioning and investigations. Structural lesions such as a nasopharyngeal carcinoma or – as in this instance – an aneurysm in the right cavernous sinus (arrow) are relatively uncommon.

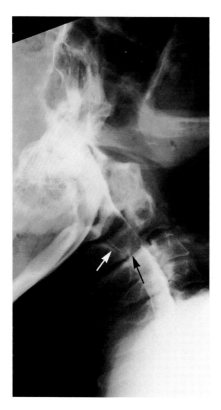

3.112 Referred pain. This elderly patient presented with a long history of left-sided deafness and a 3-year history of severe pain in the left ear. During cisternography – done because of doubts about the appearance of the cerebello-pontine angle – cervical puncture produced excruciating pain in the ear. This led to the discovery of a high cervical tumour (a meningioma) compressing the second cervical root which, as shown on 3.107, supplies the lobe of the ear. Thoracic aneurysms, hiatus hernias and bronchial carcinomas can also produce pain in this area, possibly through the auricular branch of the vagus.

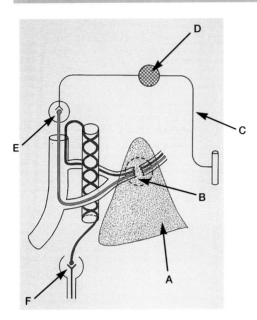

3.113 Auriculo-temporal syndrome. After injuries in the region of the parotid gland (A) with damage to the auriculotemporal branch of the mandibular nerve (B) patients may complain of perspiration on the side of the head when eating. It is thought that fibres from the tympanic branch of the glossopharyngeal nerve (C) which pass through the tympanic plexus (D), the lesser superficial petrosal nerve and the otic ganglion (E) on their way to the parotid gland regenerate into sweat fibres from the superior cervical ganglion (F) which enter the skull around the middle meningeal artery.

The facial nerve

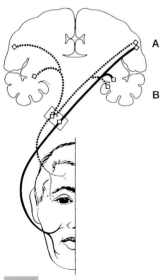

3.114 The anatomy of facial movements. When trying to understand the different forms of facial palsy it is important to remember two basic facts. The first is that the muscles of the brow (unlike those of the face) have an upper motor neurone supply from both hemispheres. The second is that, while voluntary movements are controlled from the motor strip (A), involuntary movements are controlled from more deeply placed centres (B).

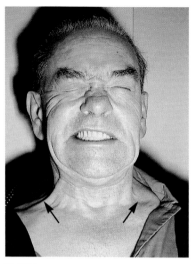 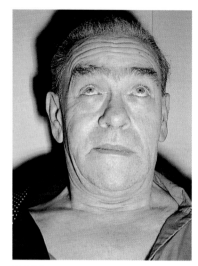

3.115   **3.116**

3.115,3.116 Upper motor neurone facial palsy. An upper motor neurone palsy, which is often associated with a hemiplegia and/or dysphasia, is characteristically mild. However, if the patient is asked to screw up his eyes, to show his teeth and to retract his jaw it is evident that the eyelashes are not buried, that the mouth droops and that the platysma (3.115 arrow) does not contract. Furrowing of the (bilaterally innervated) brow, by contrast, is normal (3.116). When paresis is due to defective control of involuntary movements (3.114B) a weakness which is evident during conversation may be difficult to demonstrate on examination.

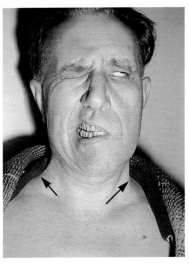
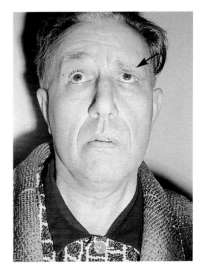

3.117 **3.118**

3.117,3.118 Lower motor neurone facial palsy. Damage to the facial nerve itself inevitably affects all the muscles supplied. In repose young patients, in whom the tissues have retained their elasticity, may look relatively normal. On testing, however, the weakness is usually more severe than that seen with upper motor neurone palsies. In particular closure of the eye is often incomplete. The patient cannot furrow his brow or raise his eyebrow on the affected side (3.118 arrow) but does *not* have ptosis. Lesions in the petrous temporal bone may also cause hyperacusis, impairment of taste and/or (with zoster) a rash in the ear. Ischaemic lesions (see 3.71,3.72) are sometimes associated with facial numbness, for the branch of the middle meningeal artery which supplies the facial nerve also supplies the second and third divisions of the trigeminus.

(Facial weakness due to lesions in the brainstem is discussed in 3.86–3.100 and lesions in the cerebello-pontine angle are discussed in 3.131–3.133.)

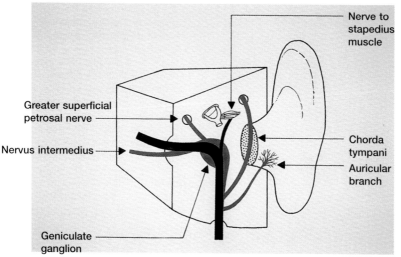

3.119 Branches of the facial nerve. The facial nerve enters the petrous temporal bone through the internal auditory meatus. It is accompanied by the nervus intermedius which contains autonomic and sensory fibres. Injury to the nerve within the bone may damage the nerve to stapedius (causing hyperacusis), the greater superficial petrosal nerve (impairing lachrymation) and/or the chorda tympani (reducing taste over the anterior two-thirds of the tongue). In geniculate herpes, in which facial palsy may sometimes be due to compression of the nerve by the swollen geniculate ganglion, a rash may be seen in the territory of the auricular branch.

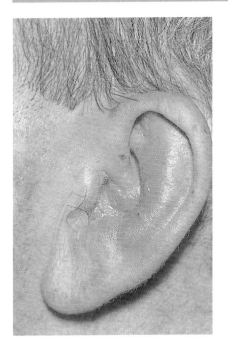

3.120 Geniculate herpes (Ramsay Hunt syndrome).
The patient complains of severe pain and is found to have a rash in the external auditory meatus. The palsy may sometimes be due to compression of the nerve by the swollen geniculate ganglion, but facial palsy is often associated with rashes far removed from the territory of the facial nerve. Pathological studies suggest that the weakness is more likely to be due to direct involvement of the nucleus of the nerve.

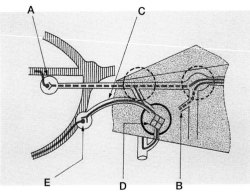

3.121 Crocodile tears.
Some months after a facial palsy patients sometimes complain of excessive lachrymation when eating. This is due to faulty re-innervation of the greater superficial petrosal nerve and the spheno-palatine ganglion (A) by fibres destined for the salivary gland. These may come from the chorda tympani (B) or from the lesser superficial petrosal nerve (C), which arises via the tympanic plexus (D) from the glossopharyngeal nerve and runs through the otic ganglion (E) to the parotid. The condition can be cured by tympanotomy.

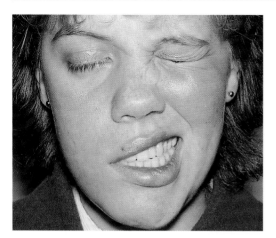

3.122

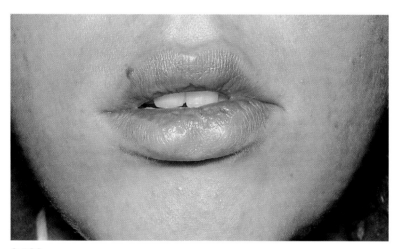

3.123

3.122,3.123 Melkersson's syndrome. The association of recurrent facial nerve palsies, recurrent swelling of the face and lips and fissuring of the tongue is known as Melkersson's syndrome. Fissuring may not be evident unless the tongue is dried and bent over at the tip. These patients have a less good prognosis than those with simple Bell's palsy and may develop scarring and deformity of the face.

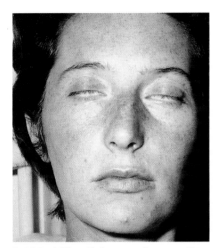

3.124 Miller Fisher syndrome. This patient with acute polyneuritis is attempting to close her eyes. Because of its symmetry the defect can easily be overlooked (see 3.46). Bilateral weakness may also occur in Bell's palsy and multiple sclerosis (3.89–3.92), as a developmental disorder (Moebius' syndrome), with basal meningitis and sarcoidosis and in myasthenia and muscular dystrophy. Bilateral facial palsies also appear to be common in Lyme disease.

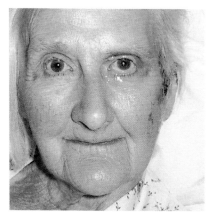

3.125

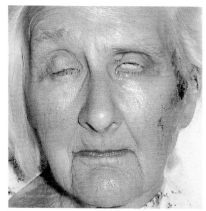

3.126

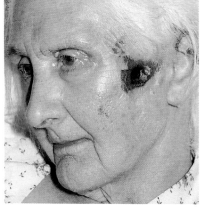

3.127

3.125–3.127 Distal lesions. An
elderly patient found on her kitchen floor
2 days after developing a hemiplegia.
She had numerous pressure sores.
Movements of the lower part of the face
were normal (3.125) but she could not
close the left eye or furrow the brow (note
position of eyebrow on 3.126). This
defect was due to compression of the
temporal branches of the nerve where
they cross the zygoma at the site of the
pressure sore on the left side of the head
(3.127). Partial palsies may also be seen
with parotid tumours and after surgery
and other injuries.

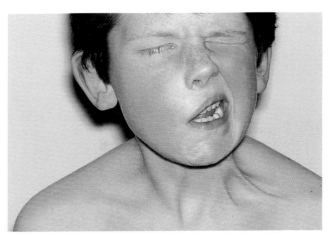

3.128 Congenital facial palsy. A child delivered by caesarean section after an attempt at forceps delivery had failed. Such palsies are usually transient. They have been attributed to forceps damage but are probably due to pressure on the head in the birth canal, for they are as common in normal deliveries and, whether or not forceps are used, nearly always affect the lowermost side of the head.

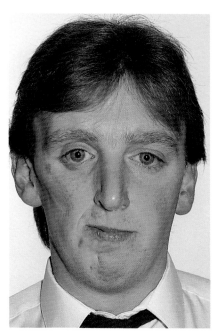

3.129

3.129, 3.130 Hemifacial atrophy (Parry–Romberg syndrome). Severe atrophy of the right side of the face which appeared suddenly 2 months before admission. There was also wasting of the tongue and palate and loss of sweating on the right. This last is of particular interest, for this mysterious condition has been attributed to damage to the sympathetic nervous system and the patient had recently had a right parietal pleurectomy for pneumothorax.

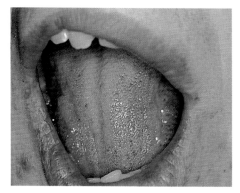

3.130

The acoustic nerve

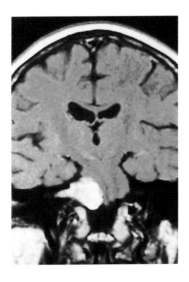

3.131 Acoustic schwannoma. Tumours in the cerebello-pontine angle, most of which are acoustic schwannomas, usually present with impairment of hearing and go on to compress the fifth (abolishing the corneal reflex) and sometimes the seventh cranial nerves, the cerebellum and the CSF pathways. Large lesions like the one shown on this MR scan cause significant displacement of the brainstem and in all but the best hands the morbidity and mortality after surgery are still significant.

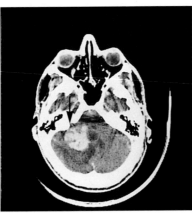

3.132 Acoustic schwannoma. The importance of early diagnosis cannot be over-emphasised. This 35-year-old man was known to have 'frequency deafness' 7 years before admission. For 1 year his writing and architectural drawings had been 'untidy' and on enquiry it transpired that he was ataxic and had morning headaches. The CT scan showed a large tumour near the widened internal auditory meatus (arrow). Although it was removed with preservation of the facial nerve, if treatment had been undertaken 7 years earlier the operation would have been easier and safer.

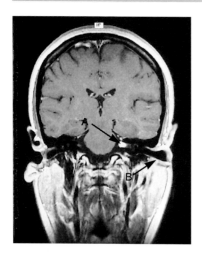

3.133 Acoustic schwannoma. The investigation of unexplained unilateral deafness therefore implies detailed scanning – preferably with a gadolinium-enhanced MR scan – which will detect a minute tumour (A) well away from the internal auditory meatus (B).

Glossopharyngeal, vagus, accessory and hypoglossal nerves

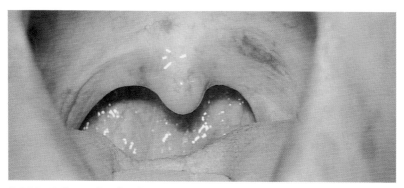

3.134 Unilateral palatal palsy. Weakness of the right side of the palate due to a lesion of the right vagus (*not* the glossopharyngeal, which for all practical purposes is a sensory nerve). The uvula moves away from the affected side as the patient says 'ah'. This weakness could be due to a lesion in the brainstem (e.g. Wallenberg's syndrome, see 7.75–7.77) or a lesion near the jugular foramen which also affects the ninth, eleventh and twelfth cranial nerves. Proximal lesions of this sort may also affect the larynx. With lesions of the recurrent laryngeal branch (due to surgery, oesophageal or bronchial carcinomas and aortic aneurysms) the palate is spared.

101

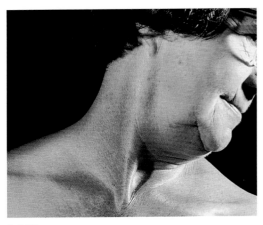

3.135

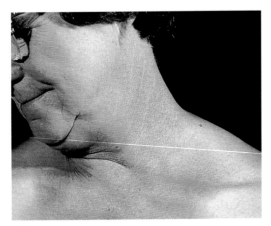

3.136

3.135–3.138 Left accessory nerve palsy. The accessory nerve may be injured individually or with the ninth, tenth and twelfth nerves as part of the jugular foramen syndrome. This is one of a series of patients in whom the nerve was avulsed in road traffic accidents. Note how the left sternomastoid and trapezius fail to contract on turning to the right (3.136) and on shrugging the shoulders (3.137). When the arms are extended there is winging of the scapula, with downward rotation due to the action of the serratus anterior (3.138).

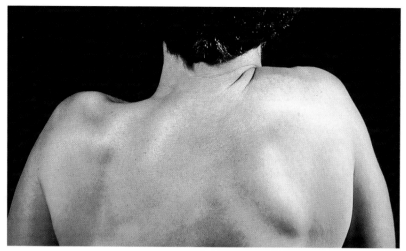

3.137

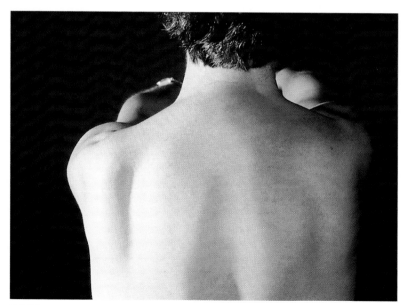

3.138

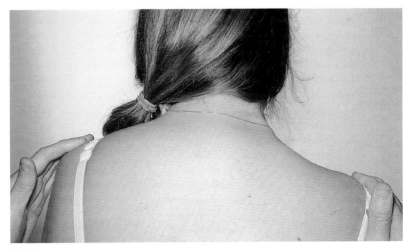

3.139

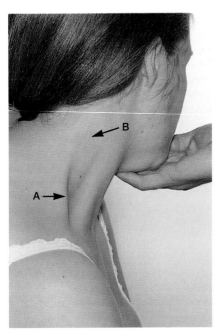

3.139,3.140 Partial accessory nerve palsy. A patient who complained of weakness of the right arm after removal of a gland from the posterior triangle. She is unable to shrug the shoulder (3.139) and wasting of the trapezius is visible (3.140A). The sternomastoid, however, is intact because the nerve was damaged by an incision (3.140B) at the point at which it emerges from that muscle. The cut ends were successfully reunited. A similar lesion has been reported as a result of a 'love bite'.

3.140

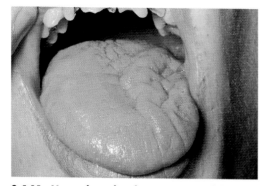

3.141 Hypoglossal palsy. Deviation of the tongue to the left with weakness and wasting on that side due to a left lower motor neurone hypoglossal palsy. An isolated twelfth nerve palsy may occur after operations on the neck, lesions of the carotid artery and fractures of the jaw.

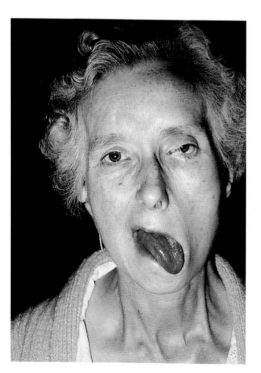

3.142 Glomus jugulare tumour. Because of the close proximity of the ninth, tenth, eleventh and twelfth nerves they can be damaged as a group by tumours, vascular lesions, carcinomatous, bacterial or sarcoid meningitis, fractures and Paget's disease of the skull. One such lesion, commonly seen in middle-aged women, is the glomus jugulare tumour, which spreads as a grape-like mass across the base of the skull and may emerge as a 'polyp' in the external auditory meatus. This patient presented with deafness and went on to develop lesions of the fifth, seventh, ninth, tenth, eleventh and twelfth nerves. Note the tarsorraphy, the smooth brow and facial palsy, and the wasting of the sternomastoid and tongue.

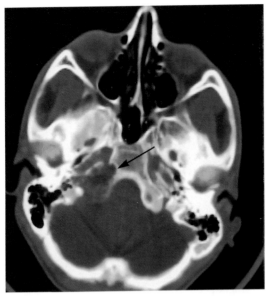

3.143

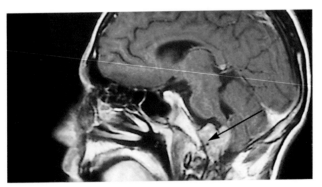

3.144

3.143,3.144 Glomus tumour. A CT scan showing erosion of bone in the region of the right jugular foramen (3.143 arrow) and an MR scan showing an extensive tumour compressing the lower part of the brainstem (3.144 arrow).

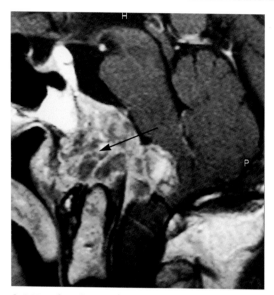

3.145 Chordoma. A patient who presented with a 12-month history of daily 5-minute attacks of 'cramp' in the tongue, during which it 'contracted like the muscles of a snail' and became a small mass at the back of the mouth. He later developed headaches made worse by coughing and straining. Examination revealed only profuse fasciculation of the tongue, but the MR scan revealed a large chordoma indenting the lower part of the brainstem (arrow).

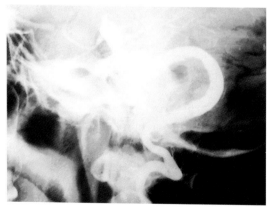

3.146 Basilar ectasia. The lower cranial nerves can be damaged by dissection or ectasia of the basilar artery. The contrast between the apparent health of the patient and the extent of the neurological lesion is often striking.

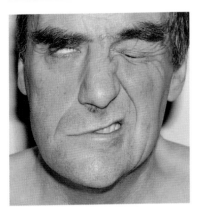

3.147

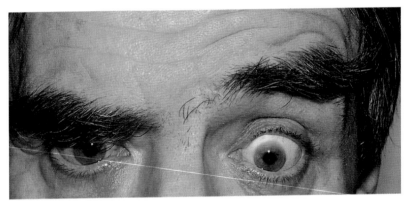

3.148

3.147–3.150 Ischaemic lesion secondary to zoster. The ninth, tenth, eleventh, and twelfth nerves are supplied by the posterior neuromuscular branch of the ascending pharyngeal artery and ischaemic lesions have been described after embolisation and with zoster. This patient presented with a 2-week history of pain in the right ear followed in quick succession by right facial weakness, dysphonia and dysphagia. Examination revealed a right lower motor neurone facial palsy (note position of the eyebrows), right-sided deafness and weakness of the right side of the palate, the right sternomastoid and the right trapezius. He had a CSF pleocytosis with large atypical cells. The cells, however, were not of epithelial origin and the CSF protein and glucose were normal. Initial fears that he might have carcinomatous meningitis were allayed by the discovery of greatly elevated varicella-zoster titres.

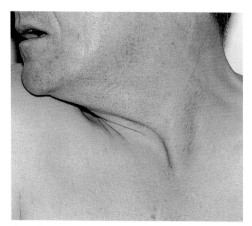

3.149

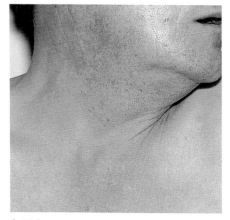

3.150

4.

Consciousness, coma and death

Consciousness exists when the cerebral cortex is stimulated by the reticular formation. This structure runs in the dorsum of the brainstem from the hypothalamus to the medulla. The upper part acts as an 'on/off' switch for consciousness and controls the sleep/wake cycle (two entirely different functions). The lower part controls respiration. Loss of consciousness can be assessed in four different ways. In the acute phase *quantitative* examination (using the Glasgow coma chart) will define the severity and progress of the patient's condition while *qualitative* examination may help to determine the cause. After a head injury it is

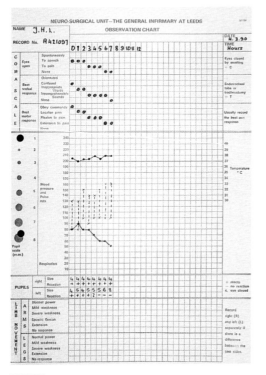

4.1 The Glasgow coma chart. Quantitative assessment is done with the Glasgow coma chart, on which serial observations of eye opening, speech, movement, the pulse, the blood pressure and the response of the pupils are made. In this instance there was cause for concern by 2 AM and by 3 AM there was clearcut evidence of serious deterioration. Note the way in which the blood pressure rises as the pulse falls and the left pupil becomes dilated and fixed.

important to establish the *duration of post-traumatic amnesia* (the length of time before the recovery of consecutive memory). This is not synonymous with the ability to talk and walk and gives some indication of the severity of the injury. In those who fail to recover *assessment of brainstem function* may indicate the site of the lesion or suggest that death has occurred.

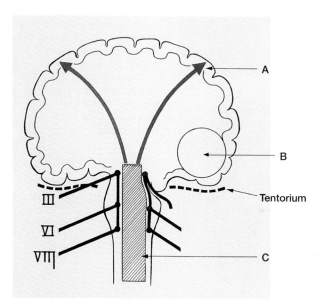

4.2 Qualitative analysis. Causes of impairment of consciousness fall into three main groups. Destruction of the cortex (A) may be caused by cardiac arrest, an anaesthetic accident, hypotension, subarachnoid haemorrhage, hepato-renal failure, hypoglycaemia, hypothermia or status epilepticus. As the whole cortex is involved signs are bilateral, more or less symmetrical and may be accompanied by fits or myoclonus. The brainstem, which is relatively resistant to such insults, is spared. Supratentorial lesions (B), which are usually associated with a contralateral hemiparesis, uncal herniation and an ipsilateral third nerve palsy, cause serial disintegration of brainstem function with dysconjugate eye movements, flexor and then extensor spasms and respiratory failure. Damage to the brainstem (C) by drugs, haemorrhage, infarction or mass lesions in the posterior fossa causes early disruption of conjugate eye movements. Structural lesions produce asymmetrical signs, often affect the pupil but tend to spare the corneal reflex. Drugs, by contrast, produce symmetrical signs, impair the corneal reflex but (with the exception of opiates) tend to spare the pupils.

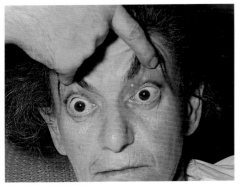

4.3

4.3–4.5 Doll's head eye movements. The reticular formation, as shown in 4.2, is surrounded by the nerves and tracts which control ocular movements. The integrity of these structures – and by inference of the reticular formation itself – can be tested in an unconscious patient by tilting and turning the head to stimulate the vestibule. With cortical lesions, as in this unconscious patient, movements tend to be normal. With brainstem lesions and with a developing uncal hernia they are disrupted.

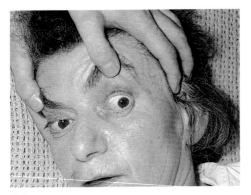

4.4

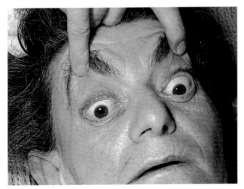

4.5

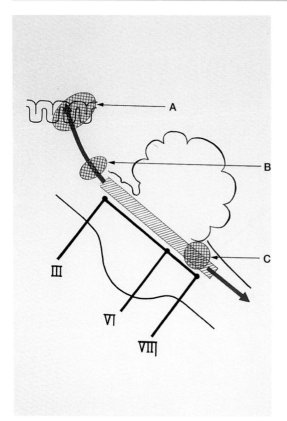

4.6 Permanent vegetative state. Patients in whom the cortex (A) or the links between the reticular formation and the cortex (B) are destroyed may lapse into a permanent vegetative state. They are unconscious but retain a normal sleep/wake cycle, eye opening, random eye movements and respiration. This is in effect the mirror image of the patient with poliomyelitis who is conscious but cannot breathe because the respiratory centre in the lowest part of the reticular formation has ceased to function (C).

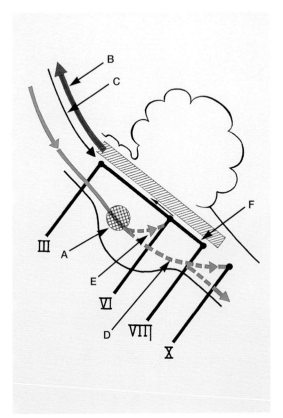

4.7 Locked-in syndrome. The permanent vegetative state must not be confused with the locked-in syndrome which is caused by a lesion in the ventral part of the pons (A). The cortex, the link with the reticular formation (B) and efferent fibres to the upper brainstem (C) are intact. The patient is therefore conscious and can look up and down to order. He is however unable to move, speak or swallow because of damage to the cortico-spinal and -bulbar tracts (D) and cannot look from side to side because the cortical control of lateral gaze is destroyed (E). Conjugate lateral movements can however be induced by turning the head and stimulating the brainstem mechanism controlling lateral gaze – which is intact – via the vestibule (F).

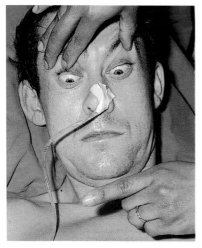

4.8

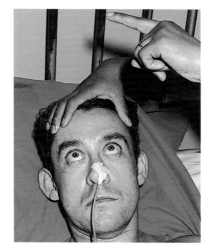

4.9

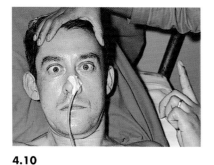

4.10

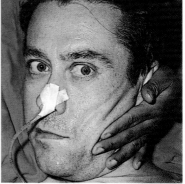

4.11

4.8–4.11 Locked-in syndrome. A 38-year-old hypertensive who suddenly complained of headache and had a fit. On recovery he was tetraplegic, dysphagic and mute. Conjugate movements in a vertical direction were intact (4.8,4.9) but he was unable to look or to follow to the side (4.10). Conjugate lateral movements could however be induced by rotating the head to stimulate the intact brainstem mechanism via the vestibular apparatus.

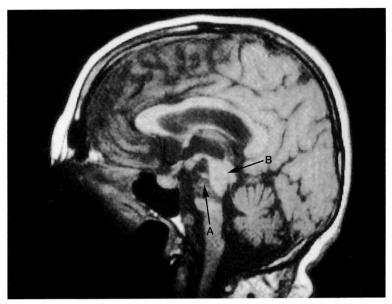

4.12 Locked-in syndrome. An MR scan of a man who, after complaining of vertigo, right facial numbness, transient left hemiparesis and transient bilateral weakness developed a locked-in syndrome. A large (dark) area of infarction is visible in the ventral midbrain and pons (A) but the area in front of the aqueduct (B) is preserved.

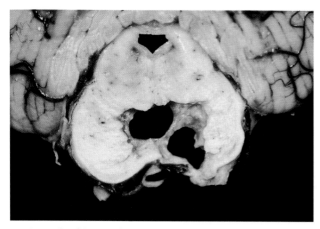

4.13 Locked-in syndrome. A 53-year-old man who suddenly complained of vertigo, collapsed and was admitted in 'coma'. He was breathing spontaneously but apart from eye opening was immobile and mute. However, an observant nurse had noticed that he cried whenever his family was mentioned. Closer examination showed that he could open his eyes to order and look up and down, thus indicating that he was not unconscious. Autopsy revealed vertebrobasilar thrombosis with massive infarction of the anterior part of the pons.

Brainstem death

Patients with the locked-in syndrome are conscious and can breathe because the cortex, its links with the reticular activating system and the respiratory centre are intact. Patients with the permanent vegetative state can breathe because the respiratory centre is intact but are rendered unconscious by destruction of the cortex or its links with the reticular activating system. By contrast, patients with bulbar poliomyelitis are conscious but are unable to breathe because the respiratory centre has been destroyed. All, however, are indisputably 'alive', having retained either consciousness or the ability to breathe (analagous, as Pallis points out, with the 'soul' and the 'breath of life', the traditional manifestations of vitality). But destruction of both upper and lower parts of the reticular formation, with consequent loss of consciousness and of the ability to breathe, leads inexorably to death of the organism as a whole. That this situation is not synonymous with death of the whole organism is sometimes shown by preservation of cortical electrical activity and spinal reflexes, but these are of no consequence as they cannot be harnessed or maintained.

5.

Blackouts

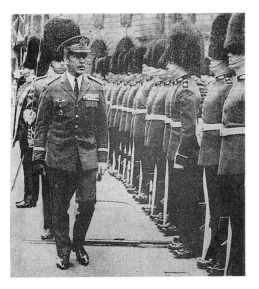

5.1 Syncope. The first and most important step when managing a patient with blackouts is to establish the cause of the attacks. The circumstances (prolonged standing, alarming or gruesome sights and jumping out of a warm bed and impeding an already diminished venous return by straining to pass water) may give an important indication that an attack was syncopal. So also do loss of vision and blurring of hearing and the ability to abort an attack by lying down. However, a sudden fall, incontinence of urine and even a considerable amount of twitching are all compatible with a diagnosis of syncope.

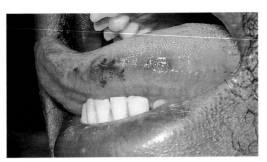

5.2 Fits. A fit is the *clinical* manifestation of a sudden disorderly discharge of brain cells. For the most part fits are stereotyped, sudden and spontaneous and can occur at any time and in any position. A report of injuries, unequivocal convulsions, laceration of the cheek or the side of the tongue and prolonged somnolence, stiffness, sickness, confusion and/or headache after the attack supports the diagnosis. Complex partial seizures can, however, look very similar to syncopal attacks and protracted syncope can cause a convulsion. Every effort should be made to establish the diagnosis before starting treatment.

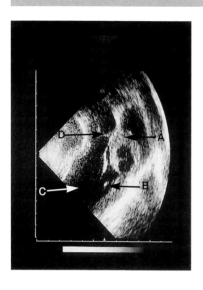

5.3 Fits due to cerebral ischaemia.

The importance of cardiovascular disease as a cause of blackouts at all ages has been increasingly appreciated and when there is doubt about the diagnosis ECG monitoring and a study of the vascular reflexes may be revealing. An atrial myxoma is much less common. This 56-year-old woman with 'rheumatic heart disease' had exclusively nocturnal fits. Her husband's statement that he could abort them by sitting her up and shaking her was viewed with scepticism until she was found to have a mass in the right atrium. The significance of her very variable murmurs and of her repeated recovery from 'terminal' heart failure then became evident. Myxomas can be demonstrated by echocardiography (A = myxoma, B = mitral valve, C = left ventricle, D = aortic valve).

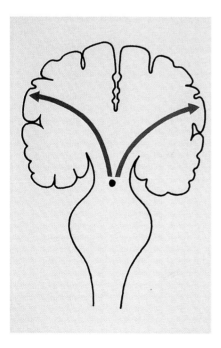

5.4 Primary generalised seizures.

The old name for generalised seizures, 'centrencephalic epilepsy', conjures up a useful picture of a discharge which starts in the reticular formation causing warningless loss of consciousness and then spreads to involve both hemispheres. Clinical manifestations may take the form of an abrupt loss of consciousness (absence or petit mal), abrupt loss of consciousness and tone (akinetic seizure), myoclonus and/or a warningless major fit. Although primary generalised epilepsy is 'idiopathic' it must be remembered that some patients with symptomatic epilepsy have no subsequent recollection of an aura.

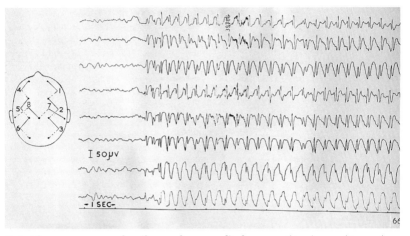

5.5 Three per second spike and wave discharge. This abnormality can be demonstrated in most patients with absences. Like absences it may be inherited, although there is some dispute about the mode of transmission. It may also be found in asymptomatic siblings. While it is important to realise that the presence of a discharge on the EEG does not mean that a patient is an epileptic it may draw attention to unnoticed seizures that are responsible for a poor performance at school. It is particularly important in distinguishing between absences and complex partial seizures, both of which can cause automatism but which require different forms of treatment.

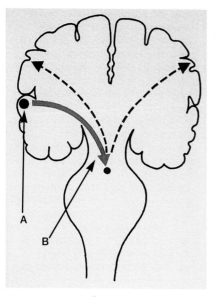

5.6 Partial seizures. Partial or focal fits start at one point on the cerebral cortex, producing symptoms of which the patient is aware (A). These may take the form of a unilateral motor (Jacksonian) or sensory disturbance or of an assortment of abnormal feelings starting in the abdomen, a *déjà vu* sensation, olfactory or gustatory hallucinations and autonomic dysfunction (temporal lobe epilepsy). Partial seizures, which may be 'symptomatic' of a tumour or of some other cortical lesion, can undergo secondary generalisation (B) resulting in loss of consciousness and a major fit. Bilateral spread, notably from a temporal lobe focus, can also result in loss of awareness and automatic behaviour (complex partial seizures).

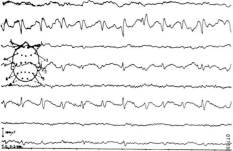

5.7 Left temporal lobe focus. A 36-year-old patient with a 2-year history of unrecognised partial (temporal lobe) seizures who presented when, after consuming a large amount of alcohol, he had his first tonic–clonic fit. (It often transpires that epileptics who have gone 'out of control' did so because they were intoxicated.) The EEG shows a sharp and slow wave discharge on the left. The late onset of the attacks and the focal nature of the problem were strong indications for further investigation to exclude a tumour.

It is now recognised that the traditional classification of fits into generalised and partial, major and minor is inadequate and that for prognostic and therapeutic purposes *syndromes* which require special management – notably benign childhood partial epilepsy and juvenile myoclonic epilepsy – have also to be identified.

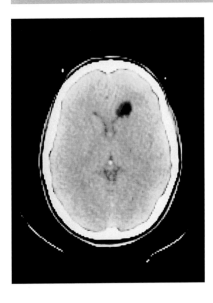

5.8 CT scanning in late onset epilepsy. There has been much debate about the place of scanning in patients presenting with late onset epilepsy (i.e. epilepsy starting after the age of 21). In an otherwise normal individual such investigations rarely reveal a remediable lesion such as a meningioma, but scans should be done routinely so that one cannot subsequently be accused of missing an assortment of indolent or irrelevant lesions that come to light. Recent examples include a heavily calcified glioma, lipomas of the corpus callosum and at the tip of the lateral ventricle (5.8), and arachnoid cysts indenting the temporal lobe or communicating with the third ventricle. By contrast, in patients who are resistant to adequate drug treatment the importance of detailed investigation with a view to surgery is being increasingly realised.

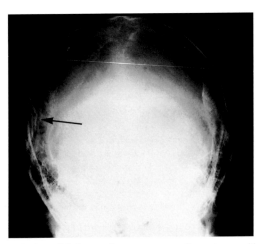

5.9 Head injury. Post-traumatic epilepsy is most likely to occur if there was an intracranial haematoma, a fit in the first week or a depressed fracture of the skull (arrow). When all are present the risk is of the order of 70%.

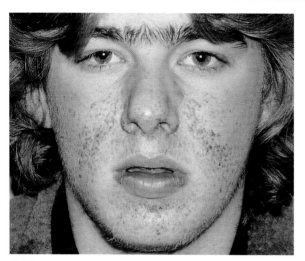

5.10

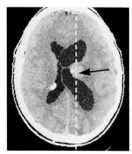

5.11

5.10,5.11 Tuberous sclerosis. The phakomatoses are genetically determined neuroectodermal lesions with a predilection for the central nervous system and the retina. They may not be evident at birth but later in life give rise to multiple tumours and cysts. In addition to tuberous sclerosis the group includes neurofibromatosis and the von Hippel–Lindau and Sturge–Weber syndromes. Patients with tuberous sclerosis, which is inherited as a Mendelian dominant, often have severe mental retardation and epilepsy. Oval white patches may be visible on the skin before angiofibromatous papules (adenoma sebaceum) develop on the nasolabial folds and around the mouth (5.10). Other findings include fibromas in the nail folds, 'shagreen' patches over the lower back, retinal and pulmonary lesions and tumours of the heart, brain and kidney which are often responsible for the patient's death. The CT scan (5.11) shows typical calcification in the wall of the lateral ventricle and a subependymal nodule (arrow) projecting into the lateral ventricle. The dilation of the ventricle and the deviation of the septum were due to a second nodule near the foramen of Monro.

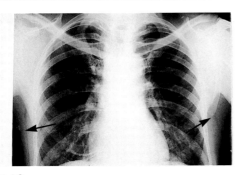

5.12

5.12–5.14 Cysticercosis.
Infection with the larval stage of *Taenia solium*, the pig tapeworm, occurs when the eggs are swallowed. A wide variety of neurological problems including epilepsy, obstructive hydrocephalus and meningitis can follow and in Mexico City, where the disease is endemic, it is responsible for 10% of hospital admissions and 33% of craniotomies. The cysts in the brain are not easily seen on a skull X-ray and those on the chest X-ray (5.12 arrow) could easily be overlooked. In the limbs – where they sometimes produce a picture of pseudohypertrophy – they are easily visible (5.13). Intracranial lesions are more easily demonstrated by scanning (5.14).

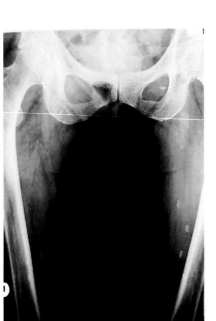

5.13

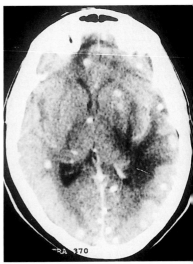

5.14

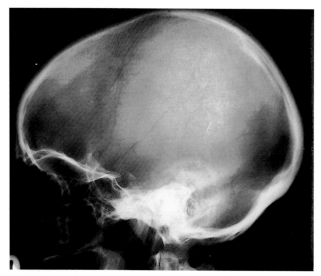

5.15

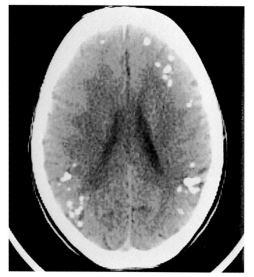

5.16

5.15,5.16 Toxoplasmosis. Toxoplasmosis also causes fits and hydrocephalus. This patient presented with a squint at the age of 3. Extensive choroidal atrophy was found and serological tests were positive. The skull X-ray and the CT scan showed flecks of calcium in both hemispheres.

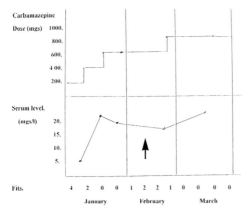

Carbamazepine
Dose (mgs) 1000.
800.
600.
400.
200.

Serum level.
(mgs/l) 20.
15.
10.
5.

Fits.   4 2 0 0 1 2 2 1 0 0 0 0
          January   February   March

Name. Joan C.   Warned about: driving.
Date of birth. 14 2 53   snooring in bath.
Date of onset. 1985   contraception.
Cause. Head injury 1982   teratogenicity.
        (? irrelevant)
E.E.G. ⊖
Scan. ⊖
Other conditions.

Date	Major	Minor	Carbamazepine	Valproate		
April 85	1 (cocb)				TCR prn	
Jan 86	2	4	200 bd			½
Feb 86	1 (cocb)	2	rash	200 tds		½
Marcb 86	—	5		400 bd		½
April 86	—	—		400 bd		³/₁₂
July 86	1	—		400 bd	? when drunk	²/₁₂
Sept 86	1	1		600 bd		²/₁₂
Nov 86	—	—		600 bd		²/₁₂

5.17 Drug treatment of epilepsy. The realisation that the dose of anticonvulsants has to be 'tailor-made' was a major therapeutic advance. This is now achieved by cautiously increasing the dose of a single drug until control is obtained or toxic symptoms appear. The regular estimation of serum anticonvulsant levels to ensure that they stay within a 'therapeutic range' is no longer advocated. Serum levels may however be useful when there are doubts about compliance or when a gradual enhancement of metabolism results in a return of seizures due to the more rapid degradation of a hitherto effective dose of (e.g.) carbamazepine (arrow).

5.18 Epilepsy data sheet. With longstanding problems such as epilepsy it is important that the salient features of the history and of past and present treatment should be easily accessible. A chart of this type, on which the patient's classification of 'major' and 'minor' fits is accepted, shows at a glance what has been done, which drugs have been used, the serum levels and important details (e.g. precipitating factors, drugs which control status, suspicions about the nature of attacks).

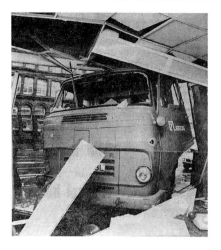

5.19 Driving. A licence holder has an obligation to inform the authorities of any condition which impairs or, in due course, is likely to impair his ability to drive. Fits, however minor, and attacks of loss of consciousness for which no cause has been found come under this heading. Civilian drivers who have had a single fit and epileptics who have attacks when awake will not be permitted to drive until they have gone for more than a year without an attack and are deemed not to be a danger. A licence may also be granted if, over the course of more than 3 years, all attacks occurred during sleep.

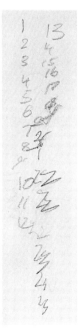

5.20 Partial seizures. For purposes of driving partial seizures, seizures with an aura and myoclonic jerks are all regarded as fits. Apart from the fact that all, sooner or later, may be associated with a major attack those with 'little attacks' often fail to realise how disabling they are. This man could often 'prevent' blackouts by concentrating on some activity when he developed premonitory symptoms. Yet in this episode – 'prevented' by writing numbers – his performance was obviously impaired after he reached the number 18.

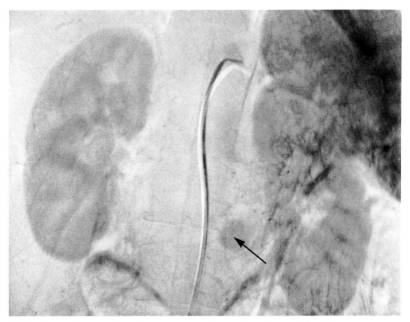

5.21 Hypoglycaemia. Diabetics on insulin and patients with insulinomas may also have road accidents. This 55-year-old woman was admitted in coma with a blood glucose of 1.6 mm/l (30 mg%). Over the previous 2 years, particularly when deprived of food, she had had ten attacks of confusion and diplopia. For example after missing tea and going for a long walk she was 'unable to understand the menu' when she got back to her hotel for dinner. On another occasion, after the late arrival of guests, she 'didn't know how to cook' the dinner she had prepared. Arteriography revealed a small insulinoma (arrow) which was successfully removed.

6.

Cerebral tumours

Tumours, unlike vascular accidents, develop gradually, presenting with symptoms that fall into one or more of four groups:

1. **Overactivity of part of the brain.** This incorporates the excessive secretion of a pituitary tumour but refers mainly to patients who present with fits. Those over the age of 45, with partial (focal) fits, in status, with neurological signs and/or with focal abnormalities on the EEG are particularly suspect.

2. **Underactivity of part of the brain.** A crossed hemiplegia due to a hemisphere lesion, ipsilateral ataxia due to a cerebellar lesion, bitemporal hemianopia and hypopituitarism due to a pituitary tumour and deafness and loss of the corneal reflex due to a cerebello-pontine angle tumour are unlikely to be overlooked. Other signs such as hemianopia, dysphasia and a change of personality are more easily missed. The point was well made by the patient who, when told 'your trouble is that you've got verbal diarrhoea' correctly replied 'no, that's my *symptom*'.

3. **Evidence of raised intracranial pressure.** Initially the headache is not severe and a mild but unfamiliar pain present for an hour or two each morning and returning if the patient has a few pints of beer or strains to lift something heavy is an alarming symptom.

4. **Evidence of a primary tumour elsewhere.** Primary *cerebral* tumours do not affect the general health or the sedimentation rate and if these are abnormal a search should be made for a primary elsewhere.

Pituitary tumours

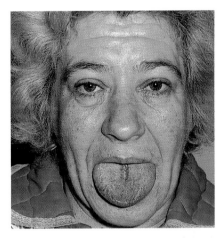

6.1 Acromegaly. Diagnosis is easy when a patient with heavy features, prognathism, a bulbous nose and a large tongue complains that she is unable to remove her wedding ring and has been obliged to increase her shoe size from 4.5 to 6.

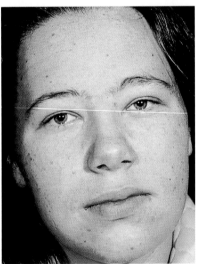

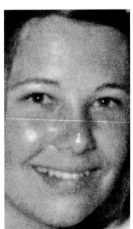

6.3

6.2

6.2,6.3 Acromegaly. Diagnosis was more difficult in this polysymptomatic patient. As she complained of diplopia and of transient loss of vision in each eye and had optic atrophy on the left the possibility of multiple sclerosis was considered. Her family was not aware that her features had changed until confronted with a photograph taken some years earlier.

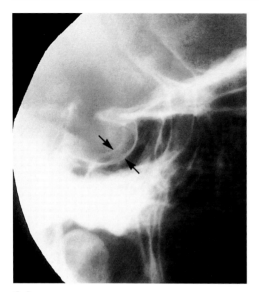

6.4

6.4,6.5 Abnormalities on plain films caused by pituitary tumours. In patients with basophil adenomas (Cushing's syndrome) the fossa is usually normal. The appearance may also be normal with acidophil adenomas (acromegaly), although closer inspection often reveals subtle abnormalities such as a double floor (6.4 arrows). More often the fossa is enlarged and the posterior clinoid process is eroded (6.5). Larger tumours, particularly chromophobe adenomas, cause extensive destruction.

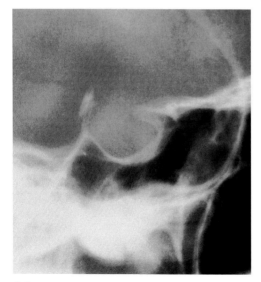

6.5

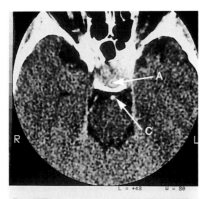

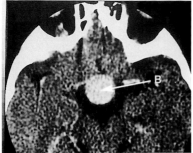

6.6

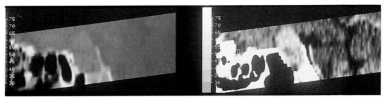

6.7

6.6,6.7 CT scan of pituitary tumour. Axial views showing a pituitary tumour, enhanced by contrast, lying within (A) and above (B) the pituitary fossa. The posterior clinoid process and the basilar artery are marked (C). The left lateral reconstructions show (on different settings) erosion of the posterior clinoid process and the tumour extending upwards and forwards.

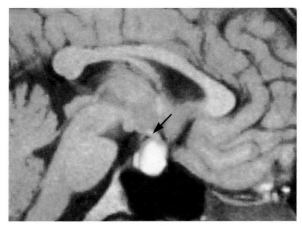

6.8 MR scan of pituitary adenoma. A post-contrast scan of a similar lesion showing the better definition obtained with MR imaging. Note how the tumour impinges on the optic chiasm (arrow).

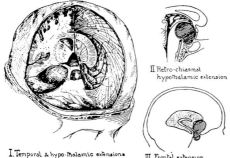

II. Retro-chiasmal hypothalamic extension

I. Temporal & hypo-thalamic extensions

III. Frontal extension.

6.9 Invasive adenomas of the pituitary. Pituitary tumours sometimes 'escape' under, in front of or behind the chiasm. Jefferson named these lesions, which can be very large, invasive adenomas. This illustration (from *Proceedings of the Royal Society of Medicine* 1940; 33: 433–458) shows: (I) extension laterally into the temporal lobe; (II) extension behind the chiasm into the third ventricle in a patient with short optic nerves and a prefixed chiasm; (III) extension in front of the chiasm in a patient with long optic nerves and a post-fixed chiasm.

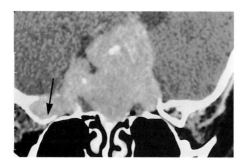

6.10 Adenoma invading the temporal lobe. A frontal view of a large pituitary tumour which is extending laterally into the temporal lobes, particularly on the right (arrow).

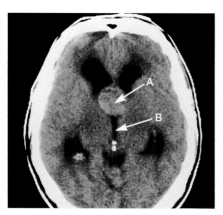

6.11

6.11,6.12 Adenoma invading the third ventricle. An axial view of a pituitary tumour (A) which has caused hydrocephalus by invading the third ventricle, the remains of which can be seen splayed across the posterior aspect of the lesion (B). On the lateral reconstruction the ventricular system can be traced from the fourth ventricle (C) through the aqueduct below the calcified pineal (D) to the remainder of the third ventricle (E) which is largely obliterated by a mass arising in the pituitary fossa (F).

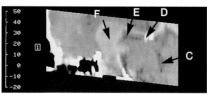

6.12

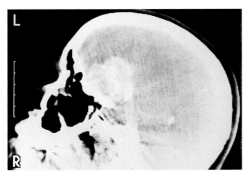

6.13 Adenoma invading the frontal lobe. A 47-year-old woman with amenorrhoea and bouts of impairment of consciousness. Following an attack of 'viral meningitis' at the age of 17 she was told that there was 'something the matter with her visual fields'. She was obese and had optic atrophy and a bitemporal hemianopia. The pituitary fossa was markedly enlarged and the calcified mass extending into the frontal lobe was thought to be a craniopharyngioma. It proved, however, to be a pituitary adenoma.

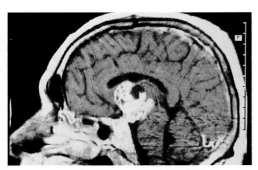

6.14 Craniopharyngioma. An MR scan showing a large lesion of mixed density in the region of the third ventricle. In younger patients calcification often suggests the nature of such tumours, but in older patients calcification is uncommon. Unlike pituitary tumours, craniopharyngiomas tend to invade the chiasm from above and the field defect is therefore most marked in the inferior quadrants. Like pituitary tumours, they can cause a change in personality by invading the frontal lobe or obstructing the flow of CSF in the third ventricle.

Meningiomas

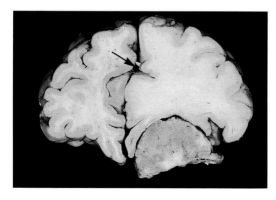

6.15 Subfrontal meningioma.

Meningiomas arise outside the substance of the brain. Although essentially benign, removal may be difficult because of inaccessibility, size, infiltration of bone or the sagittal sinus or malignant change. Subfrontal tumours may produce ipsilateral anosmia and optic atrophy with contralateral papilloedema (the Foster Kennedy syndrome (see 3.4) and/or frontal lobe signs.

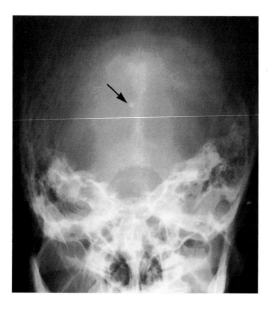

6.16 Displacement of the pineal.

The pineal gland lies on the vertical axis of the skull. Its position is not therefore altered by minor degrees of rotation and displacement of more than 3 mm is always significant. Anteriorly placed lesions, however, have little effect on its position even when large. They are more likely to displace the anterior cerebral artery and to cause herniation of the hemisphere under the falx (6.15 arrow).

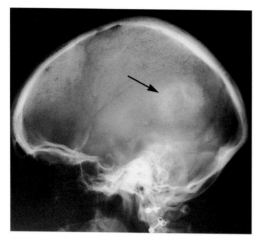

6.17

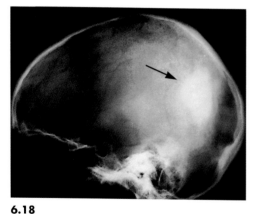

6.18

6.17, 6.18 Calcification in meningioma. Calcification, which is common, may be visible on the plain radiograph. This convexity meningioma was found by accident when the (asymptomatic) patient was X-rayed after a road accident (6.17 arrow). A similar appearance produced by an Asian patient's thick plaits (6.18 arrow) shows the importance of establishing that such 'lesions' are intracranial.

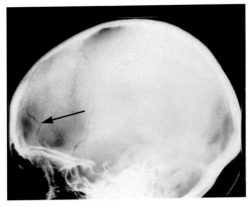

6.19

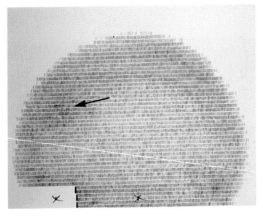

6.20

6.19,6.20 Parasagittal meningioma with vascular markings. Prominent vascular markings on the skull of a 38-year-old woman with chronic papilloedema (6.19 arrow). She gave a 6-month history of transient blurring of vision on exertion, mild headaches and occasional dizzy spells on bending. The isotope scan, a sensitive but out-dated technique for demonstrating meningiomas, showed a parasagittal lesion in the left frontal region (6.20 arrow).

(See also hyperostosis due to meningioma – 3.22, 3.23.)

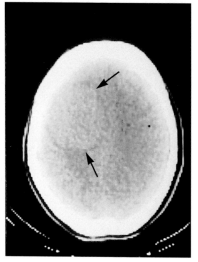 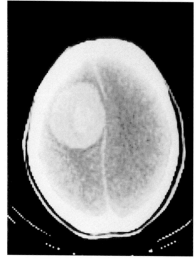

6.21 **6.22**

6.21,6.22 CT scan of meningioma. On a CT scan a meningioma usually appears as a well-defined mass adjacent to bone or the falx (6.21 arrow) which enhances vigorously with contrast (6.22).

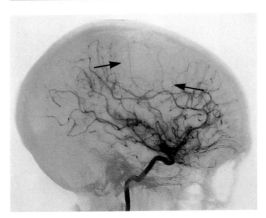

6.23

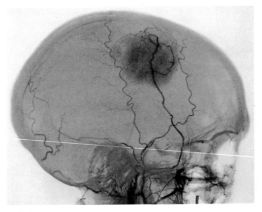

6.24

6.23,6.24 Arteriogram of meningioma. Arteriography characteristically shows displacement of vessels and a blush. On this internal carotid arteriogram the position of the tumour is shown by stretched vessels surrounding an avascular area (6.23 arrows). The blood supply, however, came from the external carotid and the tumour blush only appeared when that vessel was injected (6.24).

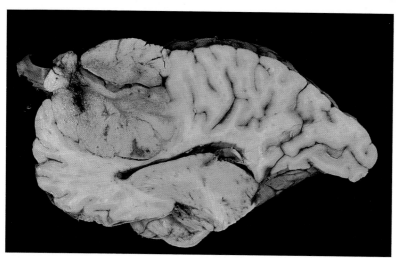

6.29 Parasagittal meningioma (cont.). Following the angiogram the patient developed a right hemiparesis and died before an attempt could be made to excise a tumour which occupied nearly a third of the left hemisphere. The fact that this enormous lesion did not cause weakness or obvious papilloedema may seem surprising, but slowly expanding tumours in the frontal lobe can be accommodated at the expense of an (often un-noticed) change of personality and a few fits. The EEG frequently fails to detect such lesions and sudden decompensation precipitated by arteriography or surgery is well recognised. In retrospect the lesion was just visible on the original (very poor) isotope scan.

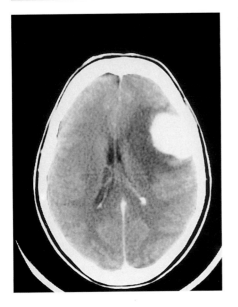

6.30 Meningioma presenting with 'transient ischaemic attacks'. Meningiomas may also present with what sound like transient ischaemic attacks. A careful history, however, often reveals that the story is in fact more complex. This lady was referred because of two transient episodes of dysphasia. It transpired, however, that she had also had great difficulty in working out how to put toothpaste on her toothbrush and how to put on her knickers – i.e. that she had ongoing dyspraxia due to a lesion in the left hemisphere.

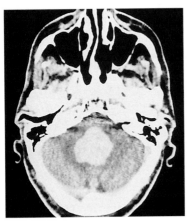

6.31 Meningioma in the fourth ventricle. Meningiomas are sometimes found in the ventricles. This 58-year-old man gave a 2-month history of headaches, ataxia and blurring of vision. He had papilloedema, diplopia and nystagmus and a CT scan revealed an enhancing lesion in the fourth ventricle which proved to be a meningioma.

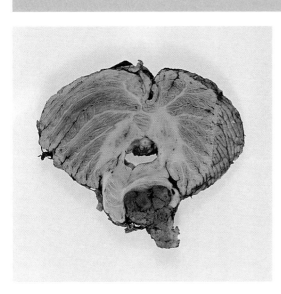

6.32 Tentorial meningioma.
Meningiomas also occur on the floor of the posterior fossa. This 60-year-old recluse had been deluded and antisocial for 5 years. When admitted she was found to have 240 tins of food and 42 pairs of new shoes in her house. An arteriogram outlined a vascular neoplasm at the tip of the left petrous temporal bone which, in retrospect, was visible on the isotope scan. To the relief of the surgeon consulted she refused an operation and at autopsy 9 months later a meningioma was found deeply impacted in the pons and lower brainstem.

(See also meningioma of optic nerve sheath – 3.10,3.20,3.21.)

Gliomas

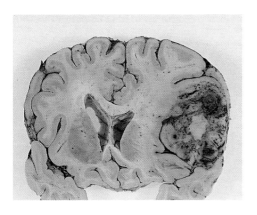

6.33 Glioma. Gliomas are tumours of varying degrees of malignancy which grow within the substance of the brain. They may expand by infiltration or form cystic or solid masses which displace midline structures. Note here how the septum and the lateral ventricle and cingulate gyrus on the right have been forced under the falx.

145

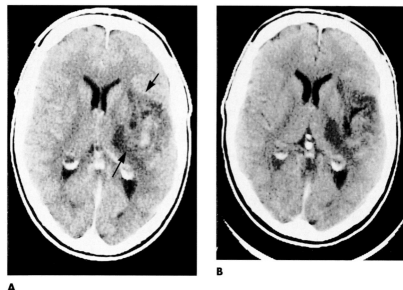

B

A

6.34A,B Slowly growing glioma. Because of their tendency to infiltrate the brain gliomas can rarely be excised. The problem of management is further increased by their unpredictable behaviour. This 52-year-old man presented with an 8-year history of right-sided fits. He was found to have a large lesion in the left hemisphere (6.34A arrows) but refused treatment. The appearance of the tumour (which by now had been present for 10 years) was unchanged 2 years later (6.34B). Histological grading, however, is of limited long-term value because some parts of the tumour may be more malignant than others and because the lesion may undergo malignant degeneration.

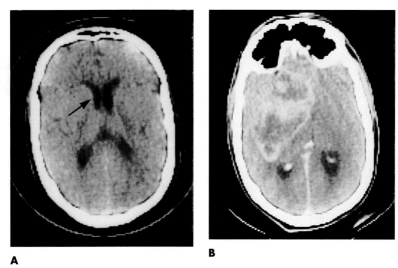

A

B

6.35A,B Rapidly growing glioma. Over the course of 6 months this 57-year-old man developed a change of personality followed by fits, morning headache and a mild left hemiparesis. He had marked inattention and other parietal lobe signs, but his fundi were virtually normal. A CT scan done 3 months before admission had been passed as normal, although in retrospect there was indentation of the right lateral ventricle (6.35A arrow). A repeat scan showed that he now had a massive lesion which caused the death of the patient within weeks (6.35B).

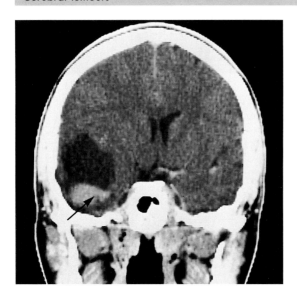

6.36 Cystic glioma.
The problems of surgery for patients with gliomas are illustrated by the two preceding cases. Treatment of the first patient could hardly have produced a better result whereas treatment of the second was clearly futile. However, for those with cystic lesions drainage can produce symptomatic relief and excision of a nubbin of tumour on the wall (arrow) may even effect a cure.

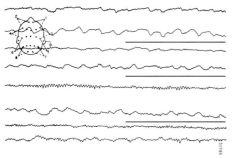

6.37 EEG abnormality due to glioma. The EEG is not an appropriate investigation for patients thought to have tumours. On the other hand, a persistent and progressive focal abnormality on the EEG is an indication for repeating the brain scan, for such changes sometimes precede obvious abnormalities on the scan.

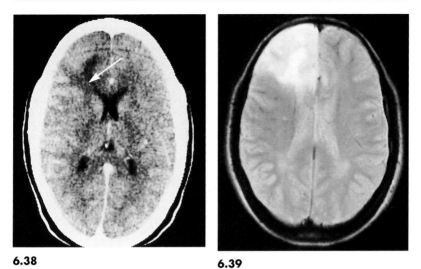

6.38

6.39

6.38,6.39 MR scan of glioma. With the introduction of MR scanning it has become less likely that gliomas will be overlooked. This 47-year-old patient presented with a single fit. Clinical examination and the EEG were normal but a lesion was found on CT (6.38 arrow). It was even more evident on the MR scan (6.39).

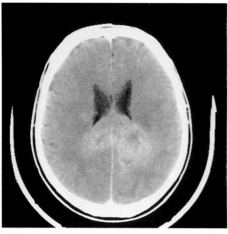

6.40

6.40, 6.41 Corpus callosum glioma. Because of the nebulous nature of their symptomatology corpus callosum gliomas are particularly difficult to diagnose. During the previous 2 months this 56-year-old man, who held a very responsible job, had undergone 'a personality change'. He had no sense of the passage of time, could no longer find his way around, had become forgetful and had lost his drive and his ability to reason. Outwardly he appeared to be well but the scan revealed a 'butterfly' glioma of the corpus callosum from which he died 3 months later. (The linear scar on 6.41 is a needle biopsy track.)

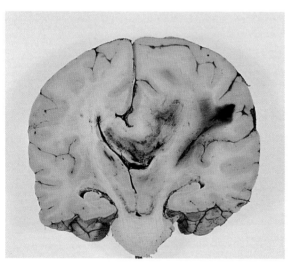

6.41

Colloid cysts and metastases

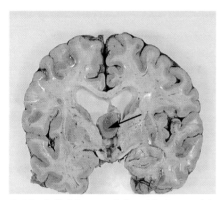

6.42 Colloid cyst of the third ventricle. This uncommon tumour obstructs the flow of CSF causing paroxysmal headache, ataxia, dementia and/or drop attacks. For 5 months this 45-year-old man had been muddled, disorientated, forgetful, casual and sleepy. He also complained of paroxysms of severe headache, in one of which he lost consciousness and died. At autopsy he was found to have marked hydrocephalus and a colloid cyst (arrow) impacted in the interventricular foramen.

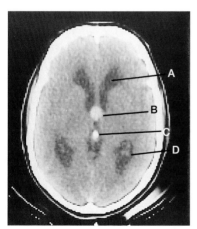

6.43 Colloid cyst of the third ventricle. Diagnosis has been simplified by the introduction of scanning. This 68-year-old man gave a 12-month history of intellectual deterioration and severe ataxia. There were no localising signs, but a scan showed marked hydrocephalus (A) and a colloid cyst in the third ventricle (B). Also shown are a calcified pineal (C) and a calcified choroid plexus in the dilated posterior horn (D).

(See also pinealoma – 3.81, 3.82.)

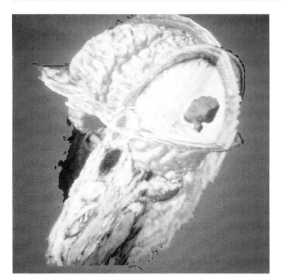

6.44 Metastases. In the United Kingdom, multiple discrete space-occupying lesions in the hemispheres usually prove to be metastases. In this colour-coded three-dimensional picture of the hemispheres the left hemisphere has been 'cut away' to show two discrete metastases in the parieto-occipital region. (By courtesy of Prof. M A Smith.)

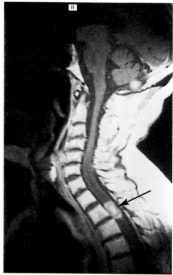

6.46

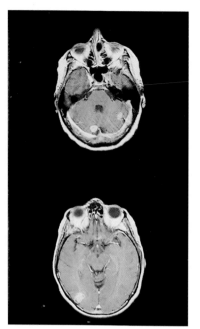

6.45

6.45,6.46 Metastases. Although the prognosis for patients with cerebral metastases is usually very poor, this is not invariably the case. This 68-year-old woman had a mastectomy in 1973. In 1982 she was noticed to have a mass in the left lung and in 1988 – when she presented with paraplegia – this mass was biopsied and found to be a malignant adenocarcinoma. She was also found to have multiple intracranial lesions – some calcified and some enhancing – and a mass in the upper thoracic cord. Serological tests for histoplasmosis, coccidioidomycosis and toxoplasmosis were negative and the lesions were not thought to be tuberculomas. She had 'palliative' radiotherapy to the spine and in 1993, when the paraplegia was complete, the spinal mass was removed. It proved to be a metastasis from a carcinoma of the breast.

Tumours in the posterior fossa

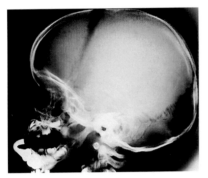

6.47

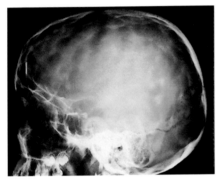

6.48

6.47,6.48 Changes on the skull X-ray. A posterior fossa tumour may cause separation of the sutures in a child (6.47), erosion of the posterior clinoid processes or 'copper beating' (6.48). Bone is constantly being remodelled and, when the intracranial pressure is high, the inner table is not replaced after it has been removed. This is most evident on the posterior clinoid processes which have dura on both surfaces. Copper beating of the vault is produced in the same way but is more difficult to assess because an identical picture may be seen in healthy individuals.

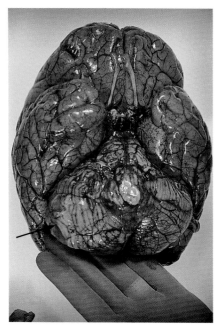

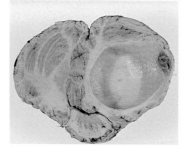

6.50

6.49

6.49,6.50 Cystic haemangioblastoma of the cerebellum. A 29-year-old woman who, over the previous 2 months, had had a brief attack of vertigo, occipital pain on movement of the head, some right-sided earache and one bout of vomiting. Apart from a trace of nystagmus and a slightly unsteady gait she had no signs and plain films, an isotope scan, an audiogram and caloric tests were normal. She was discharged, but 4 days later headache and vomiting returned and her behaviour became so extreme that a psychiatrist was asked to see her. By this time there was early swelling of the discs. A myodil ventriculogram showed that she had hydrocephalus with displacement of the aqueduct forwards and to the left.

The patient died before operation and autopsy revealed a large cyst in the right cerebellar hemisphere which seemed to be on the verge of rupture (6.49 arrow). The nodule suggested that the lesion was a glioma but it proved to be a haemangioblastoma. Although with modern methods of scanning it would have been recognised at an earlier stage, the patient was already in a critical condition at the time of presentation.

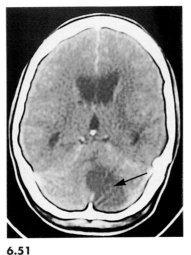

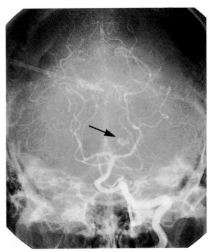

6.51

6.52

6.51,6.52 Haemangioblastoma. A 39-year-old man with a 6-week history of nausea, ataxia and occipital headache aggravated by coughing and stooping. Apart from early papilloedema he had no signs. A CT scan showed a large low-density lesion in the left cerebellar hemisphere. A small vascular nodule on the vertebral arteriogram (6.52 arrow) confirmed that the lesion was a haemangioblastoma.

Patients with large tumours in the posterior fossa often have very little in the way of symptoms and signs. A complaint of slight unsteadiness and of morning headache which, although mild, is new, persistent and aggravated by straining and alcohol should be viewed with great suspicion even when the fundi are normal. Decompensation, when it occurs, can do so with alarming speed and at this stage – as the previous case shows – treatment of a remediable lesion may be impossible.

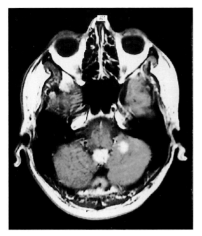

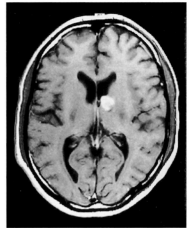

6.53

6.54

6.53–6.57 Von Hippel–Lindau syndrome. A patient who presented at the age of 23 with a history of paroxysmal headache latterly associated with nausea and transient numbness on the right side of the body. Because he had experienced similar symptoms in the past and responded to propranolol these were attributed to migraine. He returned 3 months later with the same complaint. A CT scan of the head was normal but investigation of hypertension revealed renal and pancreatic cysts. After 3 months he complained of numbness in the legs and MR scanning and myelography revealed haemangioblastomas throughout the neuraxis. The illustrations show two of the lesions in the cerebellum (6.53), a lesion in the hemisphere (6.54) and numerous lesions in the cord (6.55 arrows). The vertebral arteriogram outlines the largest of the cerebellar lesions (6.56A), the hemisphere lesion (6.56B) and the tumours at the top of the cord with their feeding vessels (6.57 arrows). Careful scrutiny revealed that there was also a peripheral lesion on the retina.

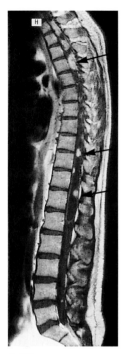

6.55

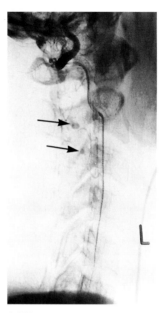

6.57

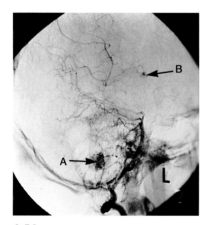

6.56

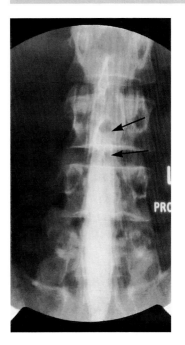

6.58 Medulloblastoma. A medulloblastoma, the other intrinsic tumour found almost exclusively in the hindbrain, occurs primarily in children. It extends into the fourth ventricle and has the characteristic of seeding throughout the rest of the neuraxis. The illustration shows droplet metastases among the roots of the cauda equina on the myelogram (arrows). Secondary deposits from tumours outside the nervous system sometimes produce a similar appearance.

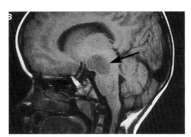

6.59 MR scan of brainstem glioma. One of the great assets of MR scanning is its ability to locate lesions in the posterior fossa safely, accurately and without distressing the patient (who is often a child). This brainstem glioma – which on CT appeared to be an extrinsic lesion compressing the brainstem – clearly lies within the substance of the midbrain (see also 9.47).

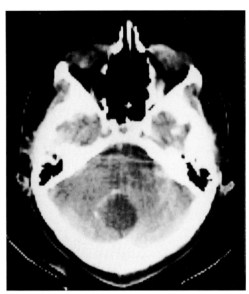

6.60 Dermoid. Midline posterior fossa dermoids appear during the process of invagination which leads to the formation of the tentorium, to which they are often attached. Some patients have a nodule or bone defect over the occiput, a sinus or a track leading down to the tumour. These lesions may present as a mass, with recurrent chemical meningitis or with more dramatic symptoms due to sudden rupture. This patient gave a 20-year history of 'things jumping up and down' (downbeat nystagmus) and mild ataxia. The diagnosis was suggested by the length of the history and the presence of a calcified mass in the middle of the posterior fossa.

(See also acoustic schwannoma – 3.131–3.133.)

7.

Cerebrovascular diseases

Cerebral haemorrhage

Cerebral haemorrhage may be traumatic or spontaneous. Spontaneous haemorrhages are usually attributable to hypertension, to the use of drugs or to aneurysmal or arteriovenous malformations. Traumatic haemorrhages may be intracerebral, subdural or extradural. A physician needs to have some knowledge of the last two, which in turn requires an understanding of the cerebral membranes.

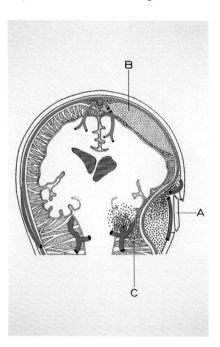

7.1 Cerebral membranes and cerebral haemorrhage. The brain is surrounded by three membranes (left of diagram). Outermost and adjacent to the skull is the dura (green) which splits to envelop the sagittal sinus. Innermost and closely adherent to the brain is the pia (black). Between the two is the arachnoid, attached to the dura but linked to the pia by web-like processes that form the subarachnoid space (stippled). An extradural haematoma occurs when the middle meningeal artery, ruptured by a fracture of the skull, rapidly pumps blood into the space between the skull and the dura (A). A subdural haematoma occurs when a vein running from the sagittal sinus to the hemisphere ruptures, allowing venous blood to collect slowly between the dura and the arachnoid (B). Haemorrhage from a berry aneurysm may go into the subarachnoid space and/or burst into the substance of the brain (C).

Extradural haematoma

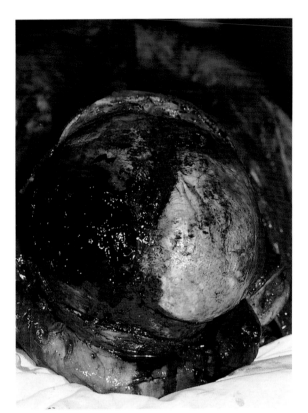

7.2 Extradural haematoma. The textbook picture of an extradural haematoma is of a significant head injury causing loss of consciousness, quickly followed by a lucid interval and a relapse into coma with subsequent dilation of the ipsilateral pupil. Survival depends on early detection and removal of the rapidly expanding clot. In practice the injury is often trivial and the lucid interval may not occur. It is therefore important that all but the most minor head injuries should be carefully monitored.

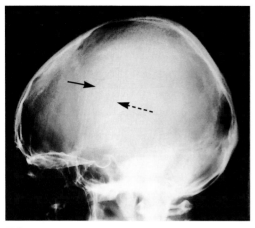

7.3

7.3–7.5 Extradural haematoma.

A 23-year-old student who was knocked off his bicycle. He was not rendered unconscious and initially attention was focused on a severe laceration of the right ear. The skull X-ray showed a fracture line (7.3 solid arrow) and a white line (7.3 dotted arrow) where the edges of a depressed fracture overlapped. A scan, done because of doubt about the appearance of the fundi, gave a better picture of the fracture (7.4) and revealed an extradural haematoma (7.5).

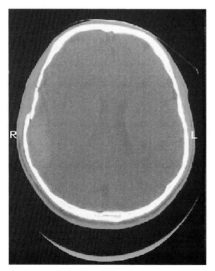

7.4

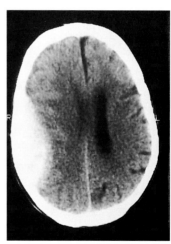

7.5

Subdural haematoma

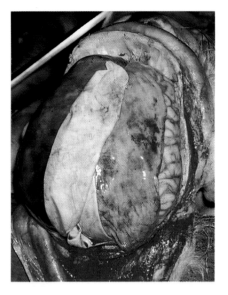

7.6 Subdural haematoma. A subdural haematoma, seen here beneath the reflected dura, is caused by minor blows to the head and often appears to be spontaneous. This lesion is commonly associated with anticoagulants, alcoholism and old age – i.e. with patients who are prone to injure themselves and in whom excessive movement of an atrophic hemisphere facilitates rupture of veins running from the sagittal sinus to the brain. The most common manifestations are headache and fluctuations in the level of consciousness which, in the elderly and alcoholics, may seem unremarkable until the patient lapses into coma.

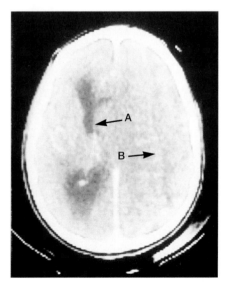

7.7 Subdural haematoma (transitional phase). For the first 10 days a subdural haematoma appears as a hyperdense mass which envelops the hemisphere (unlike an extradural which indents it). From the 10th to the 20th day the lesion becomes isodense and can easily be overlooked. Here, however, the presence of a mass is revealed by gross displacement of the ventricles (A) and by contrast enhancement of the cortex and capsule (B).

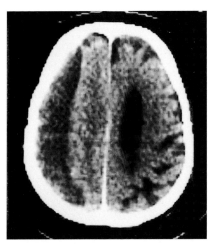

7.8 Established subdural haematoma. An established subdural which appears as a hypodense mass enveloping the right side of the brain. Note the cortical atrophy on the left which is invisible in the compressed right hemisphere.

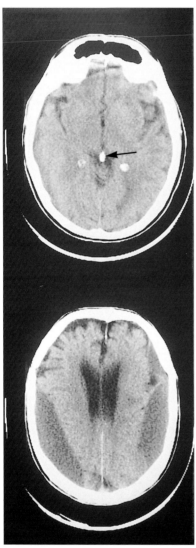

7.9 Bilateral subdural haematomas. Subdural haematomas are often bilateral, in which case the midline septum pellucidum and the calcified pineal (arrow) will not be displaced.

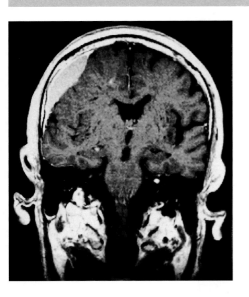

7.10 MR scan of subdural haematoma. An MR scan of a subdural haematoma, showing displacement of midline structures.

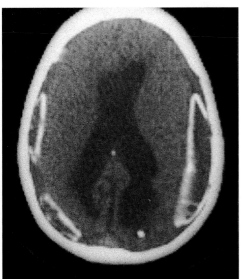

7.11 Calcified subdural haematomas. Calcification in bilateral subdural haematomas which formed in a patient with hydrocephalus after the intracranial pressure was reduced by shunting.

Spontaneous cerebral haemorrhage

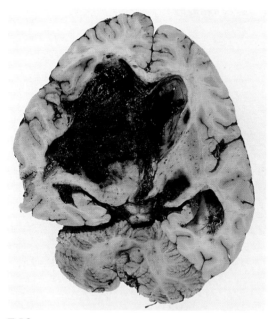

7.12

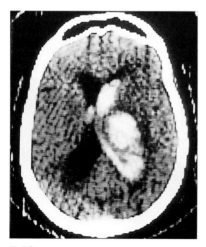

7.12,7.13 Cerebral haemorrhage.
The textbook cerebral haemorrhage
occurs suddenly during exertion in a
hypertensive patient. Signs are not
confined to the territory of one artery and
the incident is often lethal. With the
introduction of effective treatment for
hypertension such episodes have become
less common.

7.13

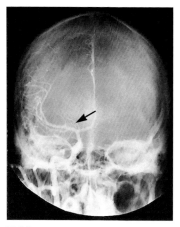

7.14

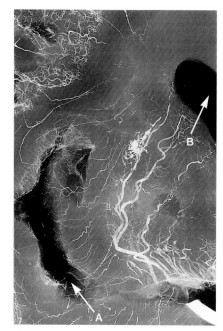

7.15

7.14, 7.15 Charcot–Bouchard aneurysms. Hypertensive cerebral haemorrhage is believed to be the result of rupture of microaneurysms, first described by Charcot and Bouchard in 1868. These lesions usually lie on perforating branches of the middle cerebral artery (7.14) in the region of the internal capsule (7.15 A = insula, B = lateral ventricle. Courtesy of Dr D G F Harriman) but may also be found beneath the parietal cortex and in the cerebellum.

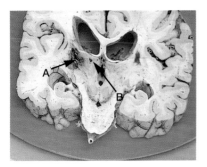

7.16 Small haemorrhage and lacunar infarct. The introduction of CT scanning showed that many minor neurological episodes attributed to infarction were in fact caused by small haemorrhages (A). Conversely, degenerative changes in the perforating vessels can cause specific neurological syndromes associated with small lesions known, because of their appearance, as lacunar infarcts (B).

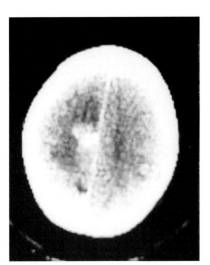

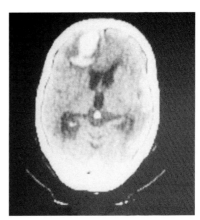

7.18

7.17

7.17,7.18 Amyloid angiopathy. In older normotensive patients cerebral amyloid angiopathy is now recognised as a cause of cerebral haemorrhages which may be subcortical, multiple and/or (as with these two lesions which appeared several weeks apart) recurrent.

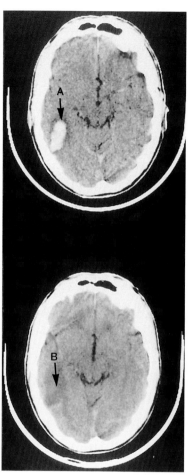

7.19 Resolution of subcortical haemorrhage. A subcortical haemorrhage in a patient with a history of transient ischaemic attacks (A) which, 3 weeks later, appears as an area of low attenuation (B). In view of the history of transient ischaemic attacks the second picture could easily be mistaken for that of an infarct. This illustrates the importance of early investigation. Although Charcot–Bouchard aneurysms do occur at this site, in younger patients a haemorrhage of this sort raises the possibility of an arteriovenous malformation. Other possibilities include amyloid angiopathy (see 7.17, 7.18), haematological disorders, venous thrombosis, alcohol and drugs such as amphetamine and cocaine – which are now a prominent cause of cerebral haemorrhage in young people.

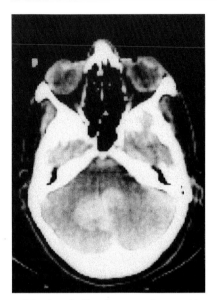

7.20 Cerebellar haemorrhage. Microaneurysms can also be found in the cerebellum where haemorrhage can cause headache, vomiting, vertigo, ataxia, dysarthria and coma. Surgical evacuation of the clot should be considered if the lesion is over 3 cm in diameter, if it is compressing the brainstem or if it is causing hydrocephalus.

(See also haemorrhage into brainstem – 3.96–3.100.)

Aneurysms

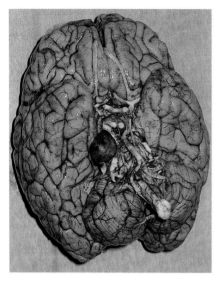

7.21 Berry aneurysm on posterior communicating artery.
Congenital or berry aneurysms occur at the bifurcations of major cerebral arteries. At this point the contour of the lumen depends entirely on the integrity of the internal elastic lamina. If, due to atheroma, age or hypertension, the wall collapses an aneurysm may form. With the exception of posterior communicating artery aneurysms which can compress the third cranial nerve, such lesions usually present when they rupture causing a subarachnoid haemorrhage.

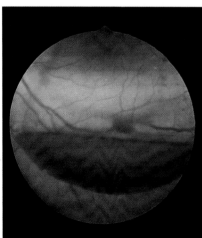

7.22 Subhyaloid haemorrhage.
The textbook picture of a subarachnoid haemorrhage is that of an adult who suddenly develops an excruciating, new and persistent headache with stiffness of the neck, vomiting and/or loss of consciousness. Occasionally, when blood tracks down to the bottom of the spinal canal, patients develop bilateral sciatica. The diagnosis can only be confirmed clinically if the patient has a subhyaloid haemorrhage. This is due to a rapid rise of intracranial pressure which suddenly obstructs the veins in the optic nerve sheath causing blood to burst through the nerve fibre layer (where it usually lies producing splinter haemorrhages) and into the subhyaloid space. Here there is no obstruction and it forms into large pools, the cells separating from the plasma to produce a fluid level.

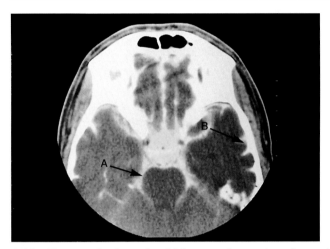

7.23 CT scan of subarachnoid haemorrhage. It is often evident that patients who have had a subarachnoid haemorrhage have had an earlier 'warning' haemorrhage that has been ignored. This greatly increases the difficulty of treatment and the risk of death. It is therefore essential that patients who present with a sudden, severe and unfamiliar headache should be investigated. In at least 90% a good CT scan done during the first 24 hours and examined by an expert will reveal evidence of subarachnoid bleeding. This rather extreme example shows the midbrain (A) and the cortical sulci (B) outlined with blood.

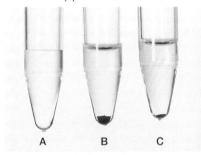

7.24 Lumbar puncture. Ideally a lumbar puncture should only be done after a CT scan has failed to show evidence of haemorrhage or an intracranial mass. However, when scanning is unavailable, the patient is conscious and there are no focal signs the risk is negligible. Normal CSF (A) and CSF from a traumatic tap (B) will be colourless provided the fluid is centrifuged *at once*. In subarachnoid haemorrhage the supernatant is xanthochromic (C). Spectrophotometry invariably reveals evidence of xanthochromia within 12 hours and it will persist for at least 2 weeks. Lumbar puncture has the added advantage that it will identify a significant number of patients with meningitis who present with symptoms suggestive of subarachnoid haemorrhage.

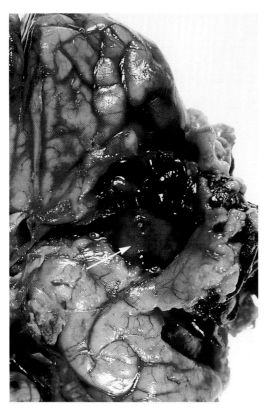

7.25 Occult haemorrhage. Blood normally appears in the spinal fluid within minutes of a haemorrhage and is nearly always present within 4 hours. Occasionally, however, no blood is found. This patient, who had had a 'stroke' 2 years earlier, was found to have an aneurysm 2 cm in diameter at the trifurcation of the middle cerebral artery (arrow). It was surrounded by clot, part of which was organised. It was therefore evident that the 'stroke' was an earlier rupture of the aneurysm into the substance of the hemisphere.

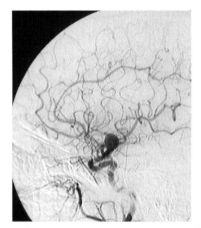

7.26

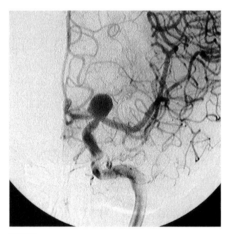

7.27

7.26,7.27 Angiography. Lateral (7.26) and PA (7.27) views of an aneurysm at the bifurcation of the left internal carotid artery. If the scan or the lumbar puncture indicate that a patient has had a subarachnoid haemorrhage angiography should be done. Current opinion seems to favour investigation and surgery within 24 hours. If angiography is negative there is a case for repeating the examination after a few weeks, particularly when the scan shows an inter-hemispheric as opposed to a perimesencephalic clot.

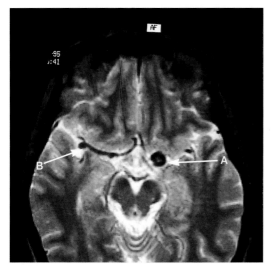

7.28

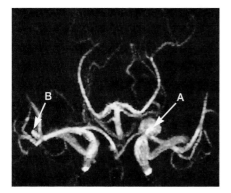

7.29

7.28, 7.29 MR scan and MR angiogram. An aneurysm may be seen on an MR scan and an MR angiogram. These films show the lesion on the left carotid artery demonstrated in 7.26, 7.27 (A) and a second smaller aneurysm at the bifurcation of the right middle cerebral artery (B).

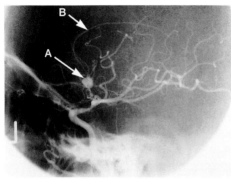

7.30

7.30, 7.31 Vasospasm and infarction due to subarachnoid haemorrhage. Vasospasm, which can be aggravated by angiography, is a major hazard of subarachnoid haemorrhage. The angiogram shows an aneurysm on the anterior communicating artery (A) with associated spasm in the anterior cerebral artery (B). The scan shows bilateral infarction of the frontal lobes induced by such an episode (arrow). Note also the blood in the inter-hemispheric fissure.

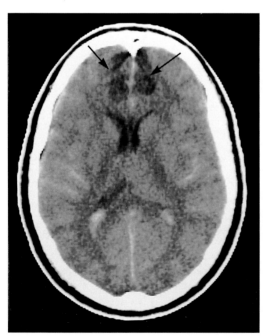

7.31

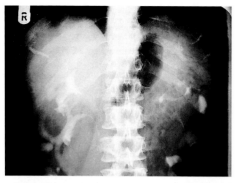

7.32 Polycystic kidney.
Berry aneurysms may be
associated with polycystic
kidneys (which can be seen on a
post-angiography pyelogram)
and with coarctation of the
aorta.

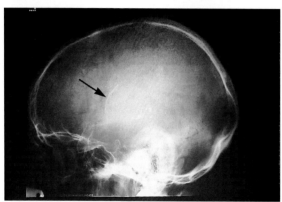

7.33

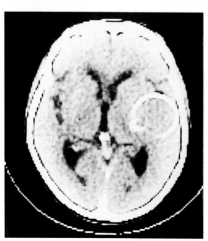

**7.33,7.34 Asymptomatic giant
aneurysm.** Aneurysms do not
always rupture. These films show
calcification in the wall of a large
aneurysm on the middle cerebral
artery found by chance in an elderly
man after a road accident.

7.34

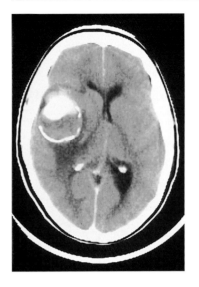

7.35 'Psychogenic' headache. A similar lesion discovered in a patient who complained repeatedly of what (even in retrospect) appeared 'obviously' to be psychogenic headaches. Sixteen per cent of patients who come to a casualty department because of headache prove to have a serious neurological disorder and it is often a great deal less embarrassing to do a scan for which there seems to be no indication than to be faced with catastrophic proof that the patient had indeed got good cause to be worried.

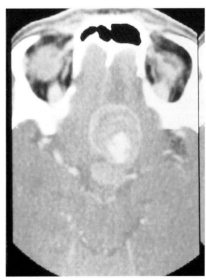

7.36 Giant globoid aneurysm. These lesions, which arise from the trunk of a main vessel, appear to be congenital and are thought to be a distinct entity. The lumen is filled with laminated clot, giving a false impression of size at angiography and reducing the risk of haemorrhage. They differ from berry aneurysms in that they cause symptoms by compression and from atherosclerotic aneurysms in that they can rupture. This 48-year-old man developed fits and euphoric, overbearing (frontal lobe) behaviour. The mass between the frontal lobes was thought to be a meningioma until it was observed that contrast was concentrated in one sector. Angiography confirmed that it was an aneurysm the lumen of which was obliterated with clot. The patient died of a cerebral haemorrhage.

(See also atherosclerotic aneurysms – 3.61–3.63,3.111.)

Arteriovenous malformations

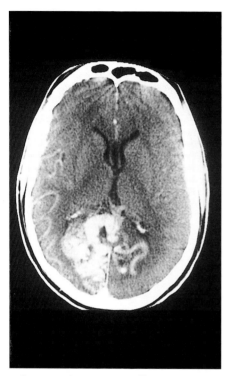

7.37 Arteriovenous malformation presenting with headache. An arteriovenous malformation may present with headache, a haemorrhage and/or (?focal) fits. Such lesions are often associated with a bruit over the skull and are usually easily demonstrated by scanning. This remarkable patient, who had a strong family history of migraine, gave a history of bouts of right hemicrania, teichopsia and transient loss of vision in the left half-field. He also gave a detailed and consistent account of three episodes of 'dream precognition' – i.e. of dreaming of a novel and complex series of events which he actually experienced a few weeks later. The 'migraine' was almost certainly in some way related to the large occipital vascular malformation. The relationship of this lesion to his bouts of dream precognition (which was not a *déjà vu* phenomenon) is a matter for debate.

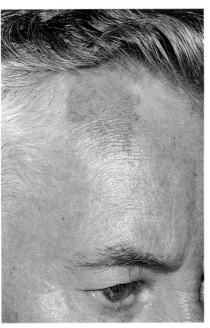

7.38,7.39 Arteriovenous malformation causing fits. A man of 54 who was woken by an attack of 'cramp' in the left arm followed soon after by a seizure. He was found to have a naevus on the right brow and a left upper quadrantic field defect. The scan shows a large right temporal arteriovenous malformation (arrow). Vascular malformations of this sort are not usually associated with naevi, but in this instance the anomaly was clearly widespread for the patient was aware that his right ear flushed when he was tense.

7.38

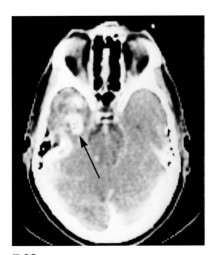

7.39

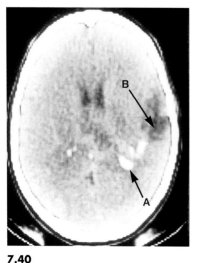

7.40

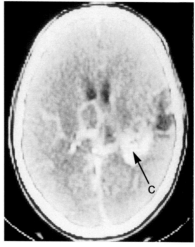

7.41

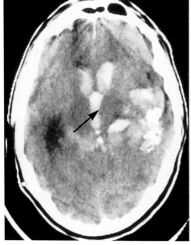

7.42

7.40–7.42 Haemorrhage from arteriovenous malformation.

Haemorrhage from an arteriovenous malformation tends to be less severe than that from an aneurysm because the blood is not under such high pressure. It has moreover been taught that patients who present with fits are unlikely subsequently to have a haemorrhage. Large series have in fact shown that the risk is virtually the same in both groups and that the annual morbidity and mortality are 1.7% and 1% respectively. This 51-year-old patient presented with a warningless fit. The skull X-ray and the scan showed an area of calcification (A) that was associated with an area of atrophy (B). The lesion enhanced with contrast (C). The patient had four further fits over 7 years and in the last recovered for long enough to tell the ambulance crew that he had 'a varicose vein in his head' before lapsing into a terminal coma. A second scan showed a haemorrhage which had ruptured into the lateral and third ventricles (7.42 arrow).

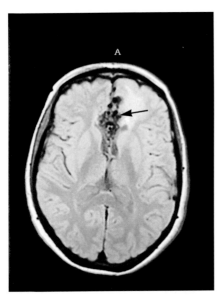

7.43

7.43, 7.44 MR scan of arteriovenous malformation.

The abnormal vessels which form the bulk of an arteriovenous malformation can easily be demonstrated on an MR scan. This is useful for, with the realisation that such lesions are potentially dangerous, there has been an increased emphasis on treatment with radiotherapy, embolisation and surgery.

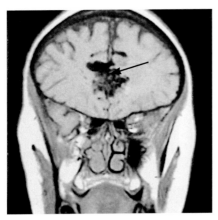

7.44

Cerebral ischaemia

In recent years therapeutic considerations have brought about a modification in the classification of cerebral ischaemia. In some instances, for example lacunar and watershed infarction, the pathogenesis of the lesion is clear. In the majority of cases, however, the relative importance of thrombosis in the carotid artery, emboli from the heart or carotid and thrombosis in situ is uncertain. To some extent, however, this problem can be side-stepped if infarcts are first divided into those in the territory of the anterior (carotid artery) and the posterior (vertebrobasilar) circulations. Anterior circulation infarcts can be further classified as total, partial and lacunar. *Clinically* a **total anterior circulation infarct** produces a 'full house' of hemiplegia, hemianopia and impairment of higher function. *Pathologically* this implies infarction of the majority of the territory supplied by the carotid due to occlusion of the internal carotid artery or of the origin of the middle cerebral artery (with or without the anterior cerebral artery). *Prognostically* it implies a mortality of 50% with little prospect of independent existence for the survivors. With doubts about the virtue of thrombolysis *treatment* is at best supportive.

Patients who have lost one component of cortical function or who have any two of the three major symptoms listed above are said to have **partial anterior circulation infarction**. *Pathologically* such lesions, which account for a third of cerebral infarcts, are likely to be an embolic phenomenon. *Prognostically* the mortality in the first year is of the order of 15% and 60% will return to independent existence. There is, however, a high risk of recurrence, particularly in the first 3 months and *treatment* is directed towards the early detection and elimination of lesions in the heart and the carotid artery.

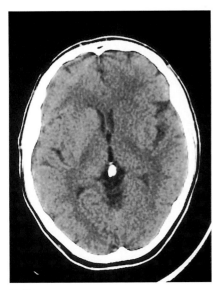

7.45,7.46 Total anterior circulation infarct. A 44-year-old patient who suddenly collapsed with a right hemiparesis. She was conscious and on admission the CT scan was unremarkable (7.45). Within 24 hours, however, she developed an extensive low-density area with oedema and displacement of midline structures in the territory of the left anterior and middle cerebral arteries, lapsed into coma and died.

7.45

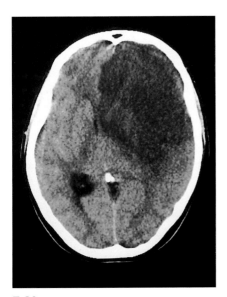

7.46

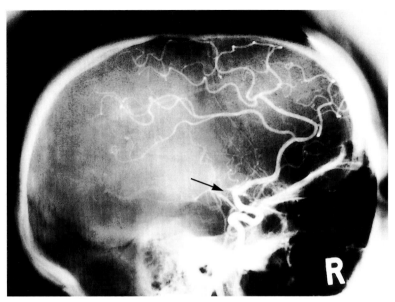

7.47

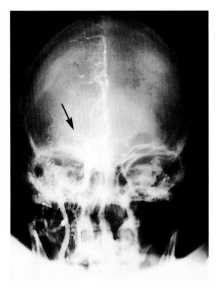

7.47,7.48 Occlusion of the origin of the middle cerebral artery. Occlusion of the origin of the middle cerebral artery can produce the picture of total anterior circulation infarction. (Compare with 7.26,7.27 on which the middle cerebral artery is visible.) Primary as opposed to embolic occlusion, once thought to be the main cause of stroke, is in fact uncommon, although it is seen as a complication of polyarteritis, cranial arteritis, meningitis, syphilis, polycythaemia and the use of oral contraceptives.

7.48

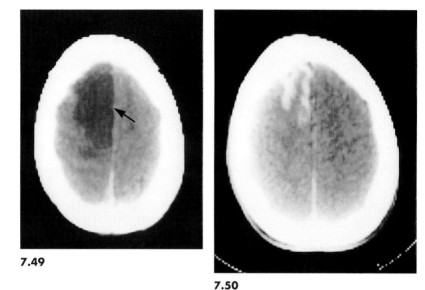

7.49

7.50

**7.49, 7.50 Partial (anterior cerebral artery) anterior circulation
infarction.** For the first 2 weeks an infarct appears as an area of low attenuation
(low density). Thereafter for about 4 weeks it takes up contrast. This patient, who
developed a left hemiparesis shortly after admission, was found to have a lesion in the
anterior part of the right hemisphere (7.49 arrow). Initially there was no uptake of
contrast, but enhancement in the territory of the anterior cerebral artery was obvious
on a second scan done 3 weeks later. (See also bilateral frontal infarction – 7.31.)

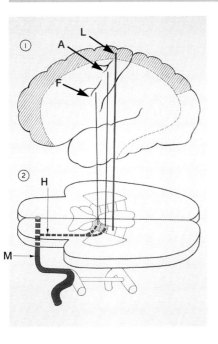

7.51 Anterior cerebral artery.

(1) Lateral view of the hemisphere to show the distribution of the cortical branches of the anterior cerebral artery (shaded) and the cortical representation of the face (F), arm (A) and leg (L). Occlusion of the cortical branches can cause weakness and loss of sensation in the lower limb, loss of bladder control and impairment of cortical function in the form of a personality change. (2) Axial view to show the distribution of the (inconstant) perforating (Heubner's) artery (H). Occlusion of this artery can cause faciobrachial weakness due to infarction of the anterior part of the internal capsule. Occlusion of the origin of the anterior cerebral artery when Heubner's artery is present (M) will cause a hemiplegia, the leg remaining flaccid but the arm (which retains an extrapyramidal supply) regaining tone.

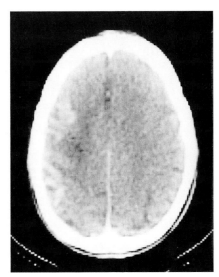

7.52 Partial (middle cerebral artery) anterior circulation infarction.

A 61-year-old man who smoked 20 cigarettes daily. Two months before admission he had a number of short bouts of left-sided numbness, after which he lost the use of his left arm. The scan shows an area of low attenuation in the right hemisphere underlying an area of cortical enhancement in the territory of the middle cerebral artery. (See also 7.66 which shows infarction in the territory of both superficial and deep branches.)

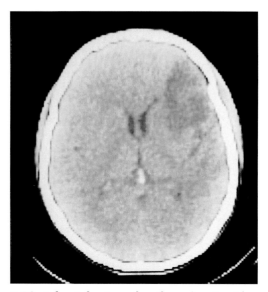

7.53 Infarct due to polycythaemia. Apart from smoking, carotid stenosis, hypertension and emboli from the heart remediable causes of cerebral infarction are rarely found. When they occur, however, they can be of great importance. This 31-year-old man gave a history of headache for 4 months, of three brief episodes of numbness and weakness on the left side and of recurrent attacks of dysphasia with numbness and weakness on the right. His blood pressure, CT scan, CSF and carotid ultrasound were normal. He discharged himself from hospital but was re-admitted 10 days later with severe dysphasia and weakness of the right arm. The scan now showed a large infarct in the territory of the left middle cerebral artery and he was found to have a haemoglobin of 18.9 g/100 ml, a haematocrit of 57.7% and a platelet count of 980 000. Even in retrospect the fact that he had polycythaemia was not evident on examination.

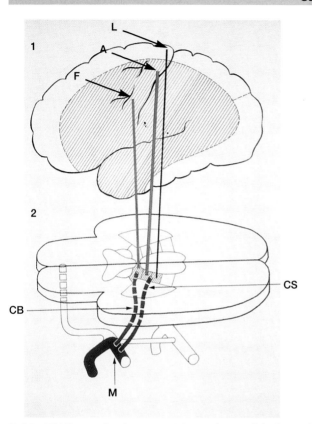

7.54 Middle cerebral artery. (1) Lateral view of the hemisphere to show the distribution of the cortical branches of the middle cerebral artery (shaded) and the cortical representation of the face (F), arm (A) and leg (L). Occlusion of the cortical branches can cause weakness and impairment of sensation in the arm and face, hemianopia and/or evidence of cortical dysfunction such as aphasia or apraxia (see 7.52). (2) Axial view to show distribution of the perforating (lenticulostriate) branches (see 7.14). Occlusion of a single branch can produce a lacunar infarct in the posterior limb of the internal capsule, destroying the cortico-spinal tract (CS) and causing a pure motor hemiplegia that involves the leg as well as the arm (see 7.15,7.72). Sensation, speech and other cortical functions are spared. An identical lesion involving the cortico-bulbar tract (CB) would be silent (because the muscles supplied are bilaterally innervated) unless the corresponding tract on the opposite side has already been damaged. Under such circumstances the patient suddenly develops a pseudobulbar palsy without having had a 'stroke'. Occlusion of the origin of the middle cerebral artery (M) causes cortical and central infarction with gross oedema, impairment of consciousness and weakness of the whole of the opposite side of the body (see 7.46).

The carotid artery

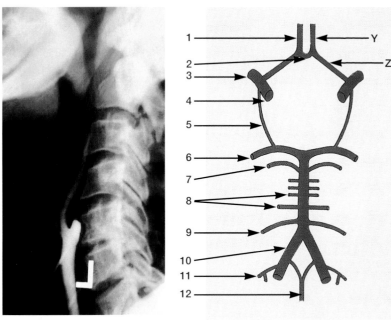

7.55

7.56

7.55,7.56 Carotid occlusion and the circle of Willis. The internal carotid artery is sometimes found to be occluded in apparently healthy patients (7.55). In others the lesion produces the picture of middle cerebral artery thrombosis. Consideration of the diagram of the circle of Willis shows why. If the carotid artery (4) is occluded the anterior and posterior cerebral arteries can still be perfused through the anterior communicating (2) and posterior cerebral (6) vessels. However, if the anterior communicating artery is absent there will also be infarction of the ipsilateral frontal lobe. If the occluded artery has to supply *both* frontal lobes because the circle is defective at (Z) there will be bilateral frontal lobe infarction. Occlusion of the distal part of the anterior cerebral artery (Y) will of course inevitably cause ipsilateral frontal lobe infarction. 1 = anterior cerebral; 2 = anterior communicating; 3 = middle cerebral; 4 = internal carotid; 5 = posterior communicating; 6 = posterior cerebral; 7 = superior cerebellar; 8 = pontine and internal auditory; 9 = anterior inferior cerebellar; 10 = vertebrobasilar; 11 = posterior inferior cerebellar; 12 = anterior spinal.

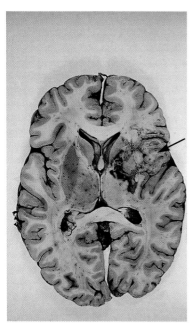 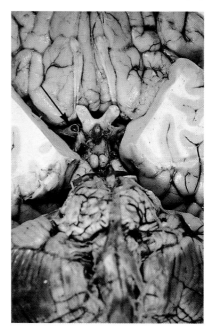

7.57   **7.58**

7.57, 7.58 Carotid occlusion causing 'middle cerebral artery thrombosis'. A 32-year-old woman with a history of migraine. Shortly after changing her oral contraceptive to a 'safer' brand she had a fit and developed a left hemiparesis. An isotope scan showed a lesion in the territory of the right middle cerebral artery. Two months later she had a fatal pulmonary embolus. Autopsy revealed a full thickness scar in the territory of the middle cerebral artery (7.57 arrow) and occlusion of the internal carotid (7.58 arrow).

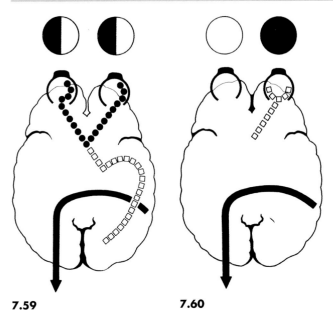

7.59   **7.60**

7.59–7.62 Carotid stenosis. Carotid stenosis, like carotid occlusion, may be a chance finding. Such patients may however present with a characteristic complaint of transient impairment of vision in the ipsilateral eye (amaurosis fugax) and transient limb symptoms on the opposite side of the body. A hemisphere lesion could cause the limb symptoms but would be associated with an homonymous hemianopia (7.59).

Impairment of vision in one eye must mean that the lesion is in the globe or the nerve on that side at a point remote from the pyramidal tract (7.60). Emboli from the carotid artery can, however, pass to the ipsilateral retina and to the motor strip on the same side (7.61). The observation of glistening emboli in the retinal arteries of such patients often confirms that this is what has happened (7.62 arrow).

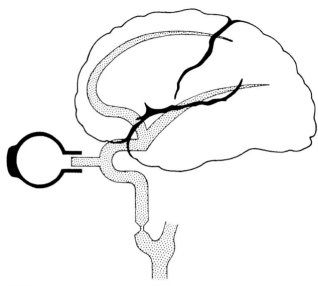

7.61

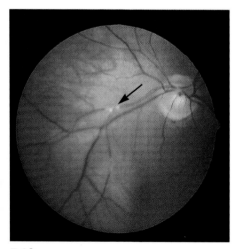

7.62

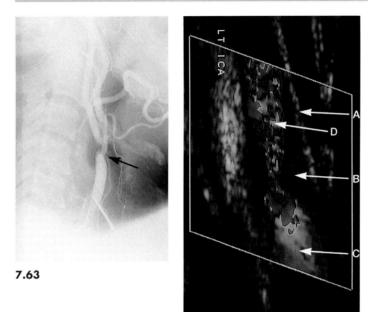

7.63

7.64

7.63,7.64 Carotid stenosis. Stenosis of the internal carotid artery (7.63 arrow) is an important and potentially remediable cause of partial anterior circulation infarction. Preliminary screening can be done with a Doppler scan (7.64 A = wall of artery; B = plaque partly occluding lumen; C (red) = normal flow proximal to plaque; D (mottled red and blue) = turbulence at and beyond stenosis). Studies have shown that the prognosis for symptomatic patients who have removal of a lesion causing narrowing of 70% or more on the appropriate side is improved after 3 months. This of course presupposes that investigation and treatment are done in a reputable unit.

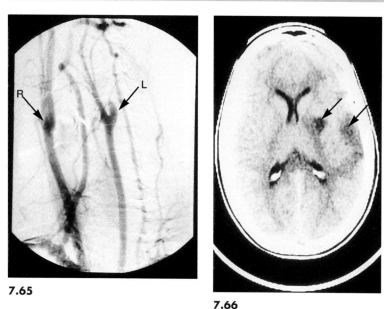

7.65

7.66

7.65,7.66 Post-traumatic occlusion of the carotid. A 30-year-old woman who was repeatedly kicked about the head and neck. She subsequently developed a hemiplegia and digital subtraction angiography showed occlusion of the internal carotid artery on the left (7.65L), the artery on the right (7.65R) being intact. A CT scan showed infarction in the territories of both superficial and deep branches of the middle cerebral artery (7.66 arrows). Post-traumatic occlusion of the carotid artery, in which the hemiplegia commonly appears 24 or more hours after the injury, may be the result of traction in a whiplash injury or of direct trauma. It has been reported after blows over the carotid, after palpation, compression and needling and in children who have fallen with pencils or lollipop-sticks in their mouths and injured the carotid artery which runs behind the tonsillar fossa.

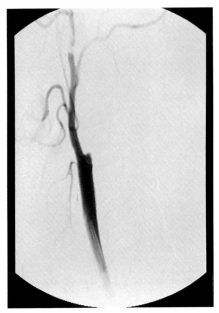

7.67 Carotid occlusion following radiotherapy. Six years before admission this 32-year-old patient had surgery and radiotherapy for a tumour of the left parotid gland. One month before admission she had a transient episode of dysphasia and right-sided incoordination and on the day of admission the dysphasia returned along with a mild right hemiparesis. Angiography revealed total occlusion of the left internal carotid artery which, in view of the patient's age and the absence of any other cause, was thought to have occurred because the vessel was damaged by radiotherapy.

Cardiac lesions as a cause of cerebral emboli

Despite the decline of rheumatic heart disease, cardiac lesions are still a significant cause of partial anterior circulation infarction. Most patients have evidence of heart disease and some may have had emboli elsewhere. Warning episodes of cerebral ischaemia are, however, uncommon and many present with a large infarct. There is a serious risk of early recurrence. Under certain circumstances (e.g. after dental extraction) the emboli in patients with rheumatic and congenital heart disease may be infected and their symptoms can be confused with those of sterile non-bacterial endocarditis. Other causes include atrial myxoma, systemic lupus erythematosus (in which emboli are the most common single cause of lesions in the central nervous system) and paradoxical emboli through septal defects.

Management is modified by the knowledge that many embolic infarcts – especially large ones – are or (spontaneously) become haemorrhagic. In patients with severe neurological deficits or large lesions on the scan it is therefore advisable to withhold anticoagulants for about 7 days, to repeat the scan and to anticoagulate slowly.

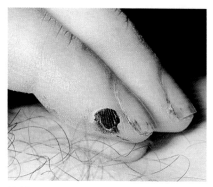

7.68

7.68–7.71 Marantic (sterile non-bacterial) endocarditis. Two days after admission with a stroke this 45-year-old man developed a fever, splinter haemorrhages and Osler's nodes (7.68) followed by gangrene of the leg (7.69). He had had an haemoptysis and Virchow's node behind the left sternomastoid was enlarged. His blood cultures were negative. Autopsy revealed cerebral, splenic and renal (7.70) infarcts and vegetations on the heart valves (7.71). Marantic endocarditis, which is particularly associated with adenocarcinomas of the pancreas, lung and (as here) stomach – tumours which cause spontaneous coagulation – can easily be confused with bacterial endocarditis. Although incurable, it is important for purposes of management that it should be recognised.

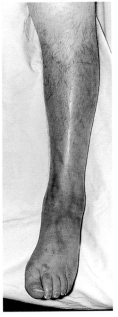

7.69

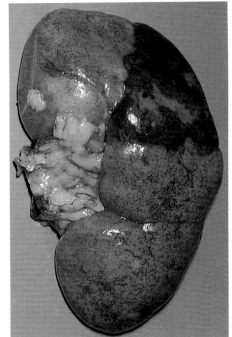

7.70

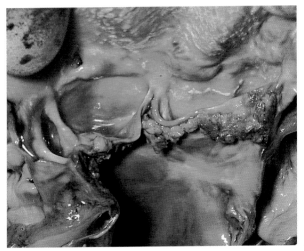

7.71

Lacunar infarcts

Degenerative changes can also result in thrombosis of perforating branches of the main cerebral arteries (see 7.14,7.54,7.72). Such incidents, which account for 25% of cerebral infarcts, produce discrete deeply placed lesions known as lacunes (see 7.16). Many, being near the confluence of the motor and sensory fibres in the internal capsule, cause an extensive unilateral motor or sensory deficit. This, however, is not associated with evidence of cortical damage such as aphasia or apraxia. Others produce ipsilateral cerebellar and pyramidal tract signs. In about a third the lesion is visible on the CT scan. Death and early recurrence are unlikely but nearly 40% will still be dependent at 12 months.

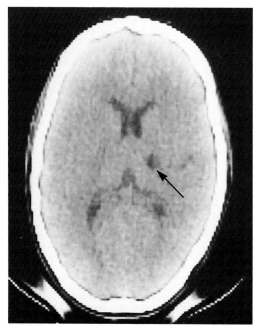

7.72 Lacunar infarct. A small deeply placed infarct due to occlusion of a perforating branch of the middle cerebral artery.

Watershed infarcts

The introduction of cardiac surgery for older patients with generalised arterial disease has focused attention on another, less common lesion – watershed infarction. This occurs when, during surgery, syncopal episodes in which the patient remains in an upright position and similar incidents, the blood pressure falls and the territory at the extremities of the main cerebral vessels is deprived of an adequate blood supply. As the most vulnerable point is that at which the territories of the three main vessels join (7.74) the most common manifestations are bilateral parieto-occipital infarction with cortical blindness, receptive aphasia, apraxia and/or inferior altitudinal hemianopia. Infarcts at the anterior/middle cerebral interface may present with weakness in both arms – the 'man in a barrel' syndrome.

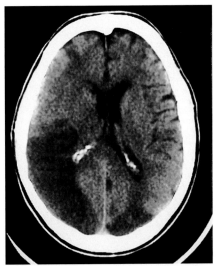

7.73 Watershed infarction. A 66-year-old patient who deteriorated soon after apparently uneventful coronary artery surgery. She was semiconscious and had bilateral weakness. The CT scan showed an extensive low-density area over the right occiput which extended outside the territory of the posterior cerebral artery and smaller lesions on the left and in both frontal poles.

The vertebrobasilar and posterior cerebral arteries

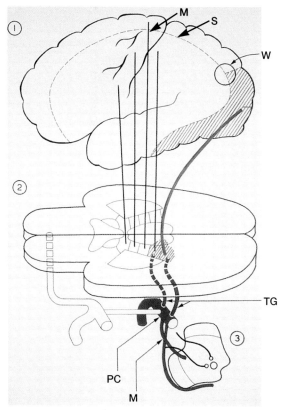

7.74 Posterior cerebral artery. An example of infarction in the territory of the posterior cerebral artery (posterior circulation infarction) has already been given (see 1.5). Such lesions, which account for about 25% of cerebral infarcts, are usually embolic, but the exact situation of the lesion is often difficult to determine. The diagram shows (1) a lateral view of the hemisphere with the motor (M) and sensory (S) strips, and the distribution of the cortical branches of the posterior cerebral artery (shaded). Occlusion will cause an homonymous hemianopia with macular sparing (see 3.19). W = watershed area where the territories of the three main vessels converge. (2) An axial view showing the posterior cerebral artery (PC) and the distribution of the perforating (thalamo-geniculate) branches (TG), occlusion of which can produce lacunar infarcts in the thalamus, the posterior limb of the internal capsule and the visual radiation with hemisensory impairment, thalamic pain and/or complete hemianopia. (3) Axial view of midbrain showing vessels (M) which supply the brainstem.

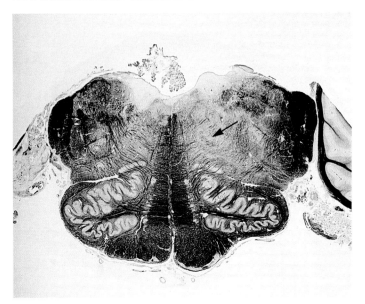

7.75

7.75–7.77 Lateral medullary syndrome. Ischaemia in the territory of the basilar artery is usually transient and may be precipitated by cervical spondylosis but eponyms have been attached to a variety of rare syndromes caused by infarction of the brainstem. Best known of these is Wallenberg's lateral medullary syndrome which, although traditionally associated with thrombosis of the posterior inferior cerebellar artery, is usually due to occlusion of the vertebral. The main features are dysphonia, dysphagia and dizziness due to damage to the the vagus, vestibular and cerebellar systems, an ipsilateral Horner's syndrome, ipsilateral impairment of pain and temperature sensation over the face and a contralateral spinothalamic deficit. The diagram and photograph show how the hypoglossal nerve, the pyramidal tract and the medial lemniscus escape. Hearing is intact because the auditory branch of the eighth nerve enters the brainstem at a higher level. Occlusion of the posterior inferior cerebellar artery can also cause extensive infarction of the cerebellar hemisphere (7.77).

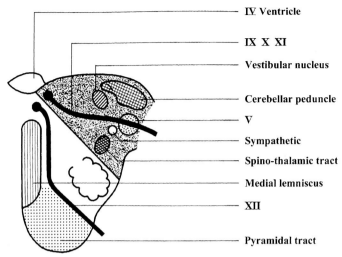

IV Ventricle

IX X XI

Vestibular nucleus

Cerebellar peduncle

V

Sympathetic

Spino-thalamic tract

Medial lemniscus

XII

Pyramidal tract

7.76

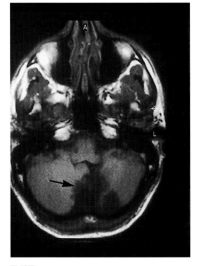

7.77

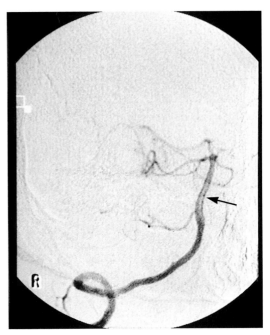

7.78 Basilar artery thrombosis. This 40-year-old patient presented with malignant hypertension and 2 months later suddenly developed a transient left hemisensory disturbance with ataxia, dizziness, dysphagia and dysphonia. After some further bouts of ataxia he developed *right* faciobrachial numbness. Angiography showed a clot (arrow) partly occluding the basilar artery.

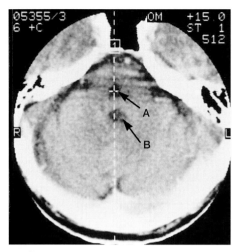

7.79

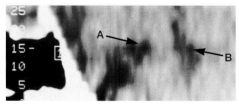

7.80

7.79,7.80 Brainstem infarct. Although brainstem infarcts are less easy to demonstrate than those in the hemispheres they can sometimes be seen on a CT scan. Two weeks after a minor head injury this 52-year-old hypertensive, who smoked heavily, suddenly complained of transient faintness, dizziness, numbness in the left hand and weakness in the legs. Three months later there was a second more severe episode of the same type. The CT scan and a lateral reconstruction showed a lacunar infarct (A) anterior to the fourth ventricle (B).

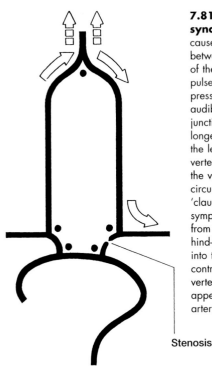

7.81–7.83 Subclavian steal
syndrome. Basilar ischaemia may also be caused by stenosis of the subclavian artery between the arch of the aorta and the origin of the vertebral artery. In such patients the pulse is delayed and weaker and the blood pressure is lower on the left, and a murmur is audible over the lesion. Pressure at the junctions of the major arteries (dots) will no longer be equal and, in particular, pressure in the left subclavian (and thus in the left vertebral) will fall when the arm is in use and the vascular bed dilates. Under such circumstances the patient may complain of 'claudication' in the arm and develop symptoms of basilar ischaemia because blood from the right vertebral is 'stolen' from the hind-brain down the left vertebral artery and into the subclavian artery. At angiography contrast medium will disappear from the right vertebral artery (7.82 arrow) before appearing in the left vertebral and subclavian arteries (7.83 arrow).

Stenosis

7.81

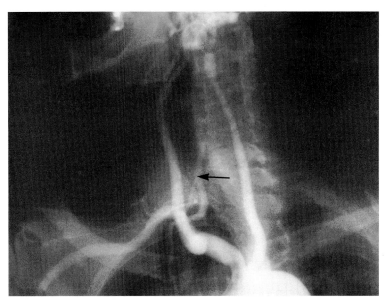

7.82

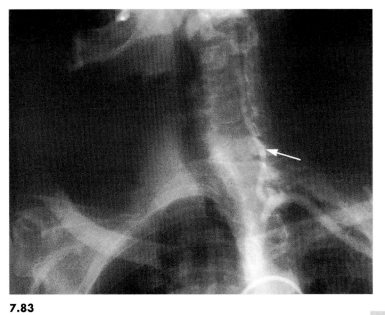

7.83

Cerebral venous thrombosis

Cerebral venous thrombosis is a complicated and somewhat neglected problem. The brunt of the damage falls on the sagittal, lateral and cavernous sinuses (see 3.30–3.33) but there is considerable overlap between the syndromes produced. Patients may present with cranial nerve palsies, raised intracranial pressure due to defective absorption of CSF, fits and/or hemiplegia. Traditional causes – infections of the face and middle ear and meningiomas of the sagittal sinus – have given way to haematological disorders, Behçet's syndrome and defects of the vessel wall.

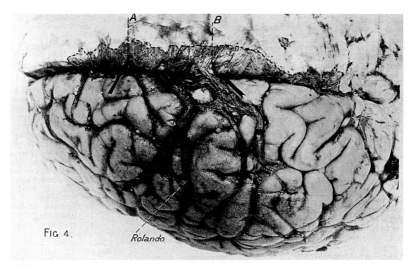

7.84 Cerebral venous thrombosis. Occlusion of the sagittal sinus causes raised intracranial pressure due to defective absorption of CSF, while associated thrombosis of cortical veins causes fits and weakness. This example – due to a bullet wound on the crown of the head – comes from the first detailed account of the condition, based on World War One battle casualties, by Holmes and Sargent (*British Journal of Surgery* 1915; 2: 493–498).

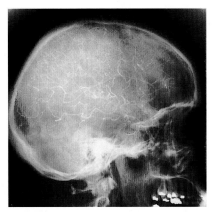

7.85

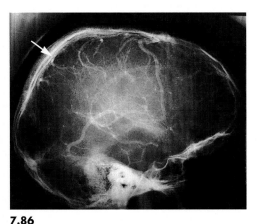

7.86

7.85,7.86 Sagittal sinus thrombosis. A 39-year-old patient who fell and injured her head shortly after delivery. She complained of headache and fits and had a left hemiparesis. The CSF was heavily bloodstained and the CT scan showed that the ventricles were small. At angiography (7.85) the sagittal sinus failed to fill even on late films. (The normal appearance is shown on 7.86.) The patient had had two previous episodes of venous thrombosis and was found to have a thrombotic tendency which, with pregnancy and trauma, resulted in occlusion of the sagittal sinus.

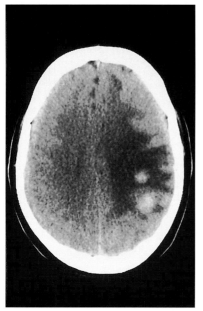 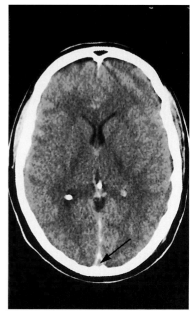

7.87   **7.88**

7.87,7.88 The delta sign. A 48-year-old patient with headache, fits and hemiparesis. A CT scan showed two hyperdense (?haemorrhagic) areas surrounded by a much larger low-density area and a filling defect (the delta sign) in the sagittal sinus produced by a clot (7.88 arrow).

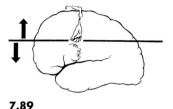

7.89

7.89–7.92 Rolandic vein thrombosis.
The cortical veins drain upwards and downwards about a horizontal line drawn through the hand area (7.89). Sagittal sinus or Rolandic vein thrombosis therefore produces an infarct in the upper half of the hemisphere (7.90). The clinical features are quite unlike those of middle cerebral artery thrombosis which develop rapidly and chiefly affect the face and the hand (7.91), sparing the leg which is in the territory of the anterior cerebral artery. In Rolandic vein thrombosis symptoms develop in a stuttering manner (due to the collateral circulation) and the hand and face, being on or below the watershed, escape (7.92). The lower limb, by contrast – and often the lower limb on the opposite side – will be severely affected because they are at the centre of the infarct.

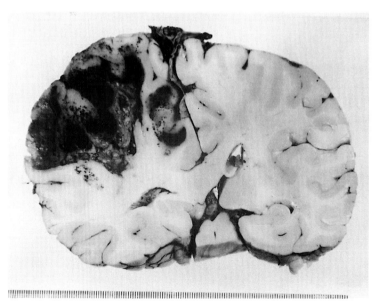

7.90

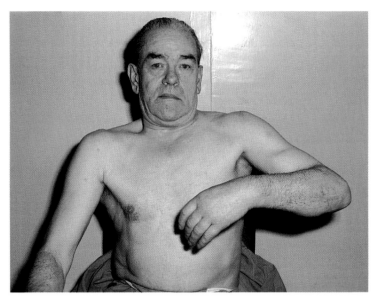

7.91

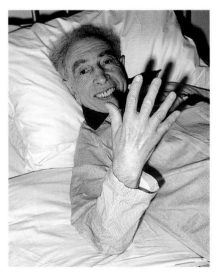

7.92

8.

Developmental disorders

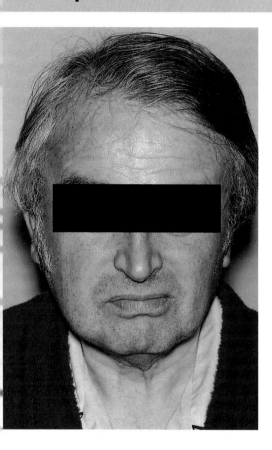

8.1 Hydrocephalus. Hydrocephalus may present in adult life as a chronic or as an acute problem. This 50-year-old man gave a 4-year history of progressive unsteadiness of gait. He had a large head (about which he had been teased at school) and a spastic paraplegia. The paraplegia was due to compression of the cortico-spinal tracts to the lower limbs as they wound round the expanded ventricles.

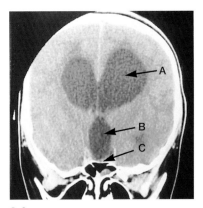

8.2

8.2–8.4 Aqueduct stenosis.
Hydrocephalus with dilation of the lateral
(8.2A) and third (8.2B) ventricles may be
caused by a stenotic lesion seen at the
bottom of the dilated aqueduct (8.4
arrow). Sudden 'decompensation' for such
a lesion, an exceedingly dangerous
condition liable to cause coning, presents
with agonising headaches and requires
urgent surgical treatment. Note how the
dilated third ventricle can compress the
pituitary fossa and the optic chiasm
(8.2C) (see 3.17).

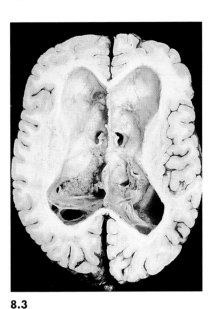

8.3

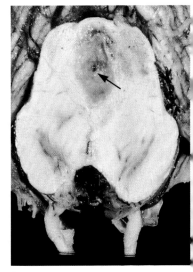

8.4

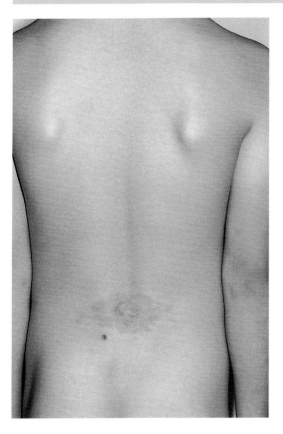

8.5 Developmental abnormalities in the lumbar region. The presence of an obvious cutaneous abnormality over the lumbar spine may indicate that impairment of bladder function or defects in the lower limbs are due to a developmental abnormality in this region.

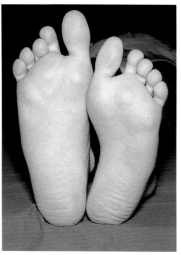

8.6

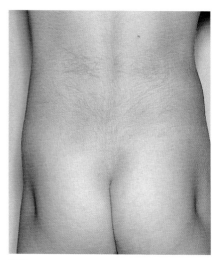

8.7

8.6–8.9 Developmental abnormalities in the lumbar region. Such
cutaneous lesions are not always immediately apparent. This 11-year-old child
presented because, despite lifelong treatment for talipes, her gait had continued to
deteriorate. The left lower limb was shorter and thinner and the left foot was smaller
than the right (8.6). There was an excessive growth of hair in the lumbar region (8.7)
and parting of the buttocks revealed a dimple in the natal cleft (8.8). The sacral arches
were defective and myelography showed that the distal part of the thecal sac was
unduly wide and that the cord was tethered to the upper part of the sacrum (8.9
arrows).

(See also lumbar lipoma – 10.23,10.24.)

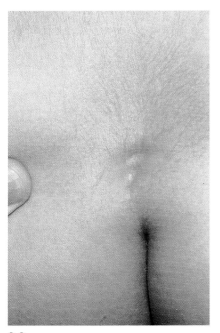

8.8

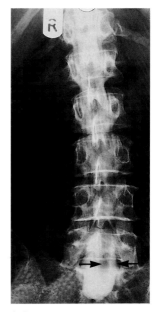

8.9

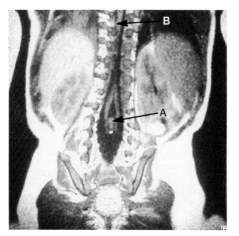

8.10

8.10–8.12
Diastematomyelia. In addition to being tethered by bands or compressed by lipomas a cutaneous lesion may indicate that the cord has been transfixed by a diastematomyelia. The MR scans show that the cord (B) is fixed to the bottom of the widened canal and transfixed and split by a spicule of bone (A). At operation (8.12) the spicule was removed from between the two halves of the cord (C) and the cord was released by cutting the lipoma that was restraining it (D).

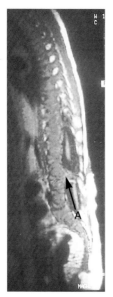

8.11

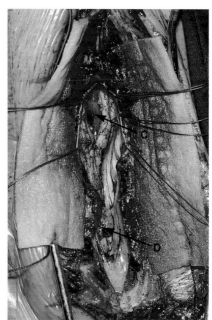

8.12

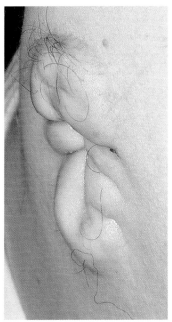

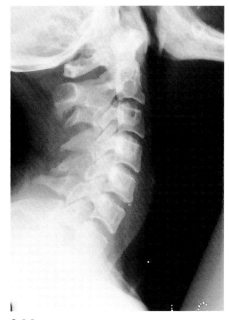

8.13

8.14

8.13,8.14 Congenital deformity of the cervical spine. A 22-year-old patient with a congenital lesion over the lower part of the cervical spine. Apart from experiencing some discomfort in the neck if she lay on her back she was asymptomatic, but there was slight hypoplasia and weakness of the right hand. A radiograph (8.14) of the cervical spine revealed widening of the canal and multiple defects in the neural arches.

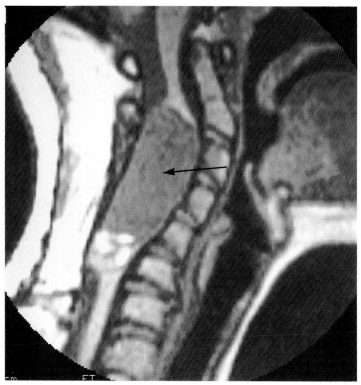

8.15 MR scan of cervical dermoid. A 20-year-old woman who presented with pain radiating from the neck into both arms and tingling in the fingers. The only significant sign was a small dimple over the sixth cervical vertebra that was connected, through a defect in the neural arch, to a large, partly calcified mass in the cervical cord (arrow). This was found to contain gelatinous material, hair and cartilage. It was evacuated on several occasions and, although there was eventually some weakness of the hands, the legs remained normal.

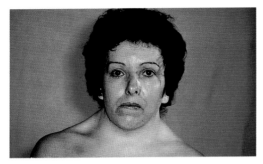

8.16

8.16–8.18 Klippel–Feil syndrome with basilar invagination. A patient with facial asymmetry, a short stiff neck, webbing and a congenital deformity of the thumbs who proved to have fusion of the cervical vertebrae and basilar invagination. She had no relevant symptoms, but in such patients injury to the neck can produce disability out of all proportion to the severity of the accident.

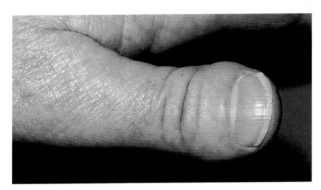

8.17

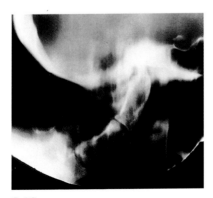

8.18

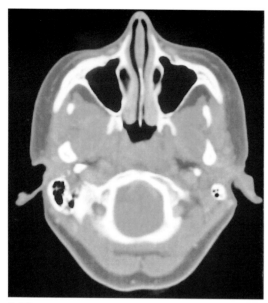

8.19

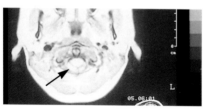

8.20

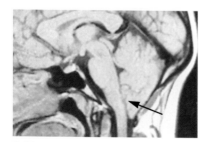

8.21

**8.19–8.22
Arnold–Chiari
malformation causing
cough headache.** A
22-year-old woman with a
5-year history of mild but
persistent headache and a
superimposed pain of
incapacitating severity
which appeared 10
seconds after coughing,
straining etc. and lasted
for 30 seconds. On one
occasion it coincided with
transient loss of vision. The
CT scan (8.19) showed
that the foramen magnum
was enlarged and the MR
scan (8.20,8.21) revealed
that in addition to the cord
it contained a tongue of
cerebellar tissue (arrow)
such as is seen on the
pathological specimen.
Anomalies of this kind are
a recognised cause of
cough headache.

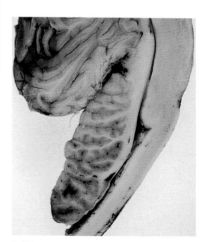

8.22

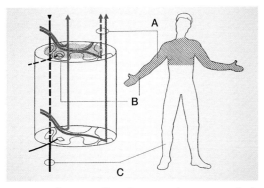

8.23 Syringomyelia. Patients with syringomyelia have a fluid-filled cavity in the centre of the cervical cord (stippled area). Pain fibres crossing at this level are destroyed (A) but fibres in the posterior columns and those which enter the spinothalamic tract at a lower level are spared. The sensory loss will therefore be 'suspended' over the upper part of the body and 'dissociated' in that only pain and temperature are affected. Further extension will damage the anterior horn cells (B), the pyramidal tracts (C) and the medulla causing wasting of the hands, a spastic paraplegia, nystagmus and a bulbar palsy.

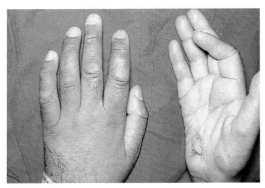

8.24 Syringomyelia. Old and recent scars resulting from painless injuries and wasting of the right thenar and hypothenar eminences in a patient who also had hemiatrophy of the tongue.

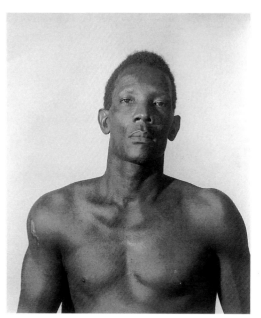

8.25

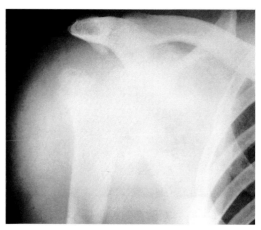

8.26

8.25, 8.26
Syringomyelia. A patient who presented with an ache in the right shoulder. He had wasting of the right pectoralis major as shown by undue prominence of the clavicle and a scar on the right shoulder resulting from a painless burn from a hot-water bottle. A radiograph of the shoulder revealed a Charcot joint.

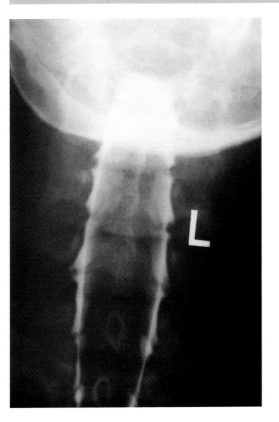

8.27 Radiology of syringomyelia.
Scoliosis is common and the cervical canal may be enlarged. (The sagittal diameter of the lower part of the canal is usually less than 19mm.) Myelography may show that the cord is widened (as here) or wasted.

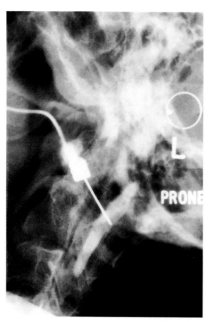

8.28

8.28,8.29 Radiology of syringomyelia. Five years before admission this 52-year-old man suddenly developed severe pain and weakness in the left upper limb. There was some subsequent improvement but wasting, fasciculation and areflexia were still present at the time of admission. At myelography (8.28) a lateral cervical puncture produced clear fluid, but when contrast was injected much of it appeared to be in a long cavity in the cervical cord which tapered to an end at about C5. This was confirmed on the CT scan (8.29) (A = theca; B = cord; C = cavity). In view of the abrupt, painful onset it is possible that this patient had a haemorrhage into the substance of the cord.

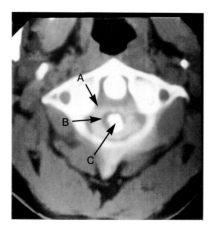

8.29

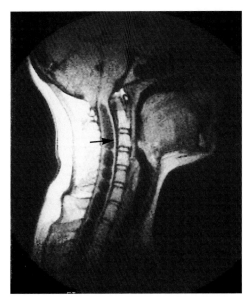

8.30 MR scan in syringomyelia. A cavity in the cord is most easily demonstrated by performing an MR scan (arrow).

9.

Diseases of the spinal cord

A neurological patient whose symptoms are confined to the legs usually has a lesion within the spine. In an adult an increase in tone, brisk reflexes, clonus and extensor plantar responses (the signs of an upper motor neurone lesion) show that it lies above L1, for the cord and therefore the pyramidal tracts end at that point. Lesions at a higher level may also produce (upper or lower motor neurone) signs in the arms, while lesions below this level produce a cauda equina syndrome (see p. 278).

The *level* of a cord lesion may be revealed by localised tenderness over the spine or by a sharp (root) pain which runs down the arm or round the trunk on coughing. Sensory levels, which often fall several segments short of the lesion, are not a reliable guide. Most patients therefore require more detailed examination.

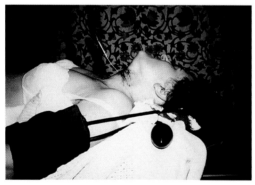

9.1

9.1,9.2 High cervical lesions. Lesions above the outflow to the upper limbs (C5–T1) result in brisk (upper motor neurone) reflexes in the arms and may produce girdle reflexes – elicited by placing the hand over the acromio-clavicular joint or the top of the chest and striking it with a hammer. With lesions at this level it is also important to examine respiratory function. This patient was conscious but tetraplegic on admission. The intercostals (T1–12), and the deltoid muscles (C5) were paralysed but the diaphragm (C3–5) was still working. The X-ray confirmed that the injury lay between C3 and C5 by showing that the blade had passed through the C3/4 interspace. It should be remembered that inability to shrug the shoulders cannot be due to a cord lesion (see 3.137) and that high cervical lesions can produce sensory impairment over the ear, the angle of the jaw and the back of the head (see 3.107, 3.112).

x

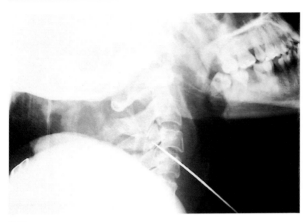

9.2

9.3,9.4 Low cervical lesions. As the fifth, sixth and seventh cervical roots (Table 1) each supply a myotome, a dermatome and a reflex, lesions in the lower part of the cervical spine are relatively easy to locate.

Table 1 Cervical roots			
	C5	**C6**	**C7**
Muscle	Deltoid	Biceps	Triceps
Reflex	Biceps	Supinator	Triceps
Sensation	Shoulder	Thumb/index	Middle finger

The practical value of this information was seen in a young woman, thought to have multiple sclerosis, who presented with weakness in all four limbs. The deltoid, biceps reflex and sensation over the shoulder (C5) were normal (9.3). So too were the biceps muscle, the supinator reflex and sensation over the thumb and index (C6). The triceps muscle, the triceps jerk and sensation over and below the middle finger were, however, impaired. She therefore had a lesion at C7 which, by damaging the pyramidal tracts, could also account for the weakness in her legs and there was no reason to believe her illness was 'disseminated'. An oblique film of the cervical spine, done to show the inter-vertebral foramina, revealed that the 5/6 foramen (arrow) was enlarged by a dumb-bell neurofibroma partly inside and partly outside the canal. The patient recovered when it was removed. This case illustrates the importance of the aphorism 'If, in "multiple sclerosis", there are no problems above the neck, do a myelogram' – or, nowadays, an MR scan of the cord.

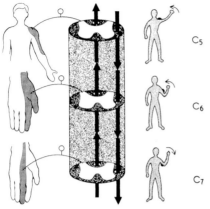

9.3

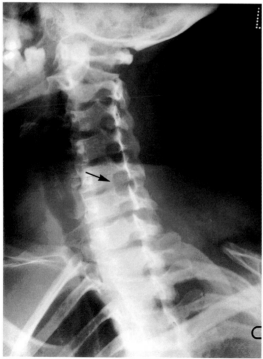

9.4

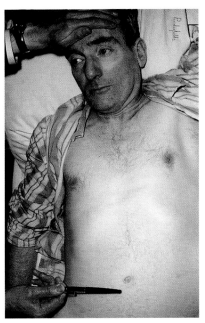

9.5, 9.6 Thoracic lesions. It is difficult to locate thoracic lesions precisely unless the patient has focal spinal tenderness or root pain. The sensory level – which commonly lies several segments lower – is most easily demonstrated by running the cold blade of a tuning fork up the back. Important levels are the nipple (T4), the costal margin (T8), the umbilicus (T10) and the groin (L1). Appropriate examination may reveal that some or all of the intercostals are inactive and weakness in the lower (T10–12) part of the rectus abdominis can be demonstrated by marking the position of the umbilicus and observing an 'umbilical shift' as the patient raises his head against resistance (9.5). It may also be possible to show that perspiration is absent below a certain level by 'towing' a teaspoon upwards over the trunk and noting the point at which it ceases to glide smoothly over the dry skin (9.6).

9.5

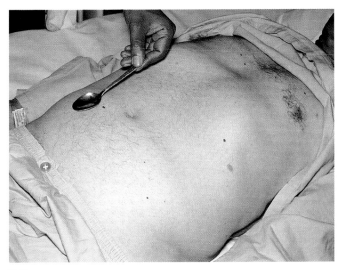

9.6

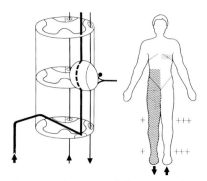

9.7 Hemisection of the cord. This case is discussed in some detail because it illustrates many aspects of the diagnosis of a spinal lesion. For 6 months the patient, a woman of 70, had complained of tripping over her left foot. For 5 months she had had a burning sensation over the *right* lower limb. She had been unable to walk for 2 months and had developed hesitancy of micturition, a shooting pain round the left costal margin on coughing and a 'spongy' feeling over the left lower limb.

Weakness confined to the legs suggested a spinal lesion and the radicular pain suggested that it was due to a lesion near the left T8 root. There were signs of damage to the left pyramidal tract and posterior column (which run directly along the cord, decussating below the medulla) explaining the tendency to trip and the spongy feeling. In the right lower limb, by contrast, pain and temperature sensation were impaired due to compression of fibres which decussated at once and ascended in the opposite (left) spino-thalamic tract. The picture was therefore one of a Brown-Séquard syndrome of hemisection of the cord.

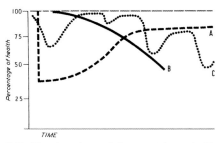

9.8 Hemisection of the cord (cont.). Timescale of neurological illness.
The timescale of an illness is important in determining its nature. Sudden deterioration with gradual but incomplete recovery suggests trauma or a vascular accident (A). Steady, progressive deterioration suggests neoplastic or degenerative disease (B). Recurrent subacute episodes, initially with full recovery, suggest demyelination (C). Patients with metastases usually deteriorate in weeks and a slowly developing lesion in the thoracic region in an elderly woman (as in this case) is more likely to be due to a meningioma.

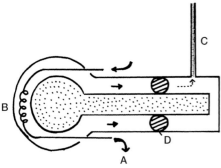

9.9 Hemisection of the cord (cont.). Queckenstedt's test. Because the
patient appeared to have a spinal tumour myelography was done. The fluid obtained
at lumbar puncture was xanthochromic (yellow) and contained a gross excess of
protein. Compression of the jugular vein (A) caused a rise in intracranial pressure due
to distension of intracranial vessels (B) but this was not transmitted to the manometer
attached to the lumbar puncture needle (C) because of the block caused by the spinal
tumour (D). (Queckenstedt's test – now rarely used – is a test for spinal block and not a
routine part of lumbar puncture, for with most intracranial lesions it is irrelevant and
potentially dangerous.)

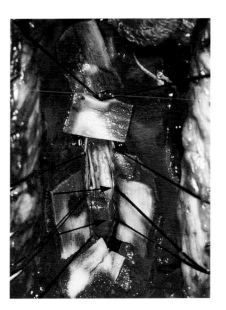

**9.10 Hemisection of the cord
(cont.). Meningioma.**
Xanthochromic fluid, a high protein
level and a positive Queckenstedt test
(Froin's syndrome) supported the
diagnosis of spinal block.
Myelography demonstrated an
obstruction at T8, with only a trickle of
contrast bypassing the predominantly
left-sided lesion. At operation this
proved to be a meningioma (A)
displacing and compressing the cord
(B) and almost obliterating the canal. It
was removed and the patient made a
good recovery.

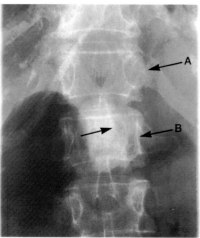

9.11

9.11,9.12 Calcified meningioma.
Calcification in a spinal tumour – a most
unusual finding – is almost diagnostic of a
meningioma. The plain film shows such
calcification opposite the body of L1
(arrow), the pedicles of which are indistinct
(compare A and B). Myelography revealed
the lower border of an ovoid tumour
blocking the spinal canal above the roots of
the cauda equina.

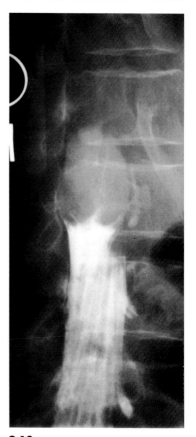

9.12

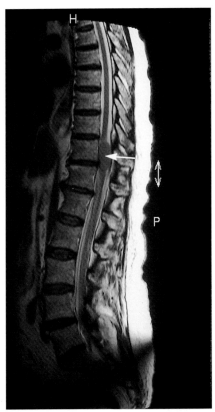

9.13 MR scan of thoracic meningioma. The investigation of spinal lesions has been simplified by the introduction of scanning and with the aid of contrast it is now possible to get an excellent picture of most tumours (arrow).

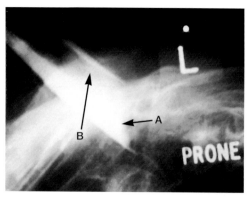

9.14

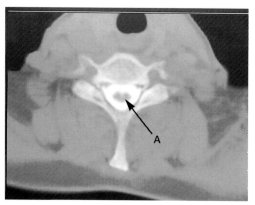

9.15A

9.14–9.16 CT myelogram of meningioma. A 60-year-old woman who presented with progressive weakness in the legs. Cervical myelography showed obstruction to the downward flow of contrast at T2 (A) and in this prone position it could be seen that the cord (B) was displaced backwards. The serial sections from the CT scan showed the centrally placed cord outlined by contrast (9.15A) being displaced backwards (9.15B) and eventually merging into the tumour at the level of the block (9.15C). At operation the dura was retracted on threads and the cord was elevated to reveal an anteriorly placed meningioma (9.16 arrow).

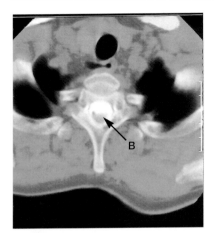

9.15B

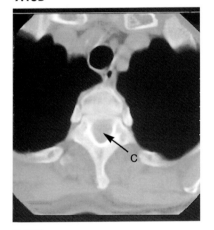

9.15C

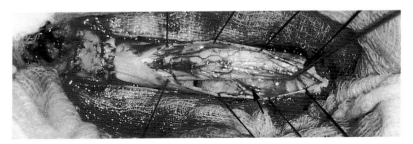

9.16

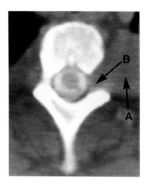

9.17 CT scan of neurofibroma. The 'dumb-bell' appearance of a neurofibroma is best seen on a CT scan where the section outside the canal (A) and the widened foramen (B) are clearly visible. In this instance the intraspinal section is not large enough to displace the theca or the cord (see also 9.4, 10.10).

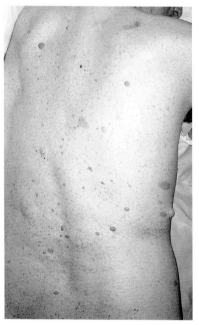

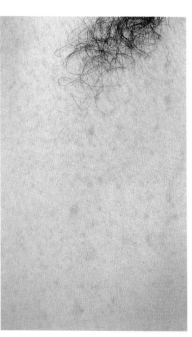

9.18   **9.19**

9.18,9.19 Neurofibromatosis. Neurofibromas may occur in isolation or as part of the syndrome of neurofibromatosis, a developmental disorder inherited as an autosomal dominant. Two main forms are recognised. The more common (NF1, previously known as peripheral neurofibromatosis or von Recklinghausen's disease) is associated with *café-au-lait* patches with a regular contour, cutaneous nodules and axillary pigmentation (9.19). NF2, previously known as central neurofibromatosis, is associated with bilateral eighth nerve tumours.

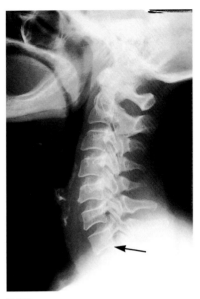 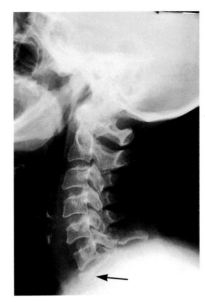

9.20   **9.21**

9.20–9.23 Secondary deposit. Six months after a radical mastectomy this 59-year-old woman complained of pain in the neck and arms and of weakness in the hands. The spine of C7 was tender and the arm pain was intensified by neck movements. Weakness of the triceps and loss of the triceps jerk supported the idea of a C7 lesion. Lateral films showed that between September 1968 and June 1969 the body of the seventh cervical vertebra had collapsed and posterior views over the same period showed that the vertebral spine had been eroded (arrows).

When treating neoplastic deposits in the spinal canal the two main errors are procrastination and an incorrect surgical approach. The disease is probably incurable, but in patients who are not near to death *rapid* intervention can prevent distressing complications such as pain, paraplegia, loss of sphincter control and bedsores. It is, however, essential that surgical advice should be sought at once. If, as is commonly the case, the lesion lies in the vertebral body it is illogical to do a laminectomy, for this destroys the only remaining column of support (the vertebral arches) and does not expose the site of the lesion. An anterolateral approach, by contrast, preserves the column of vertebral arches, allows the dura to be decompressed by the removal of damaged tissue and may even dispose of weakness which has already developed.

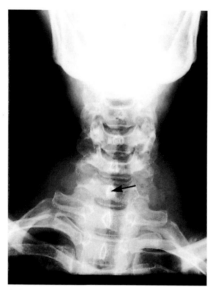

9.22

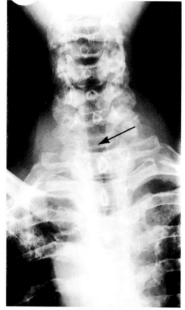

9.23

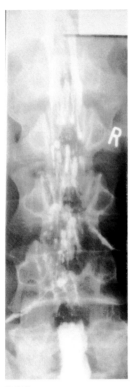

9.24

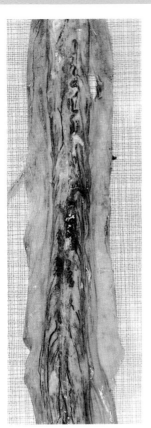

9.25

9.24,9.25 Carcinomatous meningitis. Deposits in the epidural space often cause a paraplegia without producing any abnormalities on the plain films. Much less commonly, carcinomatous infiltration of the meninges occurs. This usually affects the base of the brain, causing headache and numerous cranial nerve palsies in rapid succession. A similar lesion is sometimes seen in the spine. This 62-year-old man presented with a short history of low back pain, leg weakness and loss of sphincter control. He had a mixture of upper and lower motor neurone signs in the legs and the spinal fluid was consistently bloodstained with a lymphocytosis, a high protein level and a low glucose. There was partial obstruction to the flow of myodil at L2 the cause of which was not evident. He deteriorated rapidly and eventually developed cranial nerve palsies and confusion. At autopsy the lower part of the cord was found to be enveloped in a milky deposit which proved to be carcinomatous meningitis.

Atlanto-axial dislocation

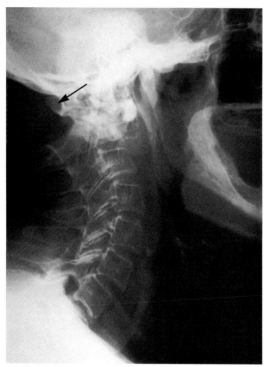

9.26 Atlanto-axial dislocation. This condition, which may be due to trauma, rheumatoid arthritis or ankylosing spondylitis, can produce horrifying radiological abnormalities with little in the way of symptoms or cause tetraparesis, vertebrobasilar ischaemia, blackouts and even sudden death. This elderly man complained of weakness in the limbs and numbness in the hands four weeks after falling downstairs. X-rays, which must be taken in flexion and extension, showed that the posterior arch of the atlas (arrow) was not in line with the other vertebral arches.

Cervical spondylosis

Degenerative changes in the neck can cause:

1. Pain in the neck due to damage to joints and soft tissues.
2. Pain in the arm due to compression of a nerve root by a (lateral) prolapse.
3. Weakness in the legs due to compression of the cord by a (central) prolapse.
4. Symptoms of basilar ischaemia due to tortuosity and loss of elasticity in the vertebral artery.

As with sciatica, the root pain is aggravated by movement, jolting and changes in CSF pressure caused by coughing, sneezing and straining. Weakness and wasting may be seen in the appropriate myotome (see 11.17), but the characteristic finding is an alteration in the arm reflexes. This may be simple loss of the triceps jerk due to a C7 lesion, or loss of the biceps or supinator jerk due to a C5/6 lesion with a brisk (triceps) jerk due to upper motor neurone damage at the level below. The hyperexcitability of reflexes below the lesion may be so great that the elbow extends when the biceps is tapped and the supinator response is replaced by finger flexion. This is known as inversion.

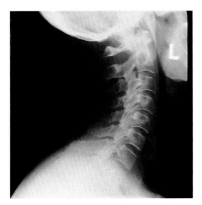

9.27 Normal cervical spine. The disc spaces are preserved and there is a smooth forward convexity. There are no spikes of bone (osteophytes) at the disc margins and the canal is of reasonable width.

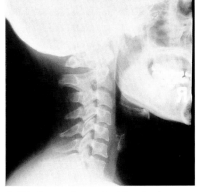

9.28 Loss of cervical lordosis. Loss of the forward convexity of the cervical spine suggests that the neck muscles are in spasm.

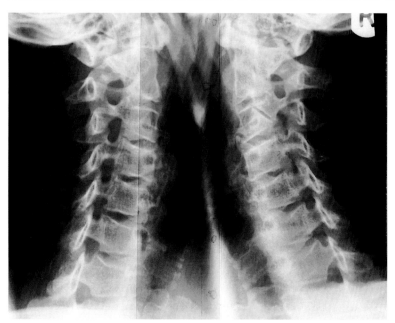

9.29 Narrowing of intervertebral foramina. Oblique films to show the foramina in a patient who complained of recurrent attacks of right-sided brachalgia some years after a serious road accident in which he was thought to be 'uninjured'. The upper intervertebral foramina on the right are markedly reduced in size.

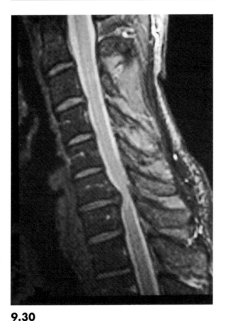

9.30

9.30, 9.31 Myelopathy due to cervical spondylosis. The cord is compressed by a prolapsed cervical disc. The forward convexity of the spine is lost and the damaged space is reduced in size with prominent osteophytes at its margins. In such patients the risk of a myelopathy is greatly increased if the spinal canal is narrow. Figure 9.31 shows the mean diameter of the canal at each level in 91 patients with spondylotic myelopathy (dots) by comparison with the range of means of normal subjects taken from various publications (vertical lines) (Nurick, *British Journal of Hospital Medicine* 1975; 14: 668–676).

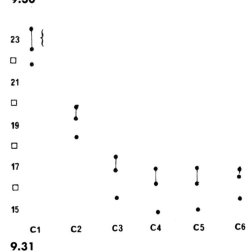

9.31

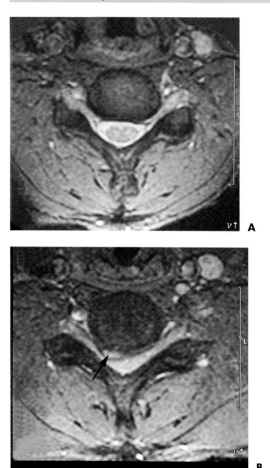

9.32A,B MR scan of prolapsed cervical disc. The normal cord and theca (9.32A) resting in the slight concavity on the posterior aspect of the normal disc in the space above, with stout root sheaths running out on either side. At the level of the prolapse (9.32B), the canal is almost obliterated by the disc (arrow) which has protruded backwards and to the right, almost obliterating the right root sheath.

Spondylolisthesis, spondylitis and prolapsed thoracic discs

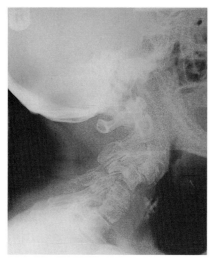

9.33,9.34 Spondylolisthesis. A 61-year-old woman with a strong family history of various joint disorders. Ten years before admission she had been treated for 'ulnar neuropathy' but soon after, when the weakness in her hands progressed, she was found to have spondylolisthesis. She also had lumbar spondylolisthesis (see 10.29) and a neuropathic (Charcot) elbow joint and went on to develop a spastic paraplegia.

9.33

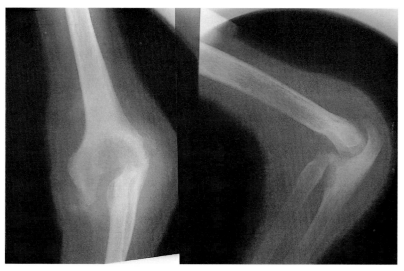

9.34

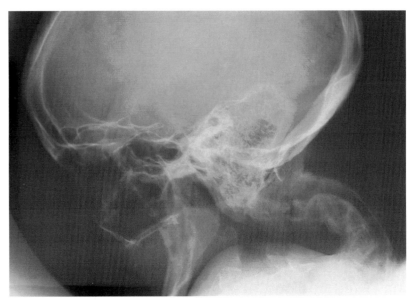

9.35 Ankylosing spondylitis. This disease, which is associated with various neurological disorders – notably a cauda equina syndrome – does not usually cause cord compression. Despite the gross deformity this patient had few neurological signs, possibly because the diameter of the canal was not reduced. There is however a serious risk of injury in a fall because of the inflexibility of the spine.

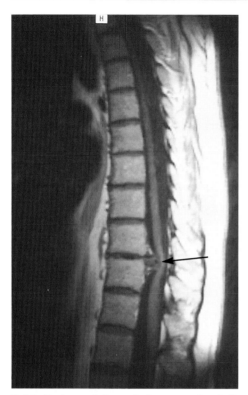

9.36 Prolapsed thoracic intervertebral disc. Prolapsed thoracic discs, which usually present with paraplegia in middle-aged men, are uncommon. Until the advent of scanning they were difficult to diagnose and the one clue sometimes found was calcification in an intervertebral space. This 51-year-old man had had a 3-month episode of weakness and numbness in the right lower limb several years earlier. He presented with similar symptoms on the left – this time extending to the costal margin – and retention of urine. He had signs of damage to the pyramidal tracts and the posterior columns but the myelogram was normal. The MR scan showed an obvious prolapse of a thoracic disc which – as is most important – was removed via an anterolateral approach.

Tuberculosis of the spine

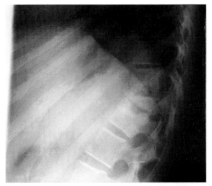

9.37

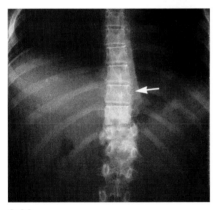

9.38

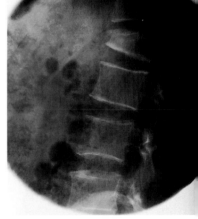

9.39

9.37–9.39 Pott's disease of the spine. Most cases of tuberculous paraplegia are caused by infections in an intervertebral space which destroy the space and the adjacent vertebral bodies, producing a wedge collapse (9.37) and possibly a paravertebral abscess (9.38). Compare the appearance with that in (9.39) in which wedge collapse due to trauma (or a secondary deposit) has left the adjacent vertebrae and disc spaces intact.

Less commonly, paraplegia due to lesions in a vertebral arch, to tuberculomas in the spinal cord and to focal low-grade meningitis around the cord is seen. Whether primary epidural tuberculomas (as opposed to tuberculomas associated with lesions in the vertebral arch hitherto undetected by relatively crude methods of investigation) exist is a matter for debate.

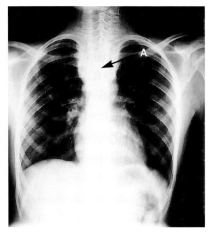

9.40

9.40, 9.41A,B Pott's disease with paraspinal abscess.

Widening of the mediastinum (A) in an 11-year-old girl. CT scanning showed destruction of vertebral bodies (cf. B and C), an extensive paravertebral mass (D) and forward displacement of the oesophagus and trachea (E). The theca is also displaced to the left (F).

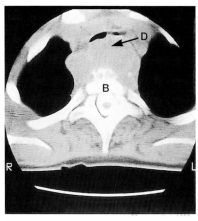

9.41A

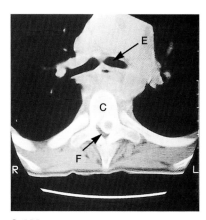

9.41B

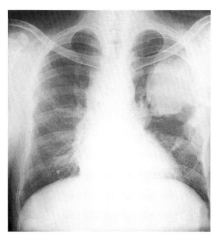

9.42 Tuberculosis mimicking carcinomatosis. Tuberculosis in immigrants may be so florid that it mimics carcinomatosis. This 41-year-old Pakistani man gave a 3-month history of back pain followed by paraplegia. He had lesions in the left lung, a widened hilum, a fractured rib and a spinal block. These were confidently attributed to carcinoma even after biopsy. However, the tough granulation tissue removed from the epidural space contained numerous giant cells typical of tuberculosis and with appropriate treatment the patient made a complete recovery.

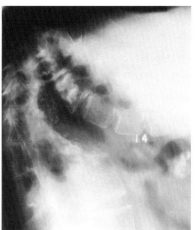

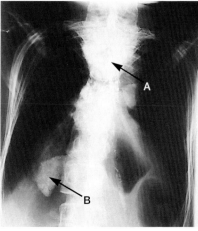

9.43   **9.44**

9.43, 9.44 Old spinal tuberculosis. A woman who had been confined to bed with spinal tuberculosis between the ages of 5 and 14. She had tuberculous meningitis at the age of 18, but gave birth to a child when she was 45. These remarkable films show the upper and lower parts of the spine running parallel. On the upper part of the chest X-ray there is a view down the length of the spinal canal (A) and calcified psoas abscesses are visible (B).

(See also Pott's disease presenting as sciatica – 10.11.)

Epidural abscess

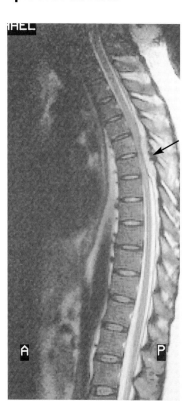

9.45 Epidural abscess. Staphylococcal infections in the epidural space are rare. They are however exceedingly dangerous and require urgent surgical treatment. There may be a history of injury to the back and of an infection there or elsewhere in the body. The spine is usually very tender and there are signs of infection. If untreated the patient rapidly develops a paraplegia which is likely to be permanent. This 43-year-old man had been febrile for 2 weeks and presented when he developed pain in the back and numbness and weakness in the legs. He was febrile, and had a tender spine and a flaccid paraplegia. An MR scan revealed an epidural mass at T5/6 which proved to be an abscess. His paraplegia was not relieved.

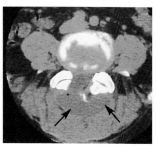

9.46 Epidural abscess. Two weeks after an apparently successful laminectomy this 51-year-old man developed malaise, vomiting, headache, photophobia, neck stiffness and extreme tenderness over the laminectomy scar. The symptoms of meningitis responded to antibiotic treatment but the scar remained tender. A CT scan revealed a large epidural abscess (arrows) which was incised and packed prior to closure a week later.

Multiple sclerosis

Multiple sclerosis, one of the most common disorders of the nervous system, is a fruitful source of errors. These are of two main types. Some patients, who have symptoms but no signs, are dismissed as 'neurotic' and are incongruously grateful when it is confirmed that there is indeed something the matter with their legs. Others, who have clearcut evidence of organic disease, acquire an incorrect diagnosis of multiple sclerosis and thereafter their problems no longer receive active consideration or treatment. Although most likely to occur with benign tumours compressing the cord, the same problem arises with such things as 'retrobulbar neuritis' due to a detached retina or a pituitary tumour and cerebellar signs due to a brainstem glioma.

These errors can to a large extent be avoided if a firm diagnosis of multiple sclerosis is only made in: (1) young white adults with (2) lesions in the *central* nervous system that are (3) disseminated in space and (4) disseminated in time. Hence a patient with retrobulbar neuritis – the presenting symptom in 25% of cases – cannot be said to have multiple

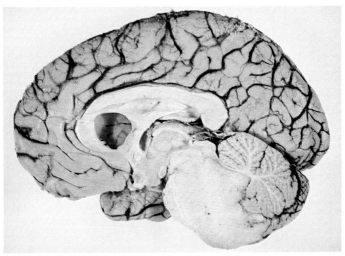

9.47 Brainstem glioma. A 34-year-old man with a 3-month history of diplopia and ataxia. Despite an uncharacteristic complaint of headache these symptoms were attributed to multiple sclerosis. The diagnosis was only revised when he began to vomit and developed a bulbar palsy. While multiple sclerosis is admittedly the most likely cause of such diplopia and ataxia, the case illustrates the danger of 'jumping to conclusions'.

sclerosis until there has been at least one subsequent episode in another part of the central nervous system. Conversely, a patient who develops multiple lesions simultaneously cannot be said to have multiple sclerosis for he may have acute disseminated encephalomyelitis.

Clinical manifestations

Patients with demyelinating lesions affecting the pyramidal tracts of the cord initially complain of heaviness or weakness in the legs and of an inability to run. At first symptoms may only appear after exertion but by degrees more persistent weakness, often exacerbated by heat and/or infections, appears. By contrast with spondylotic myelopathy signs (and especially stiffness) may be unremarkable, even in patients with quite severe disease, but the reflexes are usually brisk, vibration sense may be lost and it is often very easy to elicit an unequivocal extensor plantar response. Abnormalities in a limb which the patient regards as normal are also characteristic. Lesions in the spinothalamic tracts produce an alarming numbness that steadily spreads to other parts of the body without producing objective physical signs. Lesions in the posterior columns produce a constricting band-like sensation round the trunk or a tingling feeling that runs down the body when the neck is flexed (Lhermitte's sign). Posterior column lesions may also produce a particularly disabling loss of position sense in the upper limb (the useless hand of Oppenheim) which clears in months.

Investigations

The diagnosis of multiple sclerosis still depends primarily on clinical observation – i.e. on the discovery of clinical evidence of two separate lesions in the central nervous system of a patient aged between 10 and 59 who has had two episodes characteristic of multiple sclerosis for which there is no other explanation. 'Paraclinical' evidence of one of the lesions – for example on an MR scan – is however acceptable. An abnormal scan in a patient who has only had *one* clinical episode does not however suffice, for this could be due to an (isolated) attack of acute disseminated encephalomyelitis. The discovery of new lesions on a second scan done a month later, or the demonstration (by gadolinium injection) of lesions of two ages on a scan done after the clinical event makes the diagnosis probable. The discovery of oligoclonal bands in the spinal fluid lends further support to the diagnosis. Laboratory investigations alone, however, never suffice.

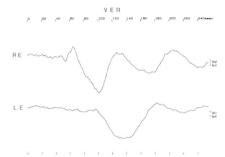

VER

9.48 Evoked responses. Defective conduction in the optic nerve, the brainstem or the spinal cord can be demonstrated by showing abnormal cerebral responses to stimulation of the eye, the ear or the body. Stimulation of one eye with a rapidly reversing chequered pattern of small black and white squares produces a response with a predictable pattern and latency (upper trace). Damage to the optic pathways causes this wave-form to be delayed and deformed. It is not, however, possible to make an aetiological diagnosis.

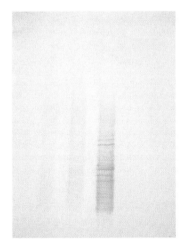

9.49 Oligoclonal bands. Discrete bands are found on electrophoresis in 50% of new cases and in 95% of established cases of multiple sclerosis. The abnormality is not, however, pathognomonic.

Conversely, recent studies indicate that the *absence* of oligoclonal bands should suggest the possibility of the antiphospholipid syndrome which, by causing multiple infarcts, can mimic the clinical and radiological features of multiple sclerosis. This is important as such patients appear to respond to treatment with anticoagulants (*Quarterly Journal of Medicine* 2000; 93: 497–499).

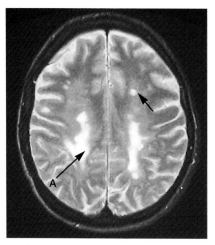

9.50,9.51 MR scan in multiple sclerosis. MR scanning is said to reveal lesions in over 90% of patients with multiple sclerosis. Although not in themselves pathognomonic, confluent lesions around the ventricles (A) and scattered lesions in the hemispheres and brainstem (arrows) are strongly suggestive of the diagnosis. The lesion (B) lying just below the aqueduct (C) probably involved the medial longitudinal bundle.

9.50

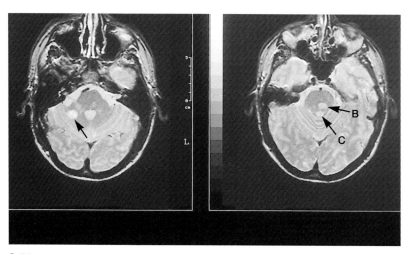

9.51

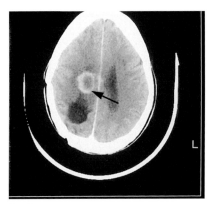

9.52

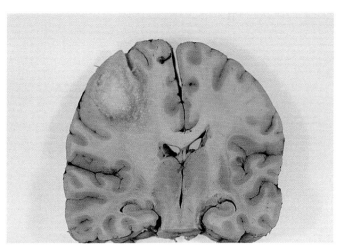

9.53

9.52,9.53 Demyelination presenting as a mass. Lesions which appear to be brain tumours or cysts sometimes prove to be areas of demyelination (9.52 arrow) which often respond to steroid treatment. In most patients this is a monophasic illness and the lesions are usually single. A history of immunisation or of an associated illness suggests that they may represent something between multiple sclerosis and acute disseminated encephalomyelitis. Others, like the patient shown in 9.53 who had previously had a mass in the cerebellum, have recurrent lesions and are thought to have multiple sclerosis.

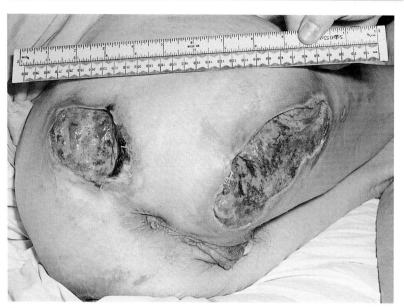

9.54 Bedsores. Immobility, incontinence, impairment of sensation, trophic changes in the skin and wasting conspire to produce bedsores in paraplegic patients with remarkable speed. This woman, whose skin was intact when discharged from hospital, returned with these lesions after a few weeks at home.

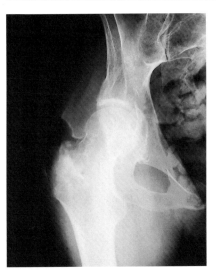

9.55

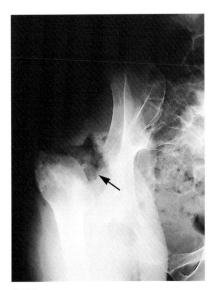

9.56

9.55, 9.56 Destruction of hip by bedsore. A young woman with paraplegia in flexion due to multiple sclerosis. Partly due to the inappropriate use of steroids an infection from a bedsore over the great trochanter extended into and demolished the hip joint. These films, taken 3 months apart, show destruction of the head of the femur and the appearance of gas in the joint (9.56 arrow).

Vascular diseases of the spinal cord

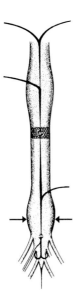

9.57 The anterior spinal artery. To understand spinal vascular disease one has to understand the anatomy of the blood supply of the spinal cord. The anterior spinal artery is formed from branches of the vertebral arteries and is joined lower down by several large radicular vessels, the residue of the segmental vessels seen in the embryo. The most important of these is the arteria magna of Adamkiewicz which usually lies on the left just above or just below the diaphragm (arrows). As the anastomosis between segments of the anterior spinal artery is often incomplete individual vessels often supply sections of the cord well above their point of entry. Occlusion, compression, ligation or avulsion of a radicular vessel may therefore result in infarction, possibly at a much higher level. Recent studies have however failed to confirm the traditional teaching that the T4 watershed (shaded) is particularly vulnerable.

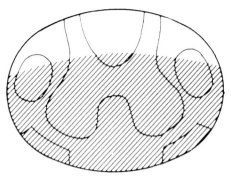

9.58 'Thrombosis of the anterior spinal artery'. The anterior spinal artery supplies the anterior two-thirds of the cord including the pyramidal and spinothalamic tracts. Occlusion therefore causes a spastic paraplegia with dissociated sensory loss (loss of pain and temperature sensation with preservation of position and vibration). Actual thrombosis of the anterior spinal artery is rare and such signs are usually caused by emboli or by occlusion of a radicular vessel.

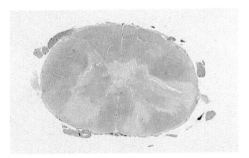

9.59 Thrombosis of the anterior spinal artery. A 76-year-old diabetic with mild hypertension who 'strained her neck' while lifting heavy curtains. The following morning she developed pain below the scapulae which quickly spread to encircle the body, and within 24 hours she was tetraplegic. She had a C7 sensory level and myelography revealed a large disc bar at C6/7. At autopsy there was histological evidence of infarction (pale areas) in the territory of the anterior spinal artery from C4 to T4, but no evidence of arterial occlusion was found.

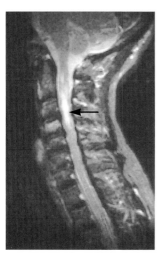
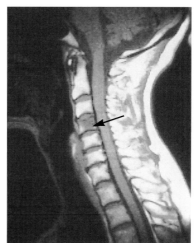

9.60   **9.61**

9.60, 9.61 Anterior spinal artery thrombosis. Since the introduction of MR scanning it has sometimes been possible to demonstrate such lesions in life. This 59-year-old woman woke with severe pain in the back and shoulders, difficulty in breathing and a paraplegia. Her arms were flaccid, her legs were spastic and she had a dissociated sensory loss with an upper limit at C4. Scanning revealed infarction of the cord and of the vertebral body at that level (arrows). With conservative treatment she made a reasonably complete recovery.

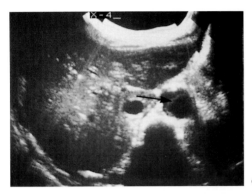

9.62

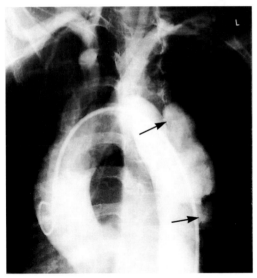

9.63

9.62, 9.63 Paraplegia due to dissecting aneurysm. Occlusion of the arteria magna by a dissecting aortic aneurysm, or during the investigation or treatment of such a lesion, is a recognised cause of paraplegia. Over the course of 3 months this 50-year-old woman had had three attacks of chest pain. In the third her legs were said to be 'hypotonic'. In the fourth episode a dissecting aneurysm was demonstrated by ultrasound (9.62 arrow) and arteriography showed an extensive lesion between the subclavian artery and the diaphragm (9.63 arrows). The sac was cleared and a prosthesis was inserted without undue difficulty, but on recovery the patient was paraplegic – presumably because the arteria magna was occluded at some stage of the illness, investigation or treatment.

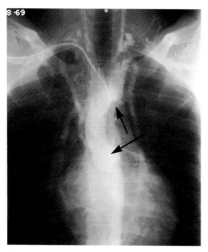

9.64

9.64, 9.65 Paraplegia due to coarctation. A 20-year-old man with coarctation who developed weakness in the legs and was found to have a spastic paraplegia. Angiography revealed severe coarctation over 3 cm just distal to the subclavian artery (9.64 arrows). A collateral circulation was provided by the internal mammary arteries and the thyro- and costo-cervical trunks which were considerably enlarged. It was surmised that the weakness was due to similar vessels within the spinal canal and resection of the lesion restored strength to the legs. Difficulty in walking may be due to claudication, to compression of the cord by an aneurysm or an angiomatous mass or to loss of a vital intercostal vessel during investigation or surgery. The vertebral bodies are very vascular and attempts to do a laminectomy may cause severe bleeding.

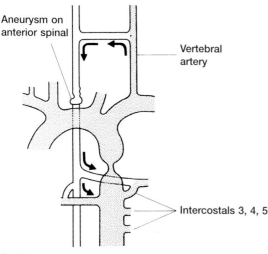

Aneurysm on anterior spinal

Vertebral artery

Intercostals 3, 4, 5

9.65

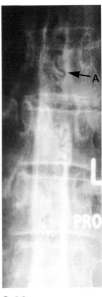

9.66

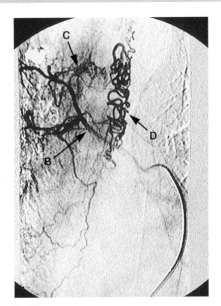

9.67

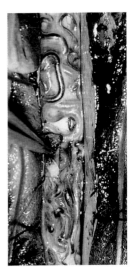

9.68

9.66–9.68 Spinal arteriovenous malformation.
Two principal types are recognised. The first, which
usually presents as a progressive paraplegia in older
patients (average age 49) is caused by a dural
arteriovenous fistula, the intradural 'angioma' consisting
of arterialised draining veins. The second, a true
arteriovenous malformation lying in or on the cord,
occurs in younger patients (average age 27) and usually
presents with severe pain in the back due to
haemorrhage. This patient complained of difficulty with
walking and proved to have a spastic paraplegia.
Myelography (9.66) revealed dilated vessels over the
surface of the cord (A) and spinal angiography (9.67)
demonstrated a vessel (B) feeding a fistula (C) which
drained into arterialised veins on the cord (D). The
lesion was resected (9.68).

10.

The lumbosacral nerve roots

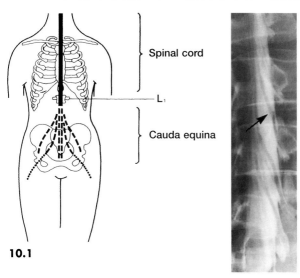

Spinal cord

L₁

Cauda equina

10.1

10.2

10.1,10.2 The cauda equina. In an adult the spinal cord, and therefore the pyramidal tracts, end just below the first lumbar vertebra. Patients with upper motor neurone signs must therefore have a lesion above that level. The rest of the canal – nearly a third of its length – is occupied by lumbar and sacral nerve roots that group together to form the cauda equina. The remarkable length of these roots, which run on into the pelvis, can be seen on the myelogram (10.2 arrow). Symptoms in this area may therefore be due to: (1) lesions in the bones, joints and soft tissues, (2) injury to a nerve root in or beyond the spinal canal or (3) compression of the cauda equina.

Pain in the back

Low back pain is usually due to degeneration of or injury to joints and/ or soft tissues in and around the spine. Such pain is clearly influenced by mechanical factors, being made worse by jolting, bending and coughing and relieved by heat and resting in certain positions. It varies in intensity from hour to hour and week to week, depending on what the patient has been doing. By contrast patients with neoplastic or inflammatory diseases (including ankylosing spondylitis) complain of pain that is largely independent of movement. It tends to be more persistent and is troublesome at night because no 'comfortable position' can be found. It is clearly important to identify, among the mass of those complaining of backache, the occasional patient with such non-mechanical pain. Those outside the 20–50 age group, those who look ill, have a history of tubercle or neoplasia or a high sedimentation rate and those with thoracic pain or severe limitation of movement should be carefully scrutinised. The possibility of referred pain due, for example, to an aortic aneurysm or a pancreatic carcinoma should also be remembered.

Pain in the leg

Pain in the leg is not necessarily due to injury to a nerve root. Damage to joints and soft tissues in and around the spine commonly causes a poorly localised, dull, aching, referred pain that may extend across the buttock and thigh to the knee. Diabetic amyotrophy and the crural counterpart of neuralgic amyotrophy can also cause proximal pain with wasting, weakness and areflexia. Pain caused by injury to a nerve root is sharper, more severe and more localised and is often associated with paraesthesiae. The pain in the *leg* is exacerbated by coughing, sneezing, jolting and straight leg raising (or, in the case of the upper lumbar roots, hip extension). Exacerbation of pain in the back or in an arthritic hip is irrelevant. Examination may reveal weakness and/or loss of reflexes in the appropriate segment. Injury to the three uppermost lumbar roots should be viewed with suspicion, for they are rarely damaged by prolapsed discs. So too should sciatic pain which is not made worse by coughing and stretching, for it is likely to be due to a lesion beyond the intervertebral foramen.

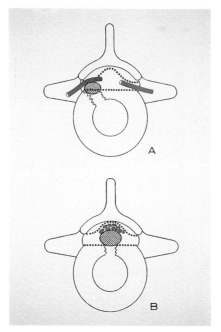

10.3 Prolapsed intervertebral disc. The most common cause of sciatica is prolapse of a lumbar intervertebral disc. Following rupture of the annulus fibrosus the nucleus pulposus may protrude in a lateral direction (A) compressing a nerve root or in a posterior direction (B) compressing the cauda equina.

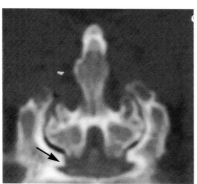

10.4 Spinal stenosis. As in the cervical region a prolapsed lumbar intervertebral disc is more likely to produce symptoms if the spine is congenitally narrow. Hypertrophic changes cause the facetal joints (arrow) to bulge into the canal, altering the normal oval shape into a triangular one (see 10.3 dotted lines) and sometimes producing the condition known as intermittent claudication of the cauda equina. The hypertrophy also elongates and narrows the lateral orifice through which the roots emerge. This is a tunnel rather than a hole and failure to relieve stenosis at this point is an important cause of failed laminectomy.

271

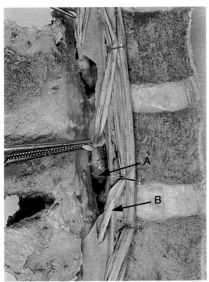

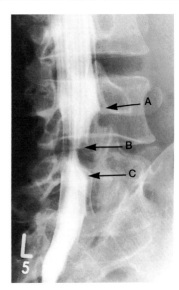

10.5

10.6

10.5,10.6 Prolapsed intervertebral disc. Surprisingly, it is usually the root at the level *below* the prolapse which is injured. Figure 10.5 shows how the ganglion on the emerging root (A) lies in the upper part of the intervertebral foramen well above the corresponding intervertebral disc. A prolapse will therefore compress the root destined for the space below (B). This is confirmed by the myelogram on which the root at the level of the prolapse is seen emerging above the filling defect (10.6A), whereas the roots destined for the following two spaces are squeezed flat (B) or grossly displaced (C). The relevant signs are given in Table 2.

Table 2 Clinical manifestations of lumbosacral root lesions

Root lesion	Disc lesion	Weakness	Reflex loss	Sensory loss	Leg pain aggravated by:
L3	2/3	Quadriceps (can't extend knee)	Knee	Knee	Hip extension
L5	4/5	Dorsiflexion (can't walk on heels)	–	Dorsum of foot	Straight leg raising
S1	5/1	Plantarflexion (can't walk on toes)	Ankle	Sole	Straight leg raising

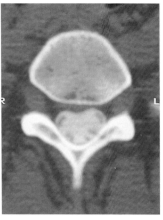

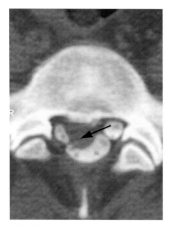

10.7A **10.7B**

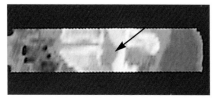

10.8

10.7A,B,10.8 CT scan of prolapsed lumbar disc. This patient developed right-sided sciatica after manipulation by an osteopath. At the level of the vertebral body (10.7A), the roots of the cauda equina are visible within the kidney-shaped theca. At the level of the disc space (10.7B), the prolapse appears as a filling defect directed backwards and to the right (arrow). The lateral reconstruction (10.8) shows displacement of the theca opposite the disc space (arrow).

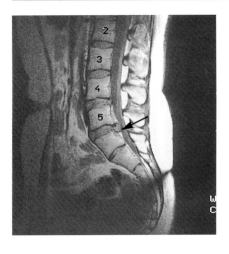

10.9 MR scan of prolapsed disc. A lesion similar to that shown on 10.8 demonstrated even more clearly by MR imaging (arrow).

Other causes of sciatica

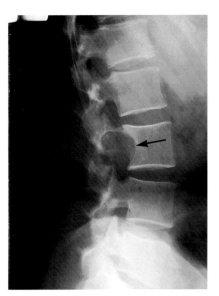

10.10 Lumbar neurofibroma. Compression by a prolapsed disc is the most common cause of injury to a lumbar nerve root, but injury anywhere on its long course will produce similar symptoms and signs. This patient complained of back pain radiating into the legs which was aggravated by coughing. The only sign was depression of the right knee jerk (L3). Investigations, done largely because prolapsed discs at this level are uncommon, revealed massive enlargement of the 3/4 intervertebral foramen (arrow) and a filling defect which, as expected, proved to be a dumb-bell neurofibroma.

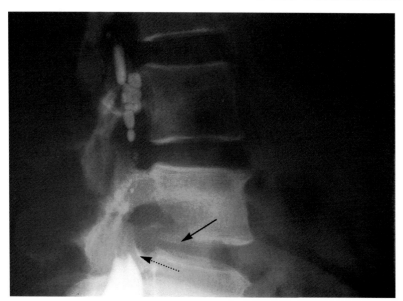

10.11 Sciatica due to spinal tuberculosis. A 49-year-old Indian lady who complained of low back pain and sciatica. Although she appeared to be improving the presence of a depressed knee jerk, a high sedimentation rate and a raised alkaline phosphatase prompted further investigation. The lower border of L4 was found to be eroded (solid arrow) at which point there was an almost complete obstruction to the flow of myodil (dotted arrow). Tubercle bacilli were grown from the body of the vertebra.

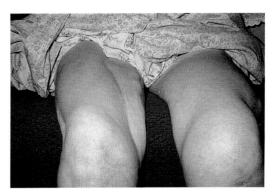

10.12

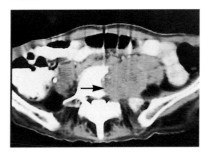

10.13

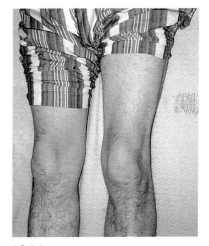

10.14

10.12–10.14 Pelvic lesions. Lesions in the pelvis which injure the lumbosacral plexus (see 11.45) can also cause sciatica. At this level, however, coughing, sneezing and stretching do not intensify the pain because the nerve root can move freely in the foramen. Three years after treatment for carcinoma of the cervix this 58-year-old woman presented with left-sided sciatica. When she tried to straighten her legs it was obvious that the left quadriceps were weak and wasted (10.12). The knee jerk was depressed and sensation over the knee was impaired. The pain was not aggravated by coughing, sneezing or tension (which with this L3 lesion implied hip *extension*). Despite normal rectal and vaginal examinations a pelvic mass was therefore suspected. The scan (10.13) showed a large lesion which had destroyed half of an adjacent vertebra. In a man wasting of the thigh can often be demonstrated by showing that the trouser-leg will slide further up one limb than the other (10.14).

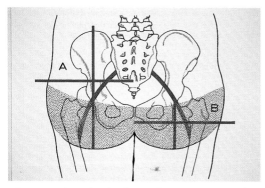

10.15 Lesions in the buttock. Injections into the upper outer quadrant of the buttock (A) are harmless provided it is understood that the buttock extends up to the iliac crest. Injections into the upper outer part of the area covered by a bikini will go straight into the sciatic nerve (B). There is a growing body of opinion which holds that it is better to avoid the risk by giving all injections into the lateral aspect of the thigh.

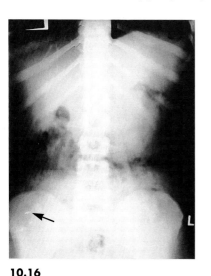

10.16

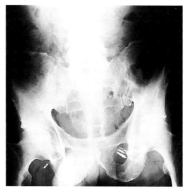

10.17

10.16, 10.17 Radio-opaque material in the buttocks. The bismuth injections once used in the treatment of syphilis are radio-opaque. Those in 10.16 are correctly sited, but the injections in 10.17 could easily damage the sciatic nerve.

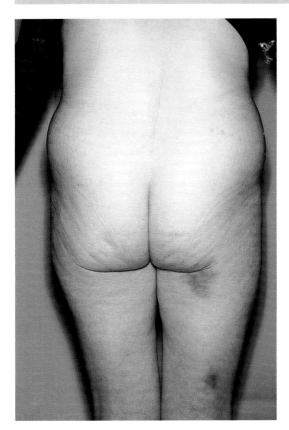

10.18 Herpes zoster. Infection of the appropriate root can cause sciatica and an incorrect diagnosis may be made if the rash is unobtrusive. However, it is worth remembering that zoster sometimes occurs in a root which is being compressed.

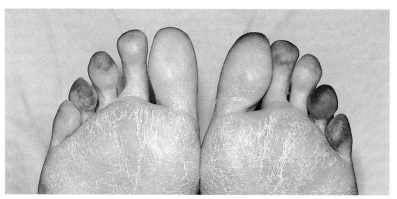

10.19

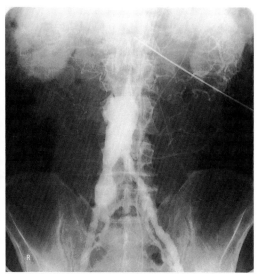

10.20

10.19, 10.20
Ischaemia. Polyarteritis may present with a severe attack of sciatica. Degenerative arterial disease may also be responsible. This 56-year-old man suddenly developed sciatica, loss of bladder control, numbness and ischaemic changes in the toes. The knee jerks were depressed and sensation over the right foot was impaired.
Arteriography showed stenosis and irregular aneurysmal dilation of the pelvic vessels.

Lesions of the cauda equina

Lesions of the cauda equina are one of the 'blind spots' of neurology. Patients present with bilateral sciatica but their other symptoms and signs – due, because of their vulnerable position, to compression of the sacral roots – are likely to be overlooked in an 'ordinary' neurological examination. Most movements, the knee jerks and sensation over the front of the lower limbs, all of which are subserved by lumbar roots, will be intact. But more careful examination will show that the ankle jerks and plantar flexion (S1), anal tone and bladder function (S2–4) and sensation over the 'saddle' area on the back of the limbs are impaired. This picture of distal weakness, numbness in the feet and absent ankle jerks must not be mistaken for peripheral neuritis in which *dorsiflexion* is more severely affected than plantarflexion. The possibility that an insidiously developing cauda equina lesion is due to infection with cytomegalovirus in a patient with AIDS must also be remembered. Most patients, however, require urgent surgical treatment.

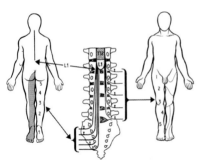

10.21

10.21,10.22 Anatomy of the cauda equina. The lumbar nerve roots, which are the first to leave, run down the side of the canal. Lesions of the cauda equina are therefore more likely to damage the sacral roots which run down the centre of the canal and subserve sensation on the back of the lower limbs, the ankle jerks, plantar flexion, sphincter and bladder control. Such defects are easily overlooked in a 'routine' neurological examination.

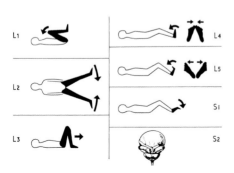

10.22

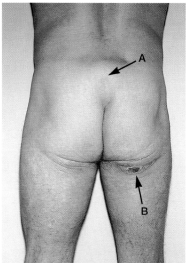

10.23

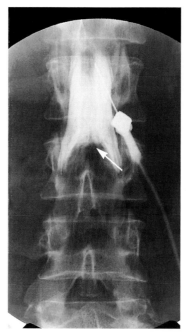

10.24

10.23,10.24 Lipoma of the cauda equina. A 51-year-old man who gave a 6-year history of 'weakness of the feet' and hesitancy of micturition. He had a fatty lump over the sacrum (10.23A) and had recently sustained painless burns on the buttocks while sitting on a radiator because he had saddle anaesthesia (10.23B). A lesion in the lumbar canal producing a complete block below L2 (10.24 arrow) proved to have the density of fat on a CT scan, thus confirming that it was an extension of the lipoma.

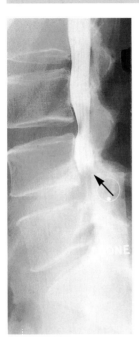

10.25 Central prolapse of lumbar intervertebral disc. A 62-year-old man who suddenly developed low back pain, followed some days later by bilateral sciatica, after pulling a rug. Myelography revealed complete obstruction to the downward flow of myodil opposite the L4/5 space. The lesion, as expected, proved to be a central disc prolapse.

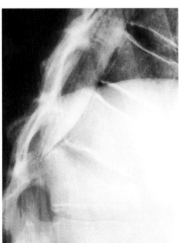

10.26 Post-traumatic compression of the cauda equina. A 58-year-old lady who sustained a wedge fracture of L1 after falling downstairs. This lesion, which was at the top of the cauda equina, produced extensive weakness in the legs, numbness below the groins, loss of the ankle jerks and loss of bladder control. The spine is angled around the collapsed vertebra and contrast introduced from above shows a block at that level. Vertebral collapse due to osteoporosis can also cause back and root pain but under these circumstances the contents of the canal usually escape injury.

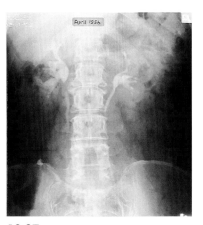

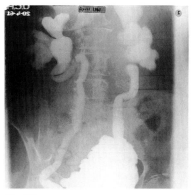

10.28

10.27

10.27,10.28 Hydronephrosis due to cauda equina lesion. These X-rays show the development of hydronephrosis, hydroureter and enlargement of the bladder over the course of 5 years in a patient who lost control of the bladder as a result of a cauda equina lesion.

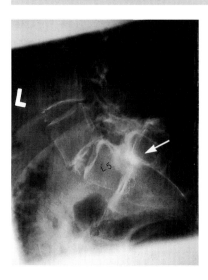

10.29 Spondylolisthesis. This condition causes pain but neurological damage is uncommon even when, as in this case, L5 lies in front of S1 (arrow) (see 9.33, 9.34).

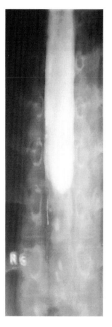

10.30 Arachnoiditis. The use of oily contrast media sometimes resulted in the development of arachnoiditis. Five years before admission this 36-year-old woman complained of non-descript backache and had a myelogram which proved to be normal. She went on to develop a spastic paraplegia. She had a spinal block with xanthochromic fluid and a gross excess of protein. Contrast introduced from above did not pass an irregular block in the lower thoracic region. At operation she was found to have extensive lumbosacral arachnoiditis which contained globules of myodil.

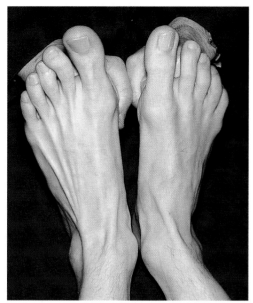

10.31 Elaboration of signs. For financial or psychiatric reasons patients with backache and sciatica often exaggerate the severity of their problem. This suspicion is often most easily tested by watching the patient's activity when he is not aware that he is being examined. Here, however, it is evident that a patient with a 'weak' left foot is using the *dorsiflexors* when he is meant to be pressing his feet downwards.

11.

Peripheral nerves

Polyneuritis

Polyneuritis has traditionally been regarded as a condition which slowly produces glove and stocking sensory loss, peripheral weakness and areflexia. It is in fact much more versatile, for symptoms may develop acutely or very insidiously, their distribution may be proximal as well as distal and damage may be confined to motor, sensory, autonomic or cranial nerve fibres. Patients may therefore present with acute respiratory failure, an indolent 'proximal myopathy', with blurred vision, facial weakness and bulbar symptoms or with hypotension, retention and impotence. This situation has been further complicated by electromyographic, serological and histological studies which have shown that entities such as peroneal atrophy and acute infectious polyneuritis are an amalgamation of conditions which may differ markedly in their pathology, prognosis and treatment. Detailed consideration of these problems is beyond the scope of this book but the main causes can be reviewed (and memorised) under alphabetical headings which cover the first eight letters of the alphabet.

Arteritis

Vasculitic lesions occur in collagen diseases, rheumatoid arthritis, diabetes and AIDS and have been shown to be responsible for 25% of cases of disabling polyneuritis in patients over 65. The most important presentation, however, is as an acute painful mononeuritis, often associated with a rash and a raised sedimentation rate, which rapidly spreads to involve other nerves (mononeuritis multiplex) and responds to immunosuppressant treatment.

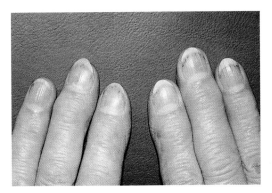

11.1,11.2 Arteritis.
A 72-year-old woman with a history of cranial arteritis who presented with swelling of the left ankle followed by intense pain and distal weakness and sensory loss in the lower limbs. A week later she developed a rash and splinter haemorrhages along with similar symptoms in the hands. Biopsy confirmed that she had an arteritis and she responded to steroids.

11.1

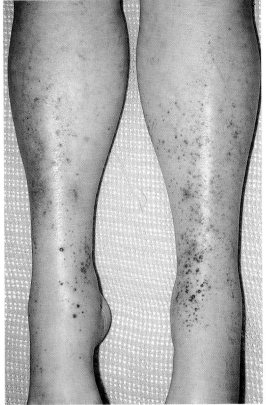

11.2

B12, B1 and other deficiencies

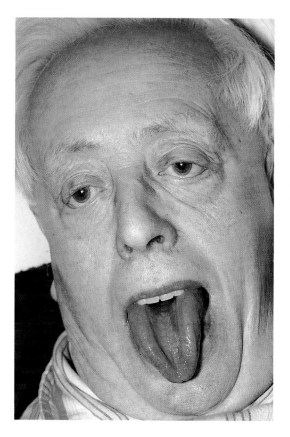

11.3 Pernicious anaemia. Patients with pernicious anaemia, the most common manifestation of vitamin B12 deficiency, are said to have fair hair, pink cheeks and sore tongues. They may develop dementia ('megaloblastic madness'), optic atrophy, subacute combined degeneration of the cord or peripheral neuritis.

Cancer

Peripheral neuritis is a well established non-metastatic complication of cancer, particularly of bronchial carcinoma. Symptoms may appear before the causative lesion is discovered and occasionally remit when it is removed.

Demyelinating polyneuritis

In recent years attention has been drawn to a chronic progressive or relapsing demyelinating polyneuropathy – possibly related to the acute form. This condition, one form of which may mimic motor neurone disease, often responds to immunosuppressants. Such treatment should certainly be considered in those with very slow conduction rates, a high CSF protein and/or a monoclonal gammopathy.

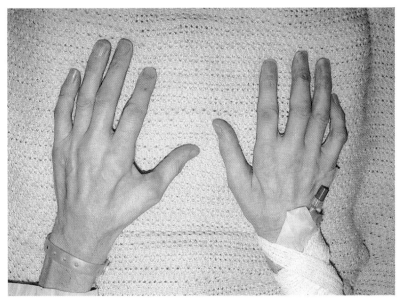

11.4 Demyelinating polyneuropathy. A 56-year-old man with an 8-month history of distal paraesthesiae and tremor followed 3 months later by wasting of the hands and clawing of the fingers. His pupils were unresponsive and he had generalised fasciculation, areflexia, hypertrophy of the peripheral nerves and glove and stocking sensory loss. The CSF protein was 1.86 g/l and the EMG showed gross slowing of conduction. A diagnosis of paraproteinaemic neuropathy (based on the tremor) could not be confirmed, but he responded to steroids.

Ethanol and other toxins

Poisoning, whether self inflicted in the form of alcohol, iatrogenic, industrial or criminal, is a medical 'blind spot', as shown by the fact that the victims of the young 'St Albans poisoner' had been seen by 43 doctors before a chemistry master stumbled across incriminating evidence.

'Fevers'

This term covers established infections such as leprosy, glandular fever and diphtheria and new infections such as AIDS and Lyme disease. It also covers the Guillain–Barré syndrome which is now known to contain at least three main subdivisions – the Miller Fisher form which affects cranial nerves, a generalised demyelinating neuropathy which has a good prognosis and an axonal neuropathy which is associated with campylobacter, affects the limbs and often has a poor prognosis.

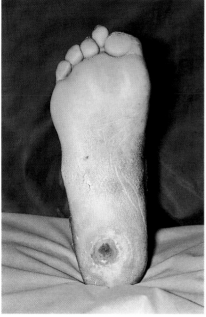

11.5–11.7 Leprosy. A 65-year-old Sikh who presented in casualty with an ulcer on his foot. It was noticed that the terminal phalanx of both great toes was eroded and that his legs were wasted.

11.5

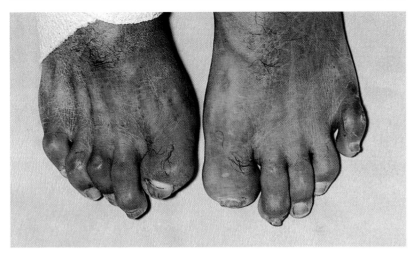

11.6

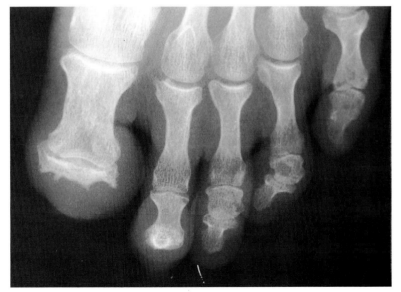

11.7

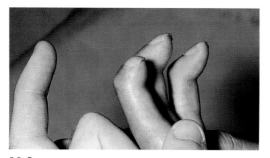

11.8

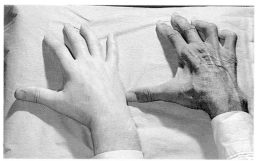

11.9

11.8–11.10 Leprosy (cont.). The tips of the fingers were also eroded and there was wasting of the first dorsal interspace with guttering on the back of the hand due to wasting of the interossei. The thenar and hypothenar masses were absent giving the palm a flat, straight-edged appearance. The patient also had flail wrists and flattening of both surfaces of the forearms. He first complained of sensory symptoms followed by weakness in the arms 22 years earlier and in the legs 10 years earlier. He had tuberculoid leprosy – the form in which resistance is good, skin lesions few in number and bacilli are rarely found.

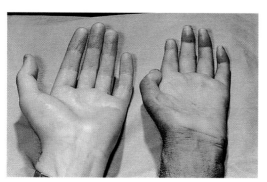

11.10

10am	1.1.l
12nD	1.3l
2pm	1 Lbc.
4pm	1 l

4Pm.	1.15
6Pm	1.25
8Pm	1.3.
10 Pm	1.15
12mn	1.05
2am	1.00
4am	0.9
6am.	0.65
8am	0.8.

Inform Dr , if below 1 litre

11.11 Acute infective polyneuritis. The most severe complication of acute infective polyneuritis is respiratory failure – a problem which, even in an advanced state, is regularly overlooked in hospital practice. It is of the utmost importance that the chest movements and vital capacity of these patients and of those with myasthenia and poliomyelitis should be examined, recorded and re-examined at frequent intervals. Patients who have severe impairment or are clearly deteriorating should be moved in anticipation so that they have immediate access to assisted ventilation should this be needed. The illustration shows an extract from the records of a patient discharged from an intensive care unit to make space for another who was more seriously ill. The nursing staff had been told, verbally and in writing, to summon assistance if the vital capacity fell below 1 litre. Having ignored a relentless fall in the readings between 8 PM and 2 AM, which in itself merited action, when the reading reached 0.9 they then decided to ignore instructions and 'wait for the ward round' – by which time the patient was moribund.

Genetic

Careful screening of patients with 'idiopathic' polyneuritis has shown that over 40% have in fact got an hereditary polyneuropathy. Skeletal deformities or a family history of skeletal deformities, arthritis or difficulty with walking may provide a clue.

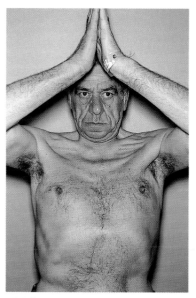 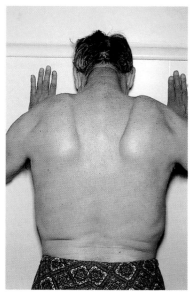

11.12   **11.13**

11.12,11.13 Scapuloperoneal atrophy. This 65-year-old man presented with a 12-month history of weakness in the legs. He had served in the army, but 20 years earlier a masseuse had said there 'was something the matter with the shoulder-blades' and he recalled a scuffle some years earlier in which he was easily beaten by a much smaller opponent. His father was said to walk with a slapping gait the sound of which was easily recognised by the family. Examination revealed winging of the scapulae, wasting of the pectoral and anterior tibial muscles, pes cavus, foot drop, absent ankle jerks and peripheral sensory loss. An EMG supported the diagnosis of polyneuritis.

11.14,11.15 Hypertrophy of nerves. In chronic demyelinating neuropathies such as hereditary motor and sensory neuropathy type 1 the peripheral nerves are often hypertrophied and palpable. In this instance the great auricular nerve is clearly seen (11.14 arrow) and enlargement of the ulnar nerve, demonstrated by the injection of thorotrast some 20 years previously, is still visible (11.15 arrows).

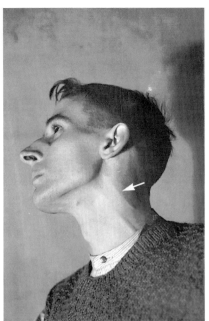

11.14

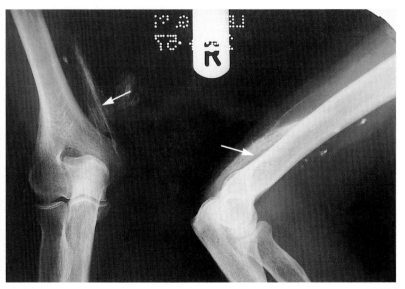

11.15

Hyperglycaemia (diabetes)

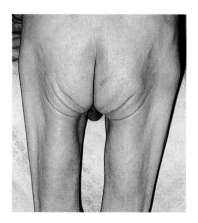

11.16 Diabetic amyotrophy. Patients with diabetes may develop 'ordinary' peripheral neuritis, proximal motor weakness, lesions in individual cranial or peripheral nerves, mononeuritis multiplex and/or an autonomic neuropathy. This patient complained of pain and weakness in the hips. He was found to be diabetic and to have marked wasting of the buttocks and thighs and absent knee jerks. This motor neuropathy – known as diabetic amyotrophy – is often asymmetrical and usually responds when the diabetes is rigorously controlled.

Anatomy of the cervical nerve roots (11.17,11.18; Table 3)

The practical importance of a knowledge of anatomy in the location of neoplastic and spondylitic lesions of the spine has already been demonstrated (see 9.1–9.4). This need not be detailed, and for routine purposes the easily memorised schemes set out below will suffice. The root values of the reflexes form a numerical sequence and if the distribution of the C5, C7 and T1 dermatomes can be established the distribution of the remaining two is evident.

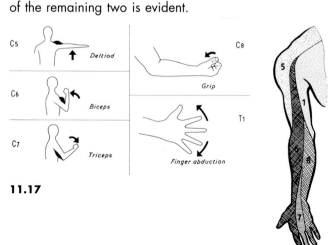

11.17

11.18

Table 3 Root value of reflexes		
Ankle jerks	(S)	1
Knee jerks	(L)	2,3,4
Biceps jerks	(C)	5
Supinator jerks	(C)	6
Triceps jerks	(C)	7
Abdominal reflexes	(T)	8,9,10,11
Cremasteric reflexes	(T)	12

The shoulder

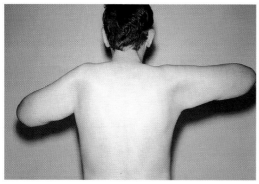

11.19

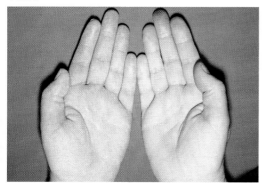

11.20

11.19,11.20 Shoulder–hand syndrome. Before assuming that inability to abduct the arm is due to a lesion in the brachial plexus or the circumflex nerve the examiner must establish that the shoulder is not 'frozen'. This 51-year-old diabetic developed pain and weakness in the left arm after an attack of zoster. The joint was virtually immobile, the left palm was flushed and he was unable to make a fist. The bones of the left hand were osteoporotic.

297

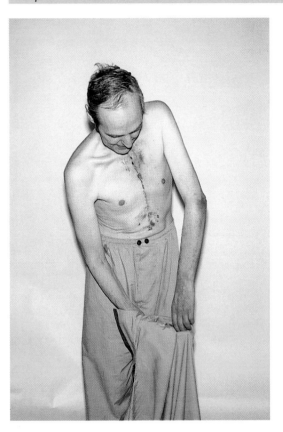

11.21 Chronic traction injuries to the brachial plexus.

The plexus can be injured by carrying heavy weights on the shoulder for long periods. It is also the nerve most commonly injured during surgery, having been compressed by the head of the humerus when the arm is rotated or stretched when it is abducted or tied to an overhead table. This patient's left arm was held in a position of forced abduction while a vein was extracted. On recovery he had an entirely flaccid 'flail' arm which he is seen trying to drop into the sleeve of a jacket. Sensation was intact. As often occurs with such lesions he made a full recovery over the next three months.

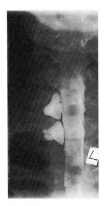

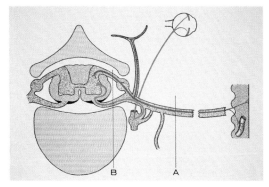

11.23

11.22

11.22,11.23 Acute traction injuries of the brachial plexus. Sudden traction injuries to the upper part of the brachial plexus during delivery or to the lower part caused by jerking the arm of a wayward child are enshrined in the literature. Similar but more extensive lesions are seen in road accidents when a motorist is flung out of a car and the shoulder is violently depressed as it hits an obstruction or a motorcyclist hangs onto the handlebars as he is hurled off his machine. Such patients present with an anaesthetic, flail arm and contrast studies show cervical diverticula formed by the avulsed nerve roots (11.22).

This condition presents an interesting exercise in anatomy. If the nerve is ruptured distally (11.23A) proximal branches – the posterior primary rami, the nerve to the rhomboids and spinati and the sympathetic – are spared. Paraspinal sensation, the proximal muscles and the eye will therefore be unaffected. Nerve conduction and the triple response (mediated through the sensory fibres) will however be lost. Because both motor and sensory roots are still in contact with their cells there is, however, a prospect of recovery. If, as is more commonly the case, the rupture is proximal (11.23B) the patient will have loss of paraspinal sensation, proximal weakness, ipsilateral diaphragmatic paralysis and a Horner's syndrome. Electrical conduction and the triple response will however be normal for the sensory fibres, although isolated and useless, are still connected to the dorsal root ganglion. Under such circumstances the prospect of recovery is remote.

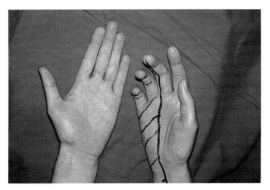

11.24

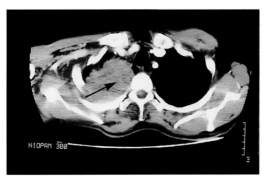

11.25
11.24,11.25 Infiltration of the brachial plexus – Pancoast's syndrome.
A patient who presented with numbness, weakness and pain in the right upper limb.
The hand was wasted and the sensory loss extended onto the middle finger and well
above the wrist on the medial side (i.e. outside the ulnar territory). The presence of a
Horner's syndrome confirmed that the lesion was in the lower roots of the brachial
plexus and, as would be expected under such circumstances, there was loss of
sweating over the brow (see 3.39–3.41). X-rays and scans revealed an apical
bronchial carcinoma. Such lesions can also infiltrate the phrenic nerve and the spinal
cord, and can be simulated by post-radiation fibrosis.

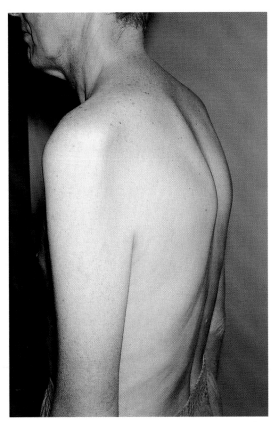

11.26 Neuralgic amyotrophy. A young man who suddenly developed excruciating pain in the left shoulder. It subsided within 48 hours, but was rapidly replaced by profound weakness and wasting of the spinati and deltoid (note angular appearance of the shoulder and scapula). This picture is characteristic of neuralgic amyotrophy which affects the muscles of the shoulder-girdle, often appearing some 10 days after an immunisation or illness. The prognosis for recovery is good but this may take a year and there is a small risk of a recurrence (see also 11.33).

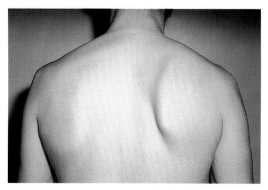

11.27

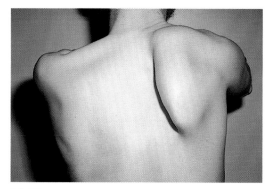

11.28

11.27, 11.28 Winging of the scapula. A 38-year-old butcher who complained of mild pain around the right shoulder for several months and then began to have difficulty with lifting. Winging of the scapula is evident at rest and the upward rotation, characteristic of weakness of the serratus anterior, becomes marked when the arms are extended. Lesions in the long thoracic nerve may be the result of operations on glands on the chest wall or of neuralgic amyotrophy, but in this instance weakness was probably caused by carrying heavy carcasses on the right shoulder. (See also winging of the scapula due to accessory nerve palsy – 3.135–3.138.)

Median nerve and thoracic outlet syndrome

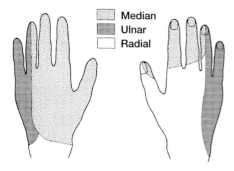

Median
Ulnar
Radial

11.29 Innervation of the hand. Sensory manifestations do not always coincide with the distribution of the nerves. Patients with a carpal tunnel syndrome often insist that all the digits are painful while those with a radial palsy may have normal sensation. Loss of feeling with an ulnar neuropathy usually coincides with the distribution of the nerve but in slowly developing lesions may be minimal.

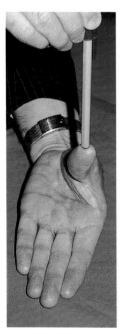

11.30

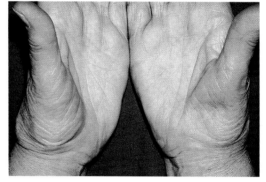

11.31

11.30,11.31 Carpal tunnel syndrome. The carpal tunnel syndrome usually appears in the dominant hand of women as a result of pregnancy or manual work. It begins with dysaesthesiae which (unlike the pain of cervical spondylosis) are characteristically worse at night. Symptoms may extend to involve *all* the digits and spread far up the arm. Eventually they become bilateral and weakness af abduction (inability to raise the thumb perpendicularly above the palm – 11.30) and wasting of the thenar eminence (11.31) become evident.

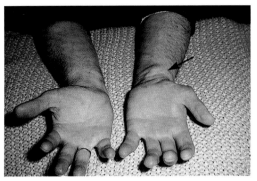

11.32 Injury to the left median nerve. Symptoms of a carpal tunnel syndrome in a man or starting in the non-dominant hand should prompt a search for predisposing factors such as acromegaly, myxoedema, amyloid, arthritis, a badly healed fracture or injury. This patient, in whom wasting of the left thenar eminence is evident, has an old laceration at the wrist (arrow).

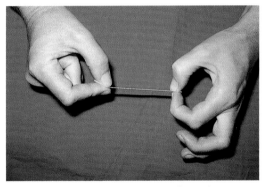

11.33 Anterior interosseous palsy. The anterior interosseous branch of the median nerve innervates the deep flexors to the medial two digits. Injury results in an inability to make a pinching movement – as when turning an ignition key to start a car. Weakness can be demonstrated by asking the patient to grip a card with the tips of the thumb and index and pull – whereupon the 'circle' on the weak (right) hand collapses. The anterior interosseous nerve is sometimes damaged in neuralgic amyotrophy. Injury to the median nerve as it traverses the pronator muscle produces a combination of (diurnal) pain in the distribution of the sensory branch and an anterior interosseous palsy – a condition known as the pronator syndrome, sometimes seen after strenuous work in men.

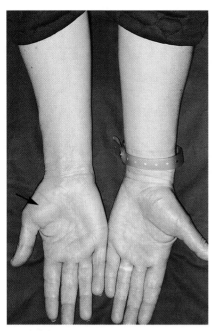

11.34,11.35 Thoracic inlet syndrome. Compression by a band or a cervical rib occasionally produces a bewildering combination of pain and impairment of sensation on the medial aspect of the forearm and wasting of the thenar eminence. Careful examination usually reveals that (as here in the forearm) the wasting is in fact more extensive. The rib is usually unobtrusive and compression of the adjacent artery may result in ischaemic changes in the hand or occasionally, as a result of retrograde embolisation into the carotid, a crossed hemiplegia.

11.34

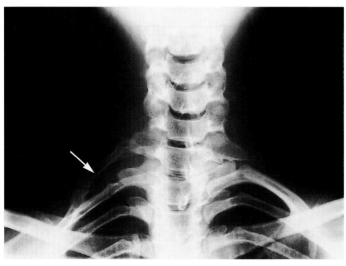

11.35

305

The ulnar nerve

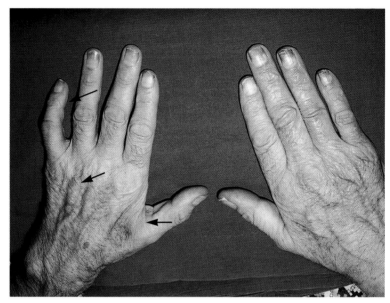

11.36 Ulnar neuropathy. Leaning on the elbow (particularly on a hard hospital mattress) and deformity of the elbow caused by injury or arthritis can damage the ulnar nerve. The sensory disturbance is confined to the medial one and a half digits and the medial aspect of the hand. Examination reveals weakness of adduction and abduction of the fingers, wasting of the hypothenar mass and the first dorsal interspace and guttering between the tendons on the back of the hand. A tendency for the medial two fingers to droop – due to weakness of the interossei and lumbricals – produces a posture known as the main apostolique. In manual workers chronic lesions may be difficult to identify because sensation, for some reason, is unaffected and the contour of the hypothenar eminence is maintained by the tough skin of the palm. On palpation, however, the softness of the hypothenar mass is still evident.

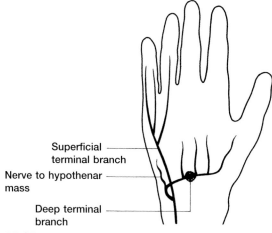

Superficial terminal branch

Nerve to hypothenar mass

Deep terminal branch

11.37

11.37–11.39 The palmar branch of the ulnar nerve.

The ulnar nerve eventually divides into a sensory branch and a deep terminal (motor) branch (11.37). Compression of the latter as it runs across the palm produces weakness and wasting in part of the thenar mass and on the dorsum of the hand without impairing sensation (11.38, 11.39). This picture, caused by the use of vibrating tools, riding drop-head cycles, driving a spade into frozen ground, using elbow crutches and other activities that apply pressure to the palm, is commonly mistaken for motor neurone disease (see 12.9).

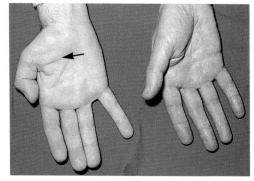

11.38

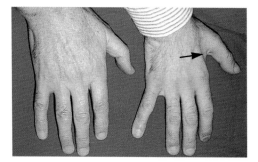

11.39

The radial nerve

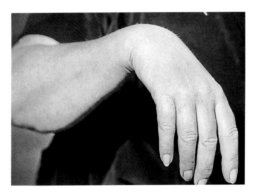

11.40 Radial nerve palsy. Damage to the radial nerve in the axilla – e.g. by incorrect use of a crutch – produces paralysis of the triceps, brachioradialis and extensors of the wrist and fingers. Injuries in the spiral groove due to fractures, misplaced injections, compression of an arm which has slipped off the side of an operating theatre table and – most commonly – resting the arm for some time around the top of an adjacent cinema seat (and its occupant) spare the triceps and simply produce a wrist drop. Because of overlap, sensory loss is usually unobtrusive.

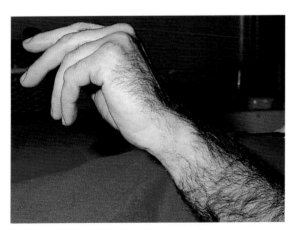

11.41 Posterior interosseous palsy. The posterior interosseous branch of the radial nerve penetrates the supinator and innervates most of the long extensor muscles. The extensor carpi radialis, however, is unaffected and as a result the patient – although unable to extend the fingers – can dorsiflex the wrist on the radial side.

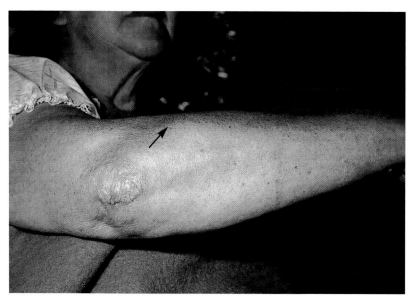

11.42

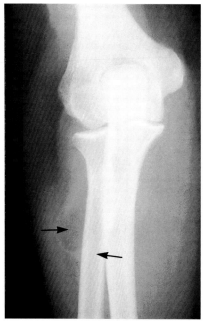

11.42,11.43 Posterior interosseous palsy. The posterior interosseous nerve can be damaged by fractures and by the prolonged and unaccustomed use of screwdrivers, paintbrushes, table tennis bats and similar activities. It can also be damaged by a lipoma which appears as a soft lump on the postero-lateral aspect of the upper third of the forearm (11.42 arrow) and can be seen on X-ray (11.43 arrows) (see 12.9).

11.43

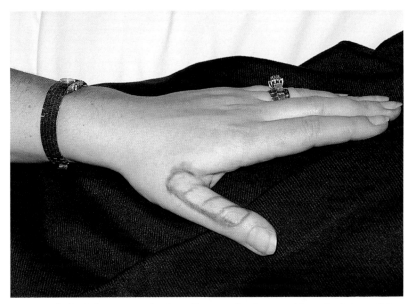

11.44 Cheiralgia paraesthetica. The superficial terminal branch of the radial nerve emerges over the distal end of the radius. Prolonged compression by a tight wristwatch band, the handle of a shopping basket, handcuffs etc. sometimes produces an unpleasant hypersensitivity in this region known as cheiralgia paraesthetica. Instruments used in laparoscopic surgery can have a similar effect at a slightly lower level.

Injury to lower limb nerves

Injury to nerves in the lower limbs

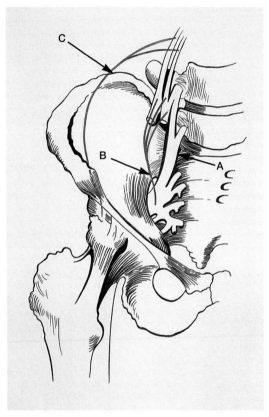

11.45 Lesions in the pelvis. Lesions in the pelvis and buttock have already been mentioned in Chapter 10, but it is worth repeating that the lumbosacral plexus can be damaged by tumours, abscesses, aneurysms, haematomas and surgical procedures. The lumbosacral trunk (A) may be compressed against the pelvis by the foetal head and the obturator nerve (B) – which lies near the uterus – can be damaged during difficult deliveries and hysterectomy. The femoral nerve may be injured during operations on the hip and operations on or catheterisation of the adjacent artery. It can also be affected by 'medical' conditions such as zoster, diabetes, arteritis and haemorrhage due to anticoagulants.

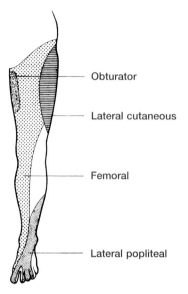

Obturator

Lateral cutaneous

Femoral

Lateral popliteal

11.46 Cutaneous nerves in the lower limb. The posterior aspect of the limb and the sole of the foot are supplied by the posterior cutaneous nerve of the thigh and the sciatic nerve. The lateral popliteal branch of the sciatic also supplies the anterolateral aspect of the leg and the dorsum of the foot. Injury to the lateral cutaneous nerve of the thigh (see 11.45C), which has been variously attributed to obesity, loss of weight and changes in posture induced by pregnancy, produces an alarming numbness on the lateral aspect of the thigh known as meralgia paraesthetica. Once the patient has been assured that it will not spread or cause paralysis and the GP has been told that it is not due to multiple sclerosis the symptom itself usually ceases to be of any importance.

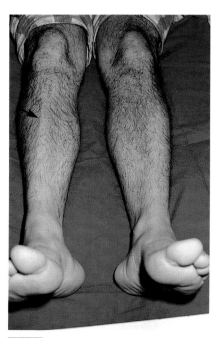

11.47 Lateral popliteal palsy. The lateral popliteal branch of the sciatic is often injured as it winds round the head of the fibula – particularly in diabetics and others predisposed to nerve damage – by sitting with the legs crossed or by squatting for long periods. As with an L5 root lesion there will be weakness of dorsiflexion and eversion and numbness on the dorsum of the foot. Inversion of the foot, however, will be spared. Note the way in which the subcutaneous border of the tibia is exposed by wasting of the anterior tibial group (arrow).

12.

Motor neurone disease, myasthenia and myopathy

Motor neurone disease

Motor neurone disease is a condition of unknown aetiology which causes progressive destruction of motor cells and tracts in the central nervous system. The majority of patients present with asymmetrical and non-anatomical weakness and wasting in the upper limbs but are also found on examination to have evidence of upper motor neurone damage in the form of brisk reflexes. This pattern of the disease is known in the United Kingdom as *amyotrophic lateral sclerosis* – a term which unfortunately is used elsewhere to describe all variants of the disease. Some patients present with lower motor neurone weakness of the tongue, palate, pharynx and larynx (*progressive bulbar palsy*) and most will ultimately develop symptoms of this sort. Patients with lesions confined to the lower or upper motor neurones (known respectively as *progressive muscular atrophy* and *progressive lateral sclerosis*) and patients with a familial form of the disease are occasionally encountered. Prolonged survival and even recovery are occasionally reported but the majority die within a few years.

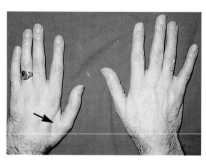

12.1

12.1,12.2 Amyotrophic lateral sclerosis. Most patients present with weakness in the hands and many complain of wasting and/or cramps. Abnormalities, which are asymmetrical, are not confined to the territory of individual nerves and sooner or later widespread fasciculation and wasting appear. Despite this evidence of lower motor neurone damage the reflexes are brisk. The illustrations show gross wasting on the left (arrows) and early wasting on the back of the right hand.

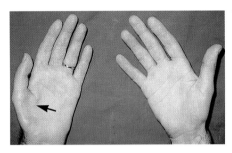

12.2

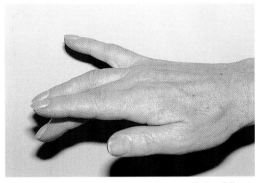

12.3 The drooping finger sign. Inability fully to extend one finger is a common early complaint.

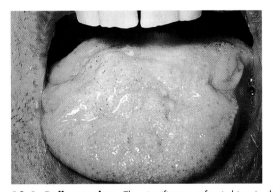

12.4 Bulbar palsy. The significance of twitching in the muscles of the tongue may be questionable until wasting appears. Patients go on to develop the (lower motor neurone) labio-palato-glosso-pharyngeal weakness of a bulbar palsy, but associated upper motor neurone damage may result in a brisk jaw jerk.

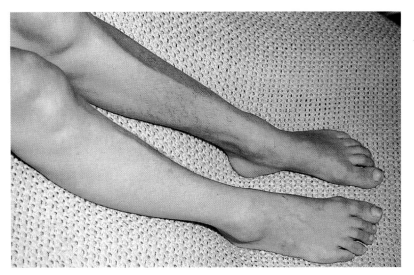

12.5 Motor neurone disease starting in the legs. Diagnosis may be difficult when the distribution of weakness is unusual – e.g. in the respiratory muscles. This 40-year-old patient gave a 12-month history of weakness and cramps in the legs. She had bilateral foot drop and prominence of the subcutaneous borders of the tibias due to gross wasting of the anterior muscle groups of the legs. Within 18 months the arms were badly affected and the diagnosis was confirmed at autopsy. Diagnosis of this uncommon but well recognised variant is often difficult because wasting and fasciculation are concealed by fat and because the tendon reflexes are absent.

Differential diagnosis

It is important that other diseases which produce fasciculation and/or (distal) wasting of the upper limbs should not be mistaken for motor neurone disease. Such errors can usually be avoided by appropriate examination. *Benign fasciculation* – particularly common in anxious individuals with a medical background – does not produce fibrillation on the EMG and twitching movements which have been present for more than 3 months without producing weakness and wasting are unlikely to be significant. *Syringomyelia* (see 8.25), which can cause wasting, weakness, fasciculation, bulbar palsy and a spastic paraplegia can be recognised because of the characteristic sensory loss and the loss of arm reflexes. *Cervical spondylosis* (see 12.6) is occasionally associated with profound weakness, wasting and fasciculation in patients with a spastic paraplegia but lower motor neurone signs are confined to certain myotomes. Wasting of the hands is occasionally an early sign of *compression of the upper cervical cord*. Wasting of the hands due to *distal spinal muscular atrophy* and *hereditary motor and sensory neuropathy* (see 12.14) is nearly always associated with gross deformity of the feet. *Demyelinating multifocal motor neuropathy* (see 11.4) and *compression of the palmar branch of the ulnar nerve* (see 12.7,12.8) – perhaps the most subtle traps for the unwary – can be eliminated by EMG studies. *Distal muscular dystrophy* is rare outside Sweden and the demonstration that the patient can 'make a fist' painlessly virtually eliminates the possibility of *wasting secondary to arthritis.*

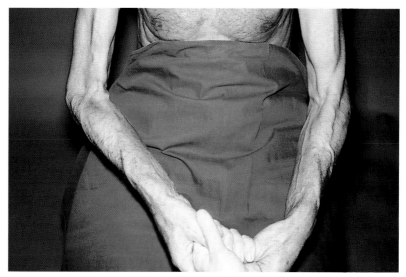

12.6 Cervical spondylosis simulating motor neurone disease. A man of 64 who presented with painless weakness in the arm. He had gross weakness, wasting and fasciculation in the right biceps and brachioradialis and the tendon reflexes on that side were unobtainable. The hand, the left arm and the leg were normal. EMG studies confirmed that he had abnormalities confined to the fifth, sixth and seventh myotomes on the right and repeated examination over a number of years showed no evidence of extension. The patient's work had imposed severe strain on his neck and the X-ray showed extensive degenerative changes.

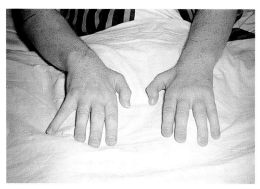

12.7

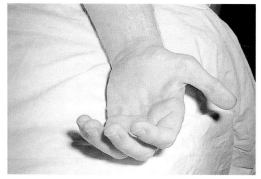

12.8

12.7–12.9 Wasting due to compression of the palmar branch of the ulnar nerve. A blind paraplegic who presented with weakness of the hands and wrists. Sensation was normal for he could still read Braille. He had profound wasting of the thenar masses and of the first dorsal interspaces but the hypothenar masses were normal. This was due to compression of the palmar branch of the ulnar nerve (see 11.37) as a result of taking his (considerable) weight on his hands when using elbow crutches. Outward pressure of the upper forearm on the collar of the crutches had also damaged the posterior interosseous nerves (12.9 arrow), resulting in weakness of extension of the fingers (see also 11.41–11.43).

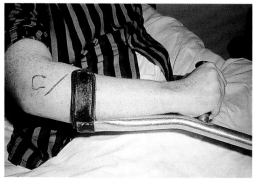

12.9

Allied disorders

The anterior horn cells may also be involved in a variety of other conditions. *Acute anterior poliomyelitis* produces rapid and potentially much more extensive destruction over the course of a few days. *Spinal muscular atrophy*, by contrast, causes insidious destruction. Four main forms are recognised. Infantile spinal muscular atrophy (Werdnig–Hoffman disease) is a major cause of the floppy baby syndrome. Inherited as a recessive, it may be recognised antepartum by the paucity of foetal movements. Most patients are unable to sit up and die within years. Juvenile, adult and distal spinal muscular atrophy are discussed below. It is worth noting that the commonly held idea that spinal atrophy does not affect bulbar muscles is incorrect, particularly in the condition known as *X-linked recessive bulbospinal neuronopathy*. This condition produces marked weakness, wasting and fasciculation of the face and tongue. It must be distinguished from bulbar palsy, which is usually fatal within a year, because these patients have a virtually normal lifespan.

Changes typical of motor neurone disease may also be seen in association with *cancer*, with dementia and extrapyramidal signs in a variety of *Creutzfeldt–Jacob disease* and in an endemic form among the *Chamorro on the island of Guam*.

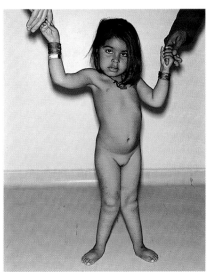

12.10 Juvenile spinal muscular atrophy (Kugelberg Welander disease). This condition presents with slowly progressive proximal weakness and wasting in childhood and early adolesence. In contrast to Duchenne dystrophy, with which it is easily confused, the sexes are equally affected, patients have fasciculation of the tongue and elsewhere and (as here) flat feet. The muscles are uniformly affected and hypertrophy does not occur. Most eventually learn to walk and many survive into adult life.

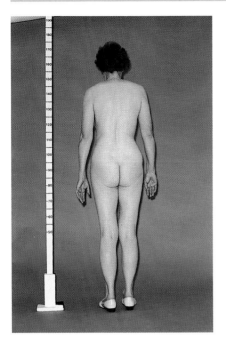

12.11 Adult spinal muscular atrophy. This condition may occur in isolation or may be inherited in various ways. It usually presents in the third decade with slowly progressive weakness. If fasciculation is evident it is mistaken for motor neurone disease until the youth of the patient, the benign course of the disease and the absence of upper motor neurone signs cast doubt on the diagnosis. If fasciculation is not present it is often mistaken for a myopathy, and it is thought that many patients formerly diagnosed as 'limb girdle dystrophy' had in fact got spinal atrophy. Electromyographic studies and biopsy have to be interpreted with care as secondary myopathic features are often present. This patient, who presented with increasing weakness in the legs proved, like her daughter, to have a significantly raised creatine kinase level.

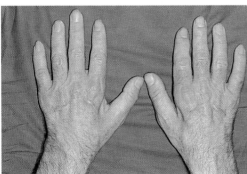

12.12

12.12–12.14 Distal spinal muscular atrophy. Patients with 'peroneal muscular atrophy', who have high arched feet and wasting below the middle third of the thighs, may also have (and may present with) wasting in the hands. Many such have an hereditary motor and sensory neuropathy. This may be demyelinating with nerve hypertrophy and profound changes on the EMG (Type 1) or axonal (Type 2). Others, however, are shown on EMG to have distal spinal muscular atrophy. In patients with pes cavus and bladder dysfunction the possibility of a developmental disorder of the spine should be considered.

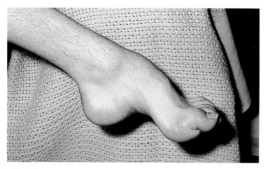

12.13

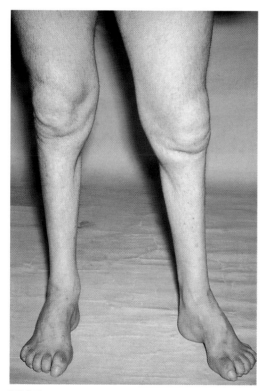

12.14

Myasthenia

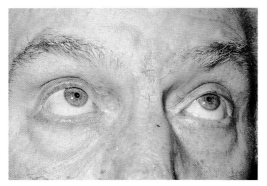

12.15

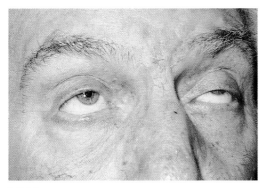

12.16

12.15,12.16 Myasthenia gravis. Myasthenia – weakness which appears with use and disappears on rest – is most commonly caused by myasthenia gravis. Typical symptoms include episodic diplopia, intermittent drooping of the eyelids, weakness of the jaw induced by chewing, of the voice induced by talking, of the neck induced by bending forwards and of the arms by hanging out washing or doing the hair. Susceptible muscles such as the neck flexors and triceps should be carefully examined and an attempt should be made to induce weakness, as in this illustration where the patient has been asked to maintain upwards gaze. If weakness is present an attempt may be made to abolish it with an injection of edrophonium (tensilon).

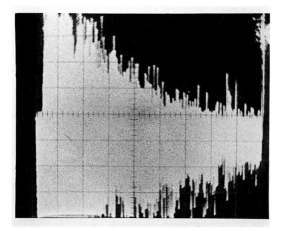

12.17

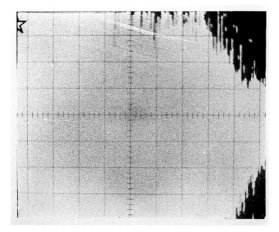

12.18

12.17,12.18 EMG in myasthenia. Myasthenic weakness can often be demonstrated by the rapid 'fade' in response to tetanic stimulation (12.17) which can be prevented with tensilon (12.18).

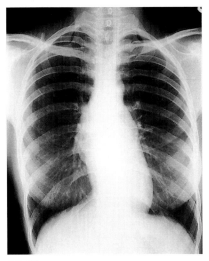

12.19

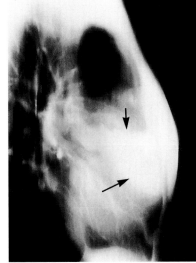

12.20

12.19, 12.20 Chest X-ray in myasthenia. Investigations include tests for anti-acetylcholine receptor antibodies (positive in 90% of patients), for anti-striated muscle antibodies (positive in 90% of those with thymomas) and for thyrotoxicosis – with which the condition is commonly associated. The chest X-ray is not a very satisfactory way of detecting a thymoma – the relatively minor widening of the mediastinum on this illustration gives no indication of the size of the tumour as seen on tomography (12.20 arrows). Contrary to expectation, thymomas are often found in the lower part of the mediastinum.

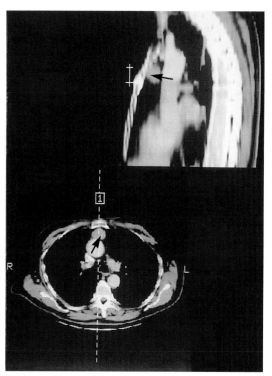

12.21 Scan of thymoma. Scans, unlike chest X-rays, usually demonstrate a thymoma clearly. In this instance the tumour can be seen in front of the aorta on the lateral and axial views (arrows). Thymectomy is indicated if the patient has a thymoma and in patients under 45 with generalised myasthenia and anti-acetylcholine receptor antibodies.

Myopathies

Diseases of muscle or myopathies, which lie outside the main stream of neurological disorders, have been rendered more difficult to understand by a welter of recent discoveries. Certain fundamentals are however obvious:

1. **Clinical presentation.** These diseases have a tendency to affect proximal (and in particular pelvic girdle) muscles. Patients may therefore walk quite well on level ground and no obvious abnormalities will be found in a 'routine' neurological examination conducted with the patient lying on a couch with his trouser legs rolled up. There is however a history of difficulty with cleaning windows, climbing stairs, boarding buses and getting out of baths and deep armchairs. Wasting, if it is present, will be around the shoulder and pelvic girdles and weakness may not be evident until the patient is asked to climb onto a low stool.

2. **Investigations.** These include estimations of the serum creatine kinase, electromyography, muscle biopsy and possibly MR scanning of muscles, genetic and metabolic tests. These investigations are not easy to interpret and, except in straightforward cases, should be left in the hands of experts.

3. **Classification.** From such investigations it has become evident that diseases of the anterior horn cell, of peripheral nerves and of the myoneural junction can (and have been) confused with myopathies. New manifestations of established disorders like limb girdle dystrophy in carriers of Duchenne dystrophy and new disorders such as the mitochondrial myopathies have also been described.

4. **Treatment.** With the notable exception of polymyositis and myopathies due to endocrine and metabolic disorders there is little to offer in the way of specific treatment.

5. **Prevention.** By contrast the recognition and prevention of genetically determined wasting diseases of muscle (muscular dystrophies) – and in particular of Duchenne dystrophy – is of paramount importance.

Muscular dystrophy

The muscular dystrophies are inherited myopathies that produce progressive degenerative changes in selected groups of muscles. For convenience they can be subdivided into pseudohypertrophic, limb girdle and facio-scapulo-humeral dystrophy, dystrophia myotonica, an ocular form (easily confused with mitochondrial myopathy) and a distal form seen mainly in Sweden.

Pseudohypertrophic (Duchenne) dystrophy

This condition is inherited as an X-linked recessive and therefore occurs in boys. It presents at about the age of 4 with clumsiness, difficulty in running and a tendency to fall. Weakness first appears in the pelvic girdle and spine and the patient develops a lordosis and a waddling gait. He is unable to place his feet flat on the floor (cf. spinal muscular atrophy – see 12.10) and when rising uses the Gower's manoeuvre of climbing up his legs. The hypertrophy from which the disease derives its name is due to fatty infiltration of certain muscles – e.g. the calf and deltoid.

With the discovery that the Duchenne dystrophy is due to absence of an (unusually large) gene on the X chromosome and that this results in absence of the sarcolemmal protein dystrophin, the accurate identification of carriers and atypical cases has become possible. This has shown that carriers, who apart from calf hypertrophy and a high creatine kinase level were thought to be normal, may in fact have a 'limb girdle dystrophy' that in some cases causes progressive disability. Conversely it shows that, while the lack of a family history in a third of cases is due to lack of information, a further third are in fact due to mutations in this large and unstable gene.

As there is no specific treatment, early diagnosis of those who have or have a high risk of developing the condition (i.e. retarded children and those who cannot walk by 18 months) and of those with 'limb girdle dystrophy' who are in fact carriers is essential. Given this information other members of the family who are carrying the gene can be identified before they give birth to children who will be confined to a wheelchair by the age of 10 and will die of pulmonary or cardiac complications in their 20s.

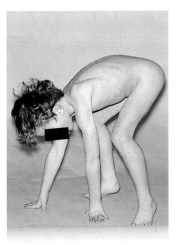

12.22

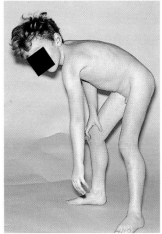

12.23

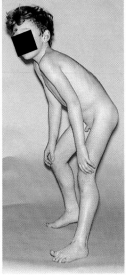

12.24

12.22–12.24 Pseudohypertrophic muscular dystrophy. A 7-year-old boy using Gower's manoeuvre of 'climbing up his legs'. Apart from the fact that he tended to run on his toes his parents had not noticed anything amiss. The calf muscles were large and firm, the ankles could not be dorsiflexed beyond 90 degrees and when lifted with hands under the armpits he tended to 'run through the hands' because he could not brace his shoulders.

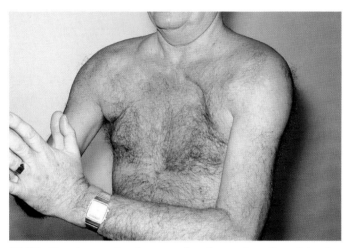

12.25 Muscle wasting in muscular dystrophy. One of the characteristic features of these disorders is their tendency to attack certain muscle groups – particularly the trapezius, serratus anterior, biceps and (as here) the sternal head of the pectoralis major. Note the well preserved deltoids.

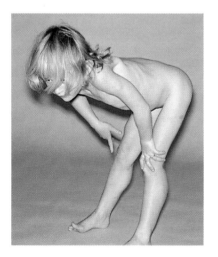

12.26 Duchenne dystrophy in a female patient. Carriers of Duchenne dystrophy may have hypertrophy of calf muscles and a raised creatine kinase, or even a limb girdle dystrophy which, in some cases, is severe and progressive. Most early reports of Duchenne dystrophy in girls were almost certainly misdiagnosed cases of the Kugelberg Welander form of spinal muscular atrophy (see 12.10) but a more benign form of the disease is sometimes transmitted as a Mendelian recessive. The patient shown in 12.22 was examined because, apart from her sex, his sister was a textbook example of the condition. Note the size of the calf and deltoid and the winging of the scapula.

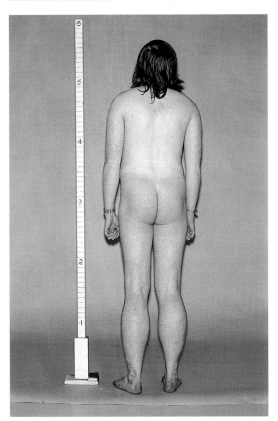

12.27 Benign pseudohypertrophic dystrophy (Becker). The genetic defect in Becker's dystrophy is the same as that in Duchenne's, but the absence of dystrophin is not complete. Clinical findings are similar save that patients present up to the age of 20, may walk up to the age of 40 and may live up to the age of 60. This 20-year-old man had never been able to run or to climb stairs in a normal manner but had only been significantly disabled in the last 12 months. Despite considerable proximal weakness the spinati, gluteal and calf muscles were hypertrophied. His mother and a younger sister were asymptomatic carriers.

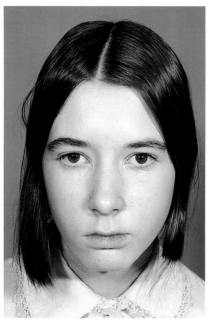

12.28

12.28–12.31
Facioscapulohumeral dystrophy.
This condition, which presents in adolescence or early adult life, is transmitted as an autosomal dominant. Weakness starts in the face and spreads downwards but the legs, in which the tibialis anterior is characteristically involved first, are seldom severely affected. This 13-year-old girl presented because her walking had deteriorated. It was evident that her surly expression was due to facial weakness of such severity that she could not close her eyes. She had a marked lordosis and was unable to raise her arms to do her hair because of wasting in the pectoral muscles (arrows) and winging of the scapulae, The creatine kinase, characteristically, was only slightly raised.

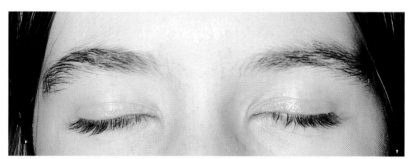

12.29

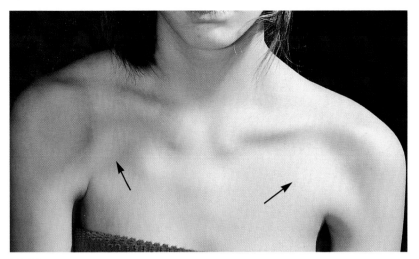

12.30

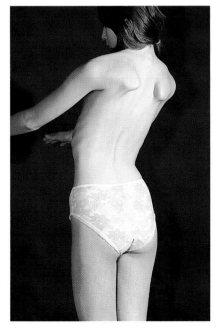

12.31

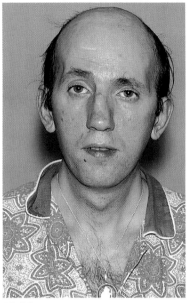

12.32

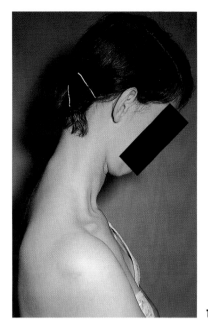

12

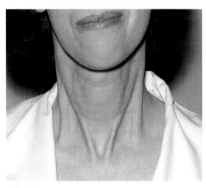

12.34

12.32–12.34 Dystrophia myotonica. Dystrophia myotonica, the most common dystrophy, is transmitted as an autosomal dominant and usually presents in the third or fourth decade. Signs include cataracts, ptosis, wasting of the temporalis muscles, facial weakness and (in men) testicular atrophy and frontal baldness that produces a monk-like appearance (12.32). Atrophy of the sternomastoids produces a 'swan neck' (12.33, 12.34). The myotonia to which the name alludes makes it difficult for the patient to release his grip rapidly, particularly in cold weather. The dystrophy, however, is the most important feature of the disease and may cause falls, confine the patient to a wheelchair and cause death from cardiac or respiratory failure in middle life. Patients should be warned of the danger of adverse reactions to anaesthetics.

Other myopathies

Weakness and wasting of muscles is also seen in association with cancer, a variety of endocrine disorders, hyper- and hypokalaemia, calcaemia and natraemia and with drugs such as alcohol, steroids, thiazide diuretics and carbenoxolone (liquorice). Myopathies associated with defects of gluconeogenesis and the mitochondrial myopathies are beyond the scope of this book.

Polymyositis

Polymyositis is a non-suppurative inflammatory disease of muscle. It is not inherited and it can occur at all ages. It may be associated with skin lesions such as dermatomyositis, scleroderma, Raynaud's phenomenon or disseminated lupus and in 25% of cases it is associated with a neoplasm – often of the gastrointestinal tract. An inflammatory myopathy may also occur in association with HIV and HTLV 1 infections and must not be confused with the myopathy sometimes caused by long-term treatment with zidovudine.

There is a wide variety of presentations, ranging from an acute and possibly fatal febrile illness with severe weakness, pain and tenderness in muscles and a high sedimentation rate through to what appears to be a mild myopathy. In the latter the correct diagnosis may again be suggested by pain and/or tenderness in muscles and by the uniform distribution of the weakness. Wasting and loss of reflexes are not usually prominent features but fasciculation and dysphagia can occur. Facial and ocular muscles are rarely affected.

Correct diagnosis is important for this is one of the few muscle diseases where treatment – in the form of steroids – is available. Changes in the creatine kinase level, the ESR and the EMG are inconstant and unreliable but the finding of subcutaneous or intramuscular calcification (see calcinosis universalis – 12.40,12.41) strongly supports the diagnosis. In most cases, however, a biopsy is required. The importance – and the complexity – of this investigation cannot be over-emphasised and when long-term treatment with an effective but dangerous drug is in question it is clearly wrong for those unfamiliar with the niceties of this technique to get involved.

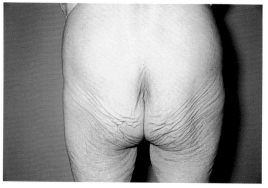

12.35

12.35–12.37 Myopathy with post-gastrectomy osteomalacia.

A 63-year-old woman who gave a 12-month history of weakness, anorexia and weight loss. She was thought to have a carcinoma but investigations revealed a low calcium, a high alkaline phosphatase and pathological fractures of the right scapula and both pubic rami (arrows). The malabsorption of calcium – and the consequent wasting of the buttocks – was attributed to a gastrectomy done 20 years earlier and she responded well to vitamin D.

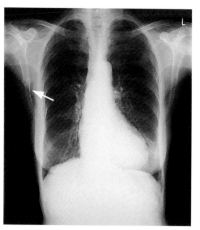

12.36

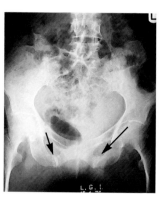

12.37

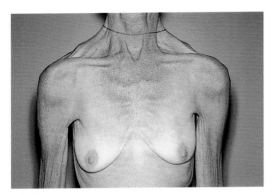

12.38

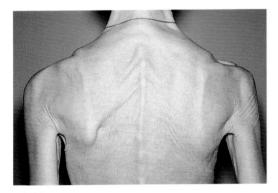

12.39

12.38,12.39 Polymyositis. A 60-year-old patient with a long history of rheumatoid arthritis and a 3-year history of weakness. By the time of admission she could no longer walk or do her hair. She had gross painless wasting of the pectoral, paraspinal, arm and gluteal muscles. The ESR was 115 mm/hr but the creatine kinase was normal. The diagnosis was confirmed by biopsy and she responded to treatment.

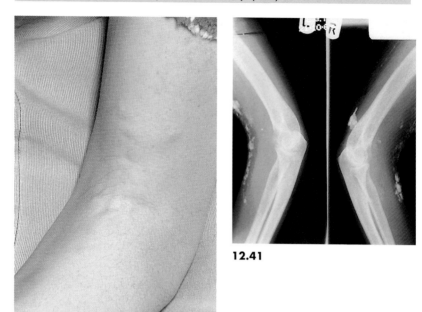

12.41

12.40

12.40, 12.41 Polymyositis. Following her first pregnancy 8 years earlier this 33-year-old woman developed weakness of such severity that she was virtually incapacitated. She later developed thyrotoxicosis and a skin rash. She improved until the birth of her second daughter when, once more, she became totally incapacitated. The muscles felt firm and there were palpable nodules of calcium around the knees, shoulders and elbows. The sedimentation rate was 30 mm/hr but the creatine kinase level was normal. Treated with steroids she made a complete recovery.

13.

Infections

Infections of the nervous system differ from other neurological disorders in that they are often amenable to specific treatment. Such infections must, however, be diagnosed and treated at once for delay commonly results in irreversible cerebral or spinal infarction. Sadly, diseases such as tuberculosis, syphilis, meningitis and cerebral abscess frequently go unrecognised because doctors are no longer familiar with these conditions particularly when – as a result of immunodeficiency due to drugs, AIDS or age – they appear in a new and unfamiliar guise. Detailed consideration of this vast topic is beyond the scope of this book but examples of the main problems will be given.

Pyogenic meningitis

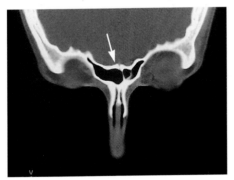

13.1 Defect in wall of frontal sinus. The mechanism whereby organisms enter the subarachnoid space is rarely established. However, in patients with recurrent meningitis or CSF rhinorrhoea detailed radiological studies sometimes reveal a defect in the wall of the frontal sinus (arrow).

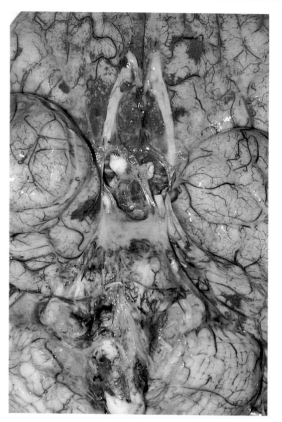

13.2 Basal exudate.
Although the classical symptoms are well known the diagnosis is often overlooked. This is usually due to failure to obtain an adequate history from patients who are young, confused or foreign or to preoccupation with a complication of the disease. Thus a fit may be regarded as a febrile convulsion without the cause of the fever being recognised and a comatose diabetic – predisposed to the disease by his condition – may be treated as a case of diabetic coma. Elderly patients may simply become confused. The main lesion in meningitis is the basal exudate which occludes blood vessels causing infarction and obstructs the flow of CSF causing hydrocephalus.

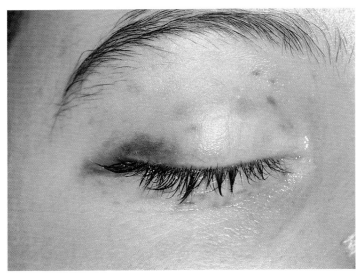

13.3 Meningococcal rash. Patients with meningococcal infections may have a rash which does not blanch on pressure. It can have the appearance of multiple pinpricks, of larger areas of haemorrhage or (as in this young woman, admitted in coma with a fever and a stiff neck) areas of bruising.

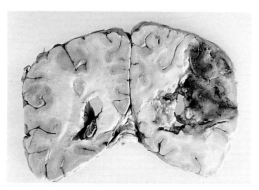

13.4 Infarction due to meningitis. Arterial occlusion resulting in (irreversible) cerebral or spinal infarction is – apart from death – the most feared complication of meningitis. If the diagnosis is suspected immediate and adequate treatment is mandatory.

Table 4 Investigation of meningitis							
Date	**White cell count**	**ESR**	**Spinal fluid**	**White cells**	**Protein (g/l)**	**Glucose (mmol/l)**	
27	14000	50	Bloody	2	5.8	0.9	Penicillin given
28	11000	52					
29	7000	25	Cloudy	305	2.2	3.4	No improvement
			75% polys				

The diagnosis of meningitis depends on examination of the spinal fluid. The efficacy of treatment may, however, have to be assessed before an organism is isolated. Emergency admission and transfer between hospitals often mean that the records available are unusually chaotic and the situation can sometimes be clarified by listing all available information in the manner shown. This patient was seen 3 days after the start of treatment. His temperature had not fallen and he remained unconscious, but it was evident from the falling white cell count, sedimentation rate and spinal fluid protein and from the rising CSF glucose that he was responding to treatment. Conversation with the referring hospital established that the initially low CSF cell count was an error and that a sensitive organism had in fact been isolated.

Cerebral abscess

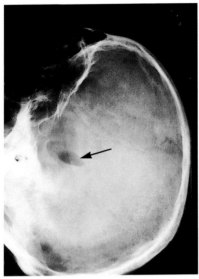

13.5,13.6 Cerebral abscess. A cerebral abscess presents subacutely as a space occupying lesion in a patient who shows evidence of an inflammation and/or a source of infection such as sinusitis, otitis, a skull fracture, bronchiectasis or congenital heart disease which allows blood to bypass the pulmonary filter. Lumbar puncture should be avoided for, despite the fact that the fundi may look normal, such patients have rapidly rising intracranial pressure. As with other rapidly developing lesions the EEG is often abnormal and the skull X-ray may show a fracture, sinusitis, mastoiditis or even a bubble of air produced by gas forming organisms (13.5 arrow). The investigation of choice, however, is a CT scan on which the fluid level may be even more evident (13.6).

13.5

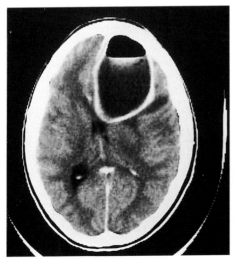

13.6

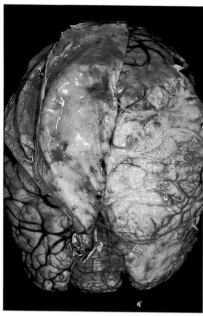

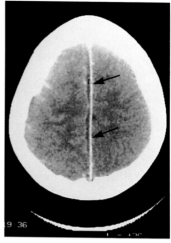

13.8

13.7

13.7, 13.8 Subdural abscess. Subdural abscesses, which are less well known and more difficult to diagnose, are even more dangerous. The lesion, which is in fact an empyema with pus spread widely over the surface of the brain (13.7), presents with severe headache and abundant evidence of infection in the form of fever, toxicity and leucocytosis. Clinical and/or radiological evidence of infection may be found in the form of sinusitis or mastoiditis. If, as is all too common, this is accepted as the root of the problem the patient will rapidly lapse into coma with fits, cranial nerve palsies and/or a hemiparesis. Initially the CT scan may appear to be normal – and may indeed *be* normal – but in patients with severe headache and obvious signs of infection it should be repeated at frequent intervals. Eventually small filling defects will appear between the brain and the vault or along the falx (13.8 arrow). Treatment is surgical, and there is a grave danger of recurrence if the extensive lesion is not fully explored.

(*See also cavernous sinus thrombosis* – 3.30–3.33; *and epidural abscess* – 9.45, 9.46.)

Tuberculosis

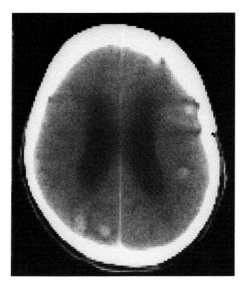

13.9

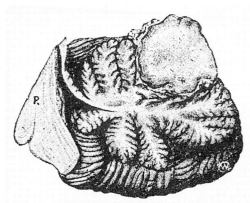

13.10

13.9, 13.10 Tubercles and tuberculomas.

Tuberculosis of the central nervous system is the result of haematogenous dissemination of organisms from a primary lesion in the lung or a quiescent focus reactivated by immunodeficiency due to drugs, AIDS or age. Multiple small lesions form within the neuraxis (13.9) and meningitis develops when such a lesion on the surface of the brain (a Rich's focus) ruptures into the subarachnoid space. Tubercles should not be confused with tuberculomas – larger masses, solitary or few in number, which present as space occupying lesions. Tuberculomas are no longer seen in the indigenous population of the United Kingdom but this illustration of a cerebellar tuberculoma (13.10) was drawn by Gowers for his textbook (*Manual of Diseases of the Nervous System*, Blakiston, Philadelphia).

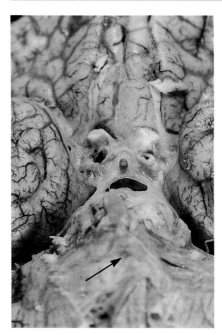

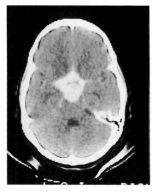

13.12

13.11

13.11,13.12 Tuberculous meningitis. The 'injection' of numerous bacilli into the subarachnoid space produces a Mantoux reaction and the symptoms of tuberculous meningitis. Elderly immunocompromised patients may, however, simply become confused. The subsequent formation of basal adhesions (13.11 arrow) obstructs the flow of CSF, causes hydrocephalus, damages cranial nerves and occludes vessels causing infarction. Figure 13.12 shows dense basal adhesions in a young Pakistani who became blind within 3 weeks of developing symptoms. Vision was restored after – and possibly as a result of – surgical decompression, but decompression at a later stage when the adhesions had become organised would not have been of value.

(See also tuberculosis of the spine – 9.37 et seq.)

Syphilis

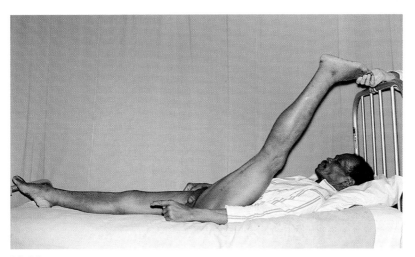

13.13

13.13–13.15 Tabes dorsalis. Despite an increase in the incidence of syphilis neurosyphilis is now uncommon – probably due to the deliberate or fortuitous administration of antibiotics. It remains to be seen whether the advent of AIDS, which hastens the onset of neurosyphilis and counteracts the effect of 'adequate' treatment, will result in a resurgence. Diagnosis has become increasingly difficult because patients who have had inadequate treatment present with an abortive form of the disease. Patients with hypotonia (13.13) which, with impairment of the senses of pain and of position leads to Charcot joints (13.14,13.15) are still however encountered. Charcot joints also occur in diabetes, syringomyelia and leprosy (see 8.26).

(See also Argyll Robertson pupil – 3.42; and bismuth injections – 10.16,10.17.)

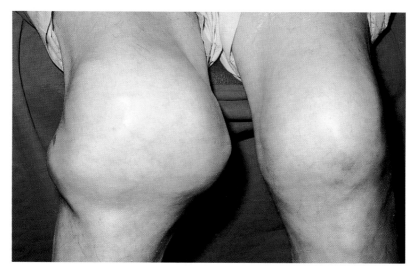

13.14

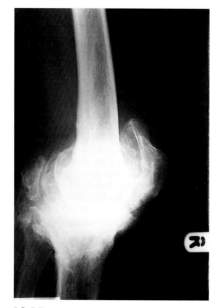

13.15

Lyme disease

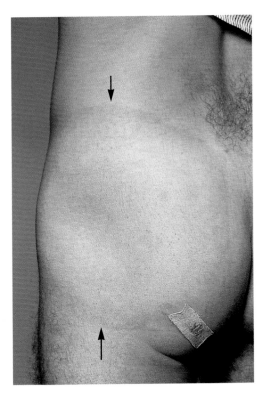

13.16 Lyme disease. In recent years infections with the tick-borne spirochaete *Borrelia burgdorferi* have frequently been reported. Patients may present with fever, headache, myalgia and an erythematous rash with an expanding margin (erythema migrans). Other complications include arthritis, myocarditis and neurological lesions such as severe and persistent headache, cranial nerve palsies (especially facial palsies which may be bilateral), radiculopathies and even polyneuritis.

Tetanus

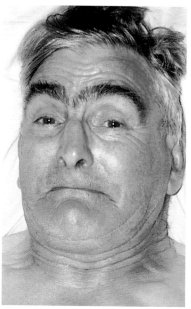 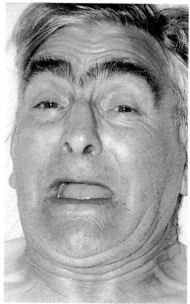

13.17   **13.18**

13.17–13.19 Tetanus. Despite extensive immunisation cases of tetanus still occur, often in patients with no history of injury. Symptoms start with dysphagia, spasm of the facial muscles which produces a risus sardonicus (13.17), and trismus ('lockjaw') which prevents the patient from opening his mouth to produce a 'three finger bite' (i.e. a 5 cm gap between the teeth (13.18). Spasm then spreads to the neck and spine, the lumbar lordosis becoming so marked that a hand can be slipped beneath the body (13.19). The abdomen is rigid but not tender but the limbs, between spasms, are remarkably supple. Most cases of 'tetanus' prove to be adverse reactions to phenothiazines or metoclopramide.

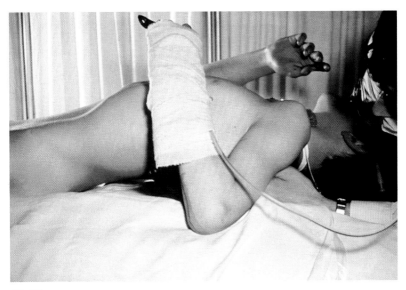

13.19

Encephalitis

Encephalitis is a non-suppurative inflammation of the brain which is usually generalised but may be mainly focal. When, as is often the case, it extends to involve the meninges, the cord and/or nerve roots compound terms such as meningo-encephalitis, encephalomyelitis and encephalo-myelo-radiculopathy are used. Manifestations vary accordingly but most patients present with a fever, headache and impairment of consciousness along with other neurological signs. Two main forms are recognised – those due to a hypersensitivity and those due to direct invasion of the brain by a virus.

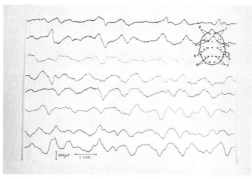

13.20

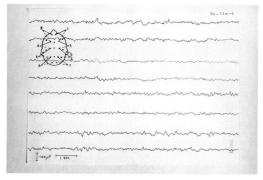

13.21

13.20, 13.21 Acute disseminated encephalomyelitis. This hypersensitivity reaction which causes widespread demyelination sometimes follows vaccination or infections such as measles, german measles and chickenpox. This 14-year-old boy became febrile, had a fit and lapsed into coma soon after an attack of german measles. Fits continued for 2 weeks but he then made a rapid recovery and his grossly abnormal EEG returned to normal. It is known that in this condition patients who appear to be gravely ill sometimes make a belated and apparently complete recovery.

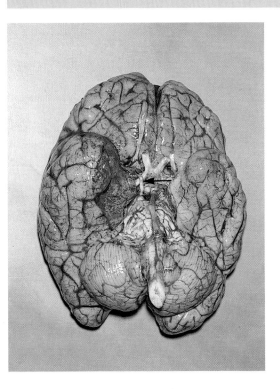

13.22 Herpes simplex encephalitis.
The most important cause of encephalitis due to direct invasion of the brain in the United Kingdom is herpes simplex encephalitis. Although, as here, the brunt of the damage usually falls on one temporal lobe (which is clearly swollen and injected – arrow) the inflammation is in fact generalised. The presentation with fever, leucocytosis, raised intracranial pressure and focal EEG abnormalities resembles that of a cerebral abscess.

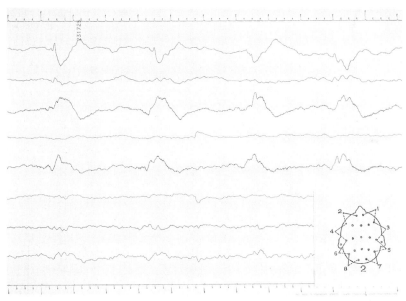

13.23

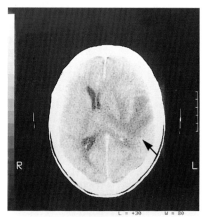

13.24

13.23,13.24 Investigation of herpes simplex encephalitis. The characteristic EEG abnormality is a distinctive periodic slow wave discharge over one temporal region. In the acute stage, however, diagnosis depends more on the CT scan which shows a low-density area in one temporal lobe with swelling and displacement of midline structures. If the diagnosis is suspected it is important that treatment with acyclovir should be started, for with early treatment there is a possibility of cure.

AIDS

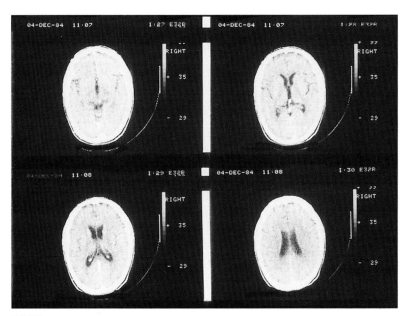

13.25

13.25,13.26 AIDS/dementia complex. Ten per cent of those with AIDS present with neurological symptoms and 75% will ultimately have lesions in the nervous system. At the time of sero-conversion the patient may develop meningitis, fits, encephalopathy, myelopathy or a neuropathy – commonly a facial palsy or mononeuritis multiplex. Although usually self-limiting, recurrent meningitis with lesions in the fifth, seventh or eighth cranial nerves and/or the long tracts has been described. Patients with established AIDS may develop a myelopathy, a cauda equina lesion, acute or chronic lesions of the cranial or peripheral nerves or muscle wasting. The most common manifestation, however, is the AIDS/dementia complex. Seen in about 15% of patients it presents with confusion, personality changes, focal signs and occasionally frank psychosis. This 35-year-old man presented with lethargy and ataxia. Within 2 years he was severely demented, incontinent and unable to walk and the mild atrophy and ventricular dilation seen on his initial scan had become severe.

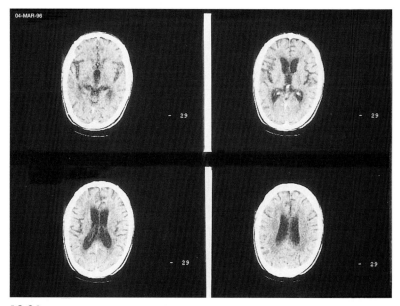

13.26

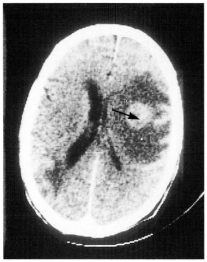
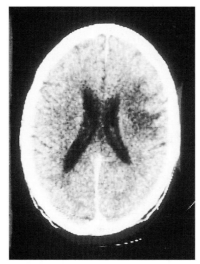

13.27   **13.28**

13.27,13.28 AIDS-related infections. Patients with AIDS are prone to infections such as zoster, simplex, tuberculosis, syphilis and progressive multifocal leucoencephalopathy – often in an unusually aggressive form and with atypical clinical and serological features. Cryptococcal infections, usually in the form of meningitis, and cytomegalovirus infections which cause retinitis or a cauda equina lesion also occur. The most common infection, however, is toxoplasmosis, which causes headache, impairment of higher functions, fits and a hemiparesis. By contrast with the AIDS dementia complex it produces impairment of consciousness at an early stage. The CT scan commonly shows multiple ring shadows in the basal ganglia and at the cortico-medullary junction but may, as in the case of this 61-year-old man, present as a focal lesion (13.27 arrow). As serological tests are unreliable diagnosis is made by therapeutic trial which eliminated the mass and improved his condition within 4 weeks (13.28).

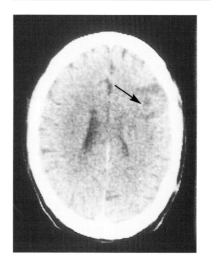

13.29 AIDS/lymphoma. Patients with AIDS are also subject to transient ischaemic attacks, infarction and haemorrhage and to certain tumours. The most common tumour is a lymphoma, usually in the brain but occasionally in the cord. Symptoms and radiological features are similar to those produced by toxoplasmosis but patients with lymphomas do not respond to a therapeutic trial. This 38-year-old man, who had a Kaposi's sarcoma, presented with intellectual impairment and a right hemiparesis. The lesion (arrow) proved to be a lymphoma.

Slow virus infections

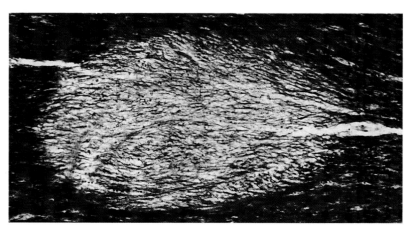

13.30

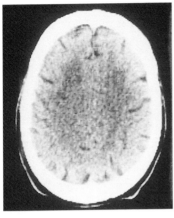

13.31

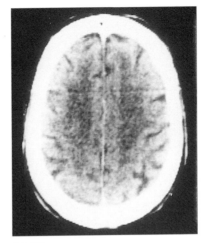

13.32

13.30–13.32 Progressive multifocal leucoencephalopathy. In recent years there has been increasing interest in certain slowly developing cerebral disorders caused by viruses and other agents. Subacute sclerosing pan-encephalitis, for example, is caused by the measles virus (see 2.23, 2.24). Progressive multifocal leuco-encephalopathy is caused by invasion of the oligodendroglia by a papovavirus (usually the JC virus, so named after the patient from whom the organism was first isolated). This causes patchy demyelination (13.30) that usually presents with hemiparesis, hemianopia and/or aphasia followed by intellectual failure and death within months. Originally seen in patients with lymphomas, sarcoidosis and on immunosuppressants it is now also associated with AIDS. This 37-year-old man presented with left-sided incoordination and ataxia. Shortly before his death 3 months later he was incontinent and unable to walk and the atrophy on his scan had become much more marked.

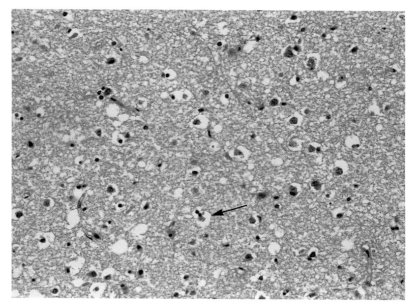

13.33 Spongiform encephalopathy. This condition, which derives its name from the microscopical appearance of the brain (arrow) usually appears between the ages of 50 and 65. Often abrupt in onset it progresses rapidly, producing a wide variety of neurological disorders including dementia, myoclonus, ataxia and cortical blindness. Death may occur in weeks and few patients live more than a year, save in the milder Gerstmann–Straussler variant. The condition is caused by prions, transmissible agents with a long incubation period which are not viruses, are hard to identify and do not cause inflammation or an immune response. They are hard to destroy and have been transmitted in preparations of growth hormone, in grafts and on electrodes. More importantly, prion infections appear to have been transmitted by mouth to cattle (causing bovine spongiform encephalopathy) and thence to humans.

Index

Praise for *The Reader*

'*The Reader* is a fine novel, as far above a Holocaust genre as *Crime and Punishment* is above the average thriller. A sensitive, daring, deeply moving book about the tragic results of fear and the redemptive power of understanding' Ruth Rendell

'Crammed with incident and analysis, and yet Schlink finds room for virtuoso passages of evocation . . . compelling'
London Review of Books

'Until I read this novel I was not convinced that there was room for many more books about the Holocaust . . . the universal appeal of his sparely told story will remain'
Sunday Telegraph

'He has thought so long and hard about German guilt that *The Reader* distils its questions, its answers, and its pure pain more simply and disturbingly than anything I've ever read'
The Spectator

'Book reviewing can be a somewhat bleak trade . . . The infrequent bonus is the arrival, almost unheralded, of a masterly work. Then, the reviewer's sole and privileged function is to say as loudly as he is able "Read this" and "read it again"'
George Steiner, *Observer*

'Achieves enormous moral force in the strength of its uncertainty . . . haunting and unforgettable' *Literary Review*

'Bernhard Schlink's extraordinary novel *The Reader* is a compelling meditation on the connections between Germany's past and present, dramatized with extreme emotional intelligence as the story of a relationship between the narrator and an older woman. It has won deserved praise across Europe for the tact and power with which it handles its material, both erotic and philosophical' *Independent* Saturday Magazine

'[Schlink] confronts the difficulty of evading (or wholly recovering) his own and his country's past. He explores the conflict between generations, wrestling with collective guilt and individual motivation. He examines the nature of understanding and tests the limits of forgiveness. He does these things with honesty, restraint and a moral precision both unsettling and rare. The result is as compelling as any thriller'

The Times

Bernhard Schlink was born in Germany in 1944. A professor of law at the University of Berlin and former judge, he is the author of the major international bestseller *Flights of Love*, and several prize-winning crime novels. His latest novel, *Homecoming*, is also available from Orion. He lives in Berlin.

By Bernhard Schlink

Homecoming
Self's Deception
Self's Punishment (with Walter Popp)
Flights of Love
The Reader

The Reader

BERNHARD SCHLINK

TRANSLATED FROM THE GERMAN BY

CAROL BROWN JANEWAY

PHOENIX

A PHOENIX PAPERBACK

First published in Great Britain by Phoenix House in 1997
This edition published by arrangement with Pantheon
Books, a division of Random House, Inc.
This paperback edition published in 1998 by Phoenix,
an imprint of Orion Books Ltd,
Orion House, 5 Upper St Martin's Lane,
London, WC2H 9EA

An Hachette UK company

Printed and bound in Great Britain by
Clays Ltd, St Ives plc

The Orion Publishing Group's policy is to use papers that
are natural, renewable and recyclable products and
made from wood grown in sustainable forests. The logging
and manufacturing processes are expected to conform to
the environmental regulations of the country of origin.

www.orionbooks.co.uk

Part One

CHAPTER ONE

WHEN I WAS FIFTEEN, I GOT HEPA-
titis. It started in the autumn and lasted
until spring. As the old year darkened and
turned colder, I got weaker and weaker. Things didn't
start to improve until the new year. January was warm,
and my mother moved my bed out onto the balcony. I
saw sky, sun, clouds, and heard the voices of children
playing in the courtyard. As dusk came one evening in
February, there was the sound of a blackbird singing.

The first time I ventured outside, it was to go from
Blumenstrasse, where we lived on the second floor of a
massive turn-of-the-century building, to Bahnhofstrasse.

That's where I'd thrown up on the way home from school one day the previous October. I'd been feeling weak for days, in a way that was completely new to me. Every step was an effort. When I was faced with stairs either at home or at school, my legs would hardly carry me. I had no appetite. Even if I sat down at the table hungry, I soon felt queasy. I woke up every morning with a dry mouth and the sensation that my insides were in the wrong place and pressing too hard against my bones. I was ashamed of being so weak. I was even more ashamed when I threw up. That was another thing that had never happened to me before. My mouth was suddenly full, I tried to swallow everything down again, and clenched my teeth with my hand in front of my mouth, but it all burst out of my mouth anyway straight through my fingers. I leaned against the wall of the building, looked down at the vomit around my feet, and retched something clear and sticky.

When rescue came, it was almost an assault. The woman seized my arm and pulled me through the dark entrance into the courtyard. Up above there were lines strung from window to window, loaded with laundry. Wood was stacked in the courtyard; in an open workshop a saw screamed and shavings flew. The woman turned on the tap, washed my hand first, and then cupped both of hers and threw water in my face. I dried myself with a handkerchief.

'Get that one!' There were two pails standing by the tap: she grabbed one and filled it. I took the other one, filled it, and followed her through the entrance. She swung her arm, the water sluiced down across the walk and washed the vomit into the gutter. Then she took my pail and sent a second wave of water across the walk.

When she straightened up, she saw I was crying. 'Hey, kid,' she said, startled, 'hey, kid' – and took me in her arms. I wasn't much taller than she was, I could feel her breasts against my chest. I smelled the sourness of my own breath and felt a sudden sweat as she held me, and didn't know where to look. I stopped crying.

She asked me where I lived, put the pails down in the entrance, and took me home, walking beside me holding my satchel in one hand and my arm in the other. It's no great distance from Bahnhofstrasse to the Blumenstrasse. She walked quickly, and her decisiveness helped me to keep pace with her. She said goodbye in front of our building.

That same day my mother called in the doctor, who diagnosed hepatitis. At some point I told my mother about the woman. If it hadn't been for that, I don't think I would have gone to see her. But my mother simply assumed that as soon as I was better, I would use my pocket money to buy some flowers, go introduce myself, and say thank you, which was why at the end of February I found myself heading for Bahnhofstrasse.

CHAPTER TWO

HE BUILDING ON BAHNHOFSTRASSE is no longer there. I don't know when or why it was torn down. I was away from my home town for many years. The new building, which must have been put up in the seventies or eighties, has five floors plus finished space under the roof, is devoid of balconies or arched windows, and its smooth façade is an expanse of pale plaster. A plethora of doorbells indicates a plethora of tiny apartments, with tenants moving in and out as casually as you would pick up and return a rented car. There's a computer shop on the ground floor where once there were a pharmacy, a supermarket, and a video shop.

The old building was as tall, but with only four floors, a first floor of faceted sandstone blocks, and above it three floors of brickwork with sandstone arches, balconies, and window surrounds. Several steps led up to the first floor and the stairwell; they were wide at the bottom, narrower above, set between walls topped with iron banisters and curving outwards at street level. The front door was flanked by pillars, and from the corners of the architrave one lion looked up Bahnhofstrasse while another looked down. The entrance through which the woman had led me to the tap in the courtyard was at the side.

I had been aware of this building since I was a little boy. It dominated the whole row. I used to think that if it made itself any heavier and wider, the neighbouring buildings would have to move aside and make room for it. Inside, I imagined a stairwell with plaster mouldings, mirrors, and an oriental runner held down with highly polished brass rods. I assumed that grand people would live in such a grand building. But because the building had darkened with the passing of the years and the smoke of the trains, I imagined that the grand inhabitants would be just as sombre and somehow peculiar – deaf or dumb or hunchbacked or lame.

In later years I dreamed about the building again and again. The dreams were similar, variations on one dream and one theme. I'm walking through a strange town and I see the house. It's one in a row of buildings in a district

I don't know. I go on, confused, because the house is familiar but its surroundings are not. Then I realize that I've seen the house before. I'm not picturing Bahnhofstrasse in my home town, but another city, or another country. For example, in my dream I'm in Rome, see the house, and realize I've seen it already in Berlin. This dream recognition comforts me; seeing the house again in different surroundings is no more surprising than encountering an old friend by chance in a strange place. I turn around, walk back to the house, and climb the steps. I want to go in. I turn the door handle.

If I see the house somewhere in the country, the dream is more long-drawn-out, or I remember its details better. I'm driving a car. I see the house on the right and keep going, confused at first only by the fact that such an obviously urban building is standing there in the middle of the countryside. Then I realize that this is not the first time I've seen it, and I'm doubly confused. When I remember where I've seen it before, I turn around and drive back. In the dream, the road is always empty, as I can turn around with my tyres squealing and race back. I'm afraid I'll be too late, and I drive faster. Then I see it. It is surrounded by fields, rape or wheat or vines in the Palatinate, lavender in Provence. The landscape is flat, or at most gently rolling. There are no trees. The day is cloudless, the sun is shining, the air shimmers and the road glitters in the heat. The firewalls make the building look unprepossessing and cut off. They could be the firewalls of any building. The house is no darker than it was on Bahnhofstrasse, but the windows are so dusty that you can't see anything inside the rooms, not even the curtains; it looks blind.

I stop on the side of the road and walk over to the entrance. There's nobody about, not a sound to be heard, not even a distant engine, a gust of wind, a bird. The world is dead. I go up the steps and turn the door knob.

But I do not open the door. I wake up knowing simply that I took hold of the knob and turned it. Then the whole dream comes back to me, and I know that I've dreamed it before.

CHAPTER THREE

I DIDN'T KNOW THE WOMAN'S NAME. Clutching my bunch of flowers, I hesitated in front of the door and all the bells. I would rather have turned around and left, but then a man came out of the building, asked who I was looking for, and directed me to Frau Schmitz on the third floor.

No decorative plaster, no mirrors, no runner. Whatever unpretentious beauty the stairwell might once have had, it could never have been comparable to the grandeur of the façade, and it was long gone in any case. The red paint on the stairs had worn through in the middle, the stamped green lino that was glued on the walls to shoulder height was rubbed away to nothing, and bits of string had been stretched across the gaps in the banisters. It smelled of cleaning fluid. Perhaps I only became aware of all this some time later. It was always just as shabby and just as clean, and there was always the same smell of cleaning fluid, sometimes mixed with the smell of cabbage or beans, or fried food or boiling laundry.

I never learned anything about the other people who lived in the building apart from these smells, the mats outside the flat doors, and the nameplates under the doorbells. I cannot even remember meeting another tenant on the stairs.

Nor do I remember how I greeted Frau Schmitz. I had probably prepared two or three sentences about my illness and her help and how grateful I was, and recited them to her. She led me into the kitchen.

It was the largest room in the flat, and contained a stove and sink, a tub and a boiler, a table, two chairs, a kitchen cabinet, a wardrobe, and a couch with a red velvet spread thrown over it. There was no window. Light came in through the panes of the door leading out onto the balcony – not much light; the kitchen was only bright when the door was open. Then you heard the scream of the saws from the carpenter's shop in the yard and smelled the smell of wood.

The flat also had a small, cramped living room with a dresser, a table, four chairs, a wing chair, and a coal stove. It was almost never heated in winter, nor was it used much in summer either. The window faced Bahnhofstrasse, with a view of what had been the railway station, but was now being excavated and already in places held the freshly laid foundations of the new courthouse and administration buildings. Finally, the flat also had a windowless toilet. When the toilet smelled, so did the hall.

I don't remember what we talked about in the kitchen. Frau Schmitz was ironing; she had spread a woollen blanket and a linen cloth over the table; lifting one piece of laundry after another from the basket, she ironed them, folded them, and laid them on one of the two chairs. I sat on the other. She also ironed her underwear, and I didn't want to look, but I couldn't help looking. She was wearing a sleeveless smock, blue with little pale red flowers on it. Her shoulder-length, ash-blonde hair was fastened with a clip at the back of her neck. Her bare arms were pale. Her gestures of lifting the iron, using it, setting it down again, and then folding and putting away the laundry were an exercise in slow concentration, as were her movements as she bent over and then straightened up again. Her face as it was then has been overlaid in my memory by the faces she had later. If I see her in my mind's eye as she was then, she doesn't have a face at all, and I have to reconstruct it. High forehead, high cheekbones, pale blue eyes, full lips that formed a perfect curve without any indentation, square chin. A broad-planed, strong, womanly face. I know that I found it beautiful. But I cannot recapture its beauty.

CHAPTER FOUR

'WAIT,' SHE SAID AS I GOT UP TO go. 'I have to leave too, and I'll walk with you.'

I waited in the hall while she changed her clothes in the kitchen. The door was open a crack. She took off the smock and stood there in a bright green petticoat. Two stockings were hanging over the back of the chair. Picking one up, she gathered it into a roll using one hand, then the other, then balanced on one leg as she rested the heel of her other foot against her knee, leaned forward, slipped the rolled-up stocking over her toes, put her foot on the chair as she smoothed the stocking up over her calf, knee, and thigh, then bent to one side as she fastened the stocking to the garter belt. Straightening up, she took her foot off the chair and reached for the other stocking.

I couldn't take my eyes off her. Her neck and shoulders, her breasts, which the petticoat veiled rather than concealed, her hips, which stretched the petticoat tight as she propped her foot on her knee and then set it on the chair, her leg, pale and naked, then shimmering in the silky stocking.

She felt me looking at her. As she was reaching for the other stocking, she paused, turned towards the door, and looked straight at me. I can't describe what kind of look it was — surprised, sceptical, knowing, reproachful. I turned red. For a fraction of a second I stood there, my face burning. Then I couldn't take it any more. I fled out of the flat, down the stairs, and into the street.

I dawdled along. Bahnhofstrasse, Häusserstrasse, Blumenstrasse — it had been my way to school for years. I knew every building, every garden, and every fence, the ones that were repainted every year and the ones that were so grey and rotten that I could crumble the wood in my hand, the iron railings that I ran along as a child, banging a stick against the posts and the high brick wall behind which I had imagined wonderful and terrible things, until I was able to climb it, and see row after boring row of neglected beds of flowers, berries, and vegetables. I knew the cobblestones in their layer of tar on the road, and the changing surface of the pavement, from flagstones to little lumps of basalt set in wave patterns, tar, and gravel.

It was all familiar. When my heart stopped pounding and my face was no longer scarlet, the encounter between the kitchen and the hall seemed a long way away. I was angry with myself. I had run away like a child, instead of staying in control of the situation, as I thought I should. I wasn't nine years old any more, I was fifteen. That didn't mean I had any idea what staying in control would have entailed.

The other puzzle was the actual encounter that had taken place between the kitchen and the hall. Why had I not been able to take my eyes off her? She had a very strong, feminine body, more voluptuous than the girls I liked and watched. I was sure I wouldn't even have noticed her if I'd seen her at the swimming pool. Nor had she been any more naked than the girls and women I had already seen at the swimming pool. And besides, she was much older than the girls I dreamed about. Over thirty? It's hard to guess ages when you're not that old yourself and won't be any time soon.

Years later it occurred to me that the reason I hadn't been able to take my eyes off her was not just her body, but the way she held herself and moved. I asked my girlfriends to put on their stockings, but I didn't want to explain why, or to talk about the riddle of what had happened between the kitchen and the hall. So my request was read as a desire for garters and high heels and erotic extravaganza, and if it was granted, it was done as a come-on. There had been none of that when I had found myself unable to look away. She hadn't been posing or teasing me. I don't remember her ever doing that. I remember that her body and the way she held it and moved sometimes seemed awkward. Not that she was particularly heavy. It was more as if she had withdrawn into her own body, and left it to itself and its own quiet rhythms, unbothered by any input from her mind, oblivious to the outside world. It was the same obliviousness that weighed in her glance and her movements when she was pulling on her stockings. But then she was not awkward, she was slow-flowing, graceful, seductive – a seductiveness that had nothing to do with breasts and hips and legs, but that was an invitation to forget the world in the recesses of the body.

I knew none of this then – if indeed I know any of it now and am not just making patterns in the air. But as I thought back then on what had excited me, the excitement came back. To solve the riddle, I made myself remember the whole encounter, and then the distance I had created by turning it into a riddle dissolved and I saw it all again, and again I couldn't take my eyes off her.

CHAPTER FIVE

A WEEK LATER I WAS STANDING AT her door again.

For a week I had tried not to think about her. But I had nothing else to occupy or distract me; the doctor was not ready to let me go back to school, I was bored stiff with books after months of reading, and although friends still came to see me, I had been sick for so long that their visits could no longer bridge the gap between their daily lives and mine, and became shorter and shorter. I was supposed to go for walks, a little further each day, without overexerting myself. I could have used the exertion.

Being ill when you are a child or growing up is such an enchanted interlude! The outside world, the world of free time in the yard or the garden or on the street, is only a distant murmur in the sickroom. Inside, a whole world of characters and stories proliferates out of the books you read. The fever that weakens your perception as it sharpens your imagination turns the sickroom into someplace new, both familiar and strange; monsters come grinning out of the patterns on the curtains and the carpet, and chairs, tables, bookcases, and wardrobes burst out of their normal shapes and become mountains and buildings and ships you can almost touch although they're far away. Through the long hours of the night you have the church clock for company and the rumble of the occasional passing car that throws its headlights across the walls and ceiling. These are hours without sleep, which is not to say that they're sleepless, because on the contrary, they're not about lack of anything, they're rich and full. Desires, memories, fears, passions form labyrinths in which we lose and find and then lose ourselves again. They are hours when anything is possible, good or bad.

This passes as you get better. But if the illness has lasted long enough, the sickroom is impregnated with it and although you're convalescing and the fever has gone, you are still trapped in the labyrinth.

I awoke every day feeling guilty, sometimes with my pyjama bottoms damp or stained. The images and scenes in my dreams were not right. I knew I would not be scolded by my mother, or the pastor who had instructed me for my confirmation and whom I admired, or by my older sister who was the confidante of all my childhood secrets. But they would lecture me with loving concern, which was worse than being scolded. It was particularly wrong that when I was not just idly dreaming, I actively fantasized images and scenes.

I don't know where I found the courage to go to Frau Schmitz. Did my moral upbringing somehow turn against itself? If looking at someone with desire was as bad as satisfying the desire, if having an active fantasy was as bad as the act you were fantasizing – then why not the satisfaction and the act itself? As the days went on, I discovered that I couldn't stop thinking sinful thoughts. In which case I also wanted the sin itself.

There was another way to look at it. Going there might be dangerous. But it was obviously impossible for the danger to act itself out. Frau Schmitz would greet me with surprise, listen to me apologize for my strange behaviour, and amicably say goodbye. It was more danger-ous not to go; I was running the risk of becoming trapped in my own fantasies. So I was doing the right thing by going. She would behave normally, I would behave nor-mally, and everything would be normal again.

That is how I rationalized it back then, making my desire an entry in a strange moral accounting, and silenc-ing my bad conscience. But that was not what gave me the courage to go to Frau Schmitz. It was one thing to tell myself that my mother, my beloved pastor, and my older sister would not try to stop me if they really thought about it, but would in fact insist that I go. Actually going was something else again. I don't know why I did it. But today I can recognize that events back then were part of a lifelong pattern in which thinking and doing have either come together or failed to come together – I think, I reach a conclusion, I turn the conclusion into a decision, and then I discover that acting on the decision is something else entirely, and that doing so may proceed from the decision, but then again it may not. Often enough in my life I have done things I had not decided to do. Something – whatever that may be – goes into action; 'it' goes to the woman I don't want to see any more, 'it' makes the remark to the boss that costs me my head, 'it' keeps on smoking although I have decided to give up, and then gives up smoking just when I've accepted the fact that I'm a smoker and always will be. I don't mean to say that thinking and reaching decisions have no influence on behaviour. But behaviour does not merely enact whatever has already been thought through and decided. It has its own sources, and is my behaviour, quite independently, just as my thoughts are my thoughts, and my decisions my decisions.

CHAPTER SIX

*S*HE WASN'T AT HOME. THE FRONT DOOR of the building stood ajar, so I went up the stairs, rang the bell, and waited. Then I rang again. Inside the flat the doors were open, as I could see through the glass of the front door, and I could also make out the mirror, the wardrobe, and the clock in the hall. I could hear it ticking.

I sat down on the stairs and waited. I wasn't relieved, the way you can sometimes be when you feel funny about a certain decision and afraid of the consequences and then relieved that you've managed to carry out the former without incurring the latter. Nor was I disappointed.

I was determined to see her and to wait until she came.

The clock in the hall struck the quarter hour, then the half hour, then the hour. I tried to follow its soft ticking and to count the nine hundred seconds between one stroke and the next, but I kept losing track. The yard buzzed with the sound of the carpenter's saws, the building echoed with voices or music from one of the flats, and a door opened and closed. Then I heard slow, heavy, regular footsteps coming up the stairs. I hoped that whoever he was, he lived on the second floor. If he saw me – how would I explain what I was doing there? But the footsteps didn't stop at the second floor. They kept coming. I stood up.

It was Frau Schmitz. In one hand she was carrying a coal scuttle, in the other a box of briquets. She was wearing a uniform jacket and skirt, and I realized that she was a tram conductor. She didn't notice me until she reached the landing – she didn't look annoyed, or surprised, or mocking – none of the things I had feared. She looked tired. When she put down the coal and was hunting in her jacket pocket for the key, coins fell out onto the floor. I picked them up and gave them to her.

'There are two more scuttles down in the cellar. Will you fill them and bring them up? The door's open.'

I ran down the stairs. The door to the cellar was open, the light was on, and at the bottom of the long cellar stairs I found a bunker made of boards with the door on the latch and a loose padlock hanging from the open bolt.

It was a large space, and the coke was piled all the way up to the ceiling hatch through which it had been poured from the street into the cellar. On one side of the door was a neat stack of briquets; on the other side were the coal scuttles.

I don't know what I did wrong. At home I also fetched the coal from the cellar and never had any problems. But then the coke at home wasn't piled so high. Filling the first scuttle went fine. As I picked up the second scuttle by the handles and tried to shovel the coal up off the floor, the mountain began to move. From the top little pieces started bouncing down while the larger ones followed more sedately; further down it all began to slide and there was a general rolling and shifting on the floor. Black dust rose in clouds. I stood there, frightened, as the lumps came down and hit me and soon I was up to my ankles in coke.

I got my feet out of the coke, filled the second scuttle, looked for a broom, and when I found it I swept the lumps that had rolled out into the main part of the cellar back into the bunker, latched the door, and carried the two scuttles upstairs.

She had taken off her jacket, loosened her tie and undone the top button, and was sitting at the kitchen table with a glass of milk. She saw me, began to choke with laughter, and then let it out in full-throated peals. She pointed at me and slapped her other hand on the table. 'Look at you, kid, just look at you!' Then I caught sight of my black face in the mirror over the sink, and laughed too.

'You can't go home like that. I'll run you a bath and beat the dust out of your clothes.' She went to the tub and turned on the tap. The water ran steaming into the tub. 'Take your clothes off carefully, I don't need black dust all over the kitchen.'

I hesitated, took off my jumper and shirt, and hesitated again. The water was rising quickly and the tub was almost full.

'Do you want to take a bath in your shoes and trousers? I won't look, kid.' But when I had turned off the tap and taken off my pants, she looked me over calmly. I turned red, climbed into the tub, and submerged myself. When I came up again she was out on the balcony with my clothes. I heard her beating the shoes against each other and shaking out my trousers and jumper. She called down something about coal dust and sawdust, someone called back up to her, and she laughed. Back in the kitchen, she put my things on the chair. Glancing quickly at me, she said, 'Take the shampoo and wash your hair. I'll bring a towel in a minute,' then took something out of the wardrobe, and left the kitchen.

I washed myself. The water in the tub was dirty and I ran in some fresh so that I could wash my head and face clean under the flow. Then I lay there, listening to the boiler roar, and feeling the cool air on my face as it came through the half-open kitchen door, and the warm water on my body. I was comfortable. It was an exciting kind of comfort and I got hard.

I didn't look up when she came into the kitchen, until she was standing by the tub. She was holding a big towel in her outstretched arms. 'Come!' I turned my back as I stood up and climbed out of the tub. From behind, she wrapped me in the towel from head to foot and rubbed me dry. Then she let the towel fall to the floor. I didn't dare move. She came so close to me that I could feel her breasts against my back and her stomach against my behind. She was naked too. She put her arms around me, one hand on my chest and the other on my erection.

'That's why you're here!'

'I . . .' I didn't know what to say. Not yes, but not no either. I turned around. I couldn't see much of her, we were standing too close. But I was overwhelmed by the presence of her naked body. 'You're so beautiful!'

'Come on, kid, what are you talking about!' She laughed and wrapped her arms around my neck. I put my arms around her too.

I was afraid: of touching, of kissing, afraid I wouldn't please her or satisfy her. But when we had held each other for a while, when I had smelled her smell and felt her warmth and her strength, everything fell into place. I explored her body with my hands and mouth, our mouths met, and then she was on top of me, looking into my eyes until I came and closed my eyes tight and tried to control myself and then screamed so loud that she had to cover my mouth with her hand to smother the sound.

CHAPTER SEVEN

*T*HE NEXT NIGHT I FELL IN LOVE with her. I could barely sleep, I was yearning for her, I dreamed of her, thought I could feel her until I realized that I was clutching the pillow or the blanket. My mouth hurt from kissing. I kept getting erections, but I didn't want to masturbate. I wanted to be with her.

Did I fall in love with her as the price for her having gone to bed with me? To this day, after spending the night with a woman, I feel I've been indulged and I must make it up somehow – to her by trying at least to love her, and to the world by facing up to it.

One of my few vivid recollections of early childhood has to do with a winter morning when I was four years old. The room I slept in at that time was unheated, and at night and first thing in the morning it was often very cold. I remember the warm kitchen and the hot stove, a heavy piece of iron equipment in which you could see the fire when you lifted out the plates and rings with a hook, and which always held a basin of hot water ready. My mother had pushed a chair up close to the stove for me to stand on while she washed and dressed me. I remember the wonderful feeling of warmth, and how good it felt to be washed and dressed in this warmth. I also remember that whenever I thought back to this afterwards, I always wondered why my mother had been spoiling me like this. Was I ill? Had my brothers and sisters been given something I hadn't? Was there something coming later in the day that was nasty or difficult that I had to get through?

Because the woman whose name I didn't even know had so spoiled me that afternoon, I went back to school the next day. It was also true that I wanted to show off my new manliness. Not that I would ever have talked about it. But I felt strong and superior, and I wanted to show off these feelings to the other kids and the teachers. Besides, I hadn't talked to her about it but I assumed that being a tram conductor she often had to work evenings and nights. How would I see her every day if I had to stay home and wasn't allowed to do anything except my convalescent walks?

When I came home from her, my parents and brother and sisters were already eating dinner. 'Why are you so late? Your mother was worried about you.' My father sounded more annoyed than concerned.

I said that I'd lost my way, that I'd wanted to walk through the memorial garden in the cemetery to Molkenkur, but wandered around who knows where for a long time and ended up in Nussloch. 'I had no money, so I had to walk home from Nussloch.'

'You could have hitched a lift.' My younger sister sometimes did this, but my parents disapproved.

My older brother snorted contemptuously. 'Molkenkur and Nussloch are in completely opposite directions.'

My older sister gave me a hard look.

'I'm going back to school tomorrow.'

'So pay attention in Geography. There's north and there's south, and the sun rises . . .'

My mother interrupted my brother. 'The doctor said another three weeks.'

'If he can get all the way across the cemetery to Nussloch and back, he can also go to school. It's not strength he's lacking, it's brains.' As small boys, my brother and I beat up on each other constantly, and later we fought with words. He was three years older than me, and better at both. At a certain point I stopped fighting back and let his attacks dissipate into thin air. Since then he had confined himself to grousing at me.

'What do you think?' My mother turned to my father. He set his knife and fork down on his plate, leaned back, and folded his hands in his lap. He said nothing and looked thoughtful, the way he always did when my mother talked to him about the children or the household. As usual, I wondered whether he was really turning over my mother's question in his mind, or whether he was thinking about work. Maybe he did try to think about my mother's question, but once his mind started going, he could only think about work. He was a professor of philosophy, and thinking was his life – thinking and reading and writing and teaching.

Sometimes I had the feeling that all of us in his family were like pets to him. The dog you take for a walk, the cat you play with and that curls up in your lap, purring, to be stroked – you can be fond of them, you can even need them to a certain extent, and nonetheless the whole thing – buying pet food, cleaning up the cat box, and trips to the vet – is really too much. Your life is elsewhere. I wish that we, his family, had been his life. Sometimes I also wished that my grousing brother and my cheeky little sister were different. But that evening I suddenly loved them all. My little sister. It probably wasn't easy being the youngest of four, and she needed to be cheeky just to hold her own. My older brother. We shared a bedroom, which must be even harder for him than it was for me, and on top of that, since I'd been ill he'd had to let me have the room to myself and sleep on the sofa in the living room. How could he not nag me? My father. Why should we children be his whole life? We were growing up and soon we'd be adults and out of the house.

I felt as if we were sitting all together for the last time around the round table under the five-armed, five-candled brass chandelier, as if we were eating our last meal off the old plates with the green vine-leaf border, as if we would never talk to each other as a family again. I felt as if I were saying goodbye. I was still there and already gone. I was homesick for my mother and father and my brother and sisters, and I longed to be with the woman.

My father looked over at me. ' "I'm going back to school tomorrow" – that's what you said, isn't it?'

'Yes.' So he had noticed that it was him I'd asked and not my mother, and also that I had not said I was wondering whether I should go back to school or not.

He nodded. 'Let's have you go back to school. If it gets to be too much for you, you'll just stay home again.'

I was happy. And at the same time I felt I'd just said my final goodbyes.

CHAPTER EIGHT

OR THE NEXT FEW DAYS, THE WOMAN was working the early shift. She came home at noon, and I cut my last class every day so as to be waiting for her on the landing outside her flat. We showered and made love, and just before half past one I scrambled into my clothes and ran out the door. Lunch was at one-thirty. On Sundays lunch was at noon, but her early shift also started and ended later.

I would have preferred to skip the shower. She was scrupulously clean, she showered every morning, and I liked the smell of perfume, fresh perspiration, and tram that she brought with her from work. But I also liked her wet, soapy body; I liked to let her soap me and I liked to soap her, and she taught me not to do it bashfully, but with assurance and possessive thoroughness. When we made love, too, she took possession of me as a matter of course. Her mouth took mine, her tongue played with my tongue, she told me where to touch her and how, and when she rode me until she came, I was there only because she took pleasure in me and on me. I don't mean to say that she lacked tenderness and didn't give me pleasure. But she did it for her own playful enjoyment, until I learned to take possession of her too.

That came later. I never completely mastered it. And for a long time I didn't miss it. I was young, and I came quickly, and when I slowly came back alive again afterwards, I liked to have her take possession of me. I would look at her when she was on top of me, her stomach which made a deep crease above her navel, her breasts, the right one the tiniest bit larger than the left, her face and open mouth. She would lean both hands against my chest and throw them up at the last moment, as she gave a toneless sobbing cry that frightened me the first time, and that later I eagerly awaited.

Afterwards we were exhausted. She often fell asleep on top of me. I would listen to the saws in the yard and the loud cries of the workers who operated them and had to shout to make themselves heard. When the saws fell silent, the sound of the traffic echoed faintly in the kitchen. When I heard children calling and playing, I knew that school was out and that it was past one o'clock. The neighbour who came home at lunchtime scattered birdseed on his balcony, and the doves came and cooed.

'What's your name?' I asked her on the sixth or seventh day. She had fallen asleep on me and was just waking up. Until then I avoided saying anything to her that required me to choose either the formal or the familiar form of address.

She stared. 'What?'

'What's your name?'

'Why do you want to know?' She looked at me suspiciously.

'You and I . . . I know your last name, but not your first. I want to know your first name. What's the matter with . . .'

She laughed. 'Nothing, kid, there's nothing wrong with that. My name is Hanna.' She kept on laughing, didn't stop, and it was contagious.

'You looked at me so oddly.'

'I was still half asleep. What's yours?'

I thought she knew. At that time it was the in thing not to carry your schoolbooks in a satchel but under your arm, and when I put them on her kitchen table, my name was on the front. But she hadn't paid any attention to them.

'My name is Michael Berg.'

'Michael, Michael, Michael.' She tried out the name. 'My kid's called Michael, he's at college.'

'At secondary school.'

'At secondary school, he's what, seventeen?'

I was proud at the two extra years she'd given me, and nodded.

'He's seventeen and when he grows up he wants to be a famous . . .' She hesitated.

'I don't know what I want to be.'

'But you study hard.'

'Sort of.' I told her she was more important to me than school and my studies. And I wished I were with her more often. 'I'll have to repeat a year in any case.'

'What class?' It was the first real conversation we'd had with each other.

'Fifth form. I've missed too much in the last months while I was ill. If I still wanted to move up next year I'd have to work like a lunatic. I'd also have to be in school right now.' I told her I was missing lessons.

'Out.' She threw back the blanket. 'Get out of my bed. And if you don't want to do your work, don't come back. Your work is idiotic? Idiotic? What do you think selling and punching tickets is?' She got out of bed, stood naked in the kitchen being a conductor. With her left hand she opened the little holder with the blocks of tickets, using her left thumb, covered with a rubber thimble, to pull off two tickets, flipped her right hand to get hold of the punch that hung from her wrist, and made two holes. 'Two to Rohrbach.' She dropped the punch, reached out her hand for a bill, opened the purse at her waist, put the money in, snapped it shut again, and squeezed the change out of the coin holder that was attached to it. 'Who still doesn't have a ticket?' She looked at me. 'Idiotic – you don't know what idiotic is.'

I sat on the edge of the bed. I was stunned. 'I'm sorry. I'll do my work. I don't know if I'll make it, school only has another six weeks to go. I'll try. But I won't get through it if I can't see you any more. I . . .' At first I wanted to say, I love you. But then I didn't. Maybe she was right, of course she was right. But she had no right to demand that I do more at school, and make that the condition for our seeing each other again. 'I can't not see you.'

The clock in the hall struck one-thirty. 'You have to go.' She hesitated. 'But tomorrow I'm working the main shift. I'll be home at five-thirty and you can come. Provided you work first.'

We stood facing each other naked, but she couldn't have seemed more dismissive if she'd had on her uniform. I didn't understand what was going on. Was she thinking of me? Or of herself? If my schoolwork is idiotic, that makes her work even more so – that's what upset her? But I hadn't ever said that my work or hers was idiotic. Or was it that she didn't want a failure for a lover? But was I her lover? What was I to her? I dressed, dawdling, and hoped she would say something. But she said nothing. Then I had all my clothes on and she was still standing there naked, and as I kissed her goodbye, she didn't respond.

CHAPTER NINE

*W*HY DOES IT MAKE ME SO SAD WHEN I think back to that time? Is it yearning for past happiness – for I was happy in the weeks that followed, in which I really did work like a lunatic and passed the class, and we made love as if nothing else in the world mattered. Is it the knowledge of what came later, and that what came out afterwards had been there all along?

Why? Why does what was beautiful suddenly shatter in hindsight because it concealed dark truths? Why does the memory of years of happy marriage turn to gall when our partner is revealed to have had a lover all those years?

Because such a situation makes it impossible to be happy? But we were happy! Sometimes the memory of happiness cannot stay true because it ended unhappily. Because happiness is only real if it lasts forever? Because things always end painfully if they contained pain, conscious or unconscious, all along? But what is unconscious, unrecognized pain?

I think back to that time and I see my former self. I wore the well-cut suits which had come down to me from a rich uncle, now dead, along with several pairs of two-tone shoes, black and brown, black and white, suede and calf. My arms and legs were too long, not for the suits, which my mother had let down for me, but for my own movements. My glasses were a cheap over-the-counter pair and my hair a tangled mop, no matter what I did. In school I was neither good nor bad; I think that many of the teachers didn't really notice me, nor did the students who dominated the class. I didn't like the way I looked, the way I dressed and moved, what I achieved and what I felt I was worth. But there was so much energy in me, such belief that one day I'd be handsome and clever and superior and admired, such anticipation when I met new people and new situations. Is that what makes me sad? The eagerness and belief that filled me then and exacted a pledge from life that life could never fulfil? Sometimes I see the same eagerness and belief in the faces of children and teenagers and the sight brings back the same sadness I feel in remembering myself. Is this what sadness is all about? Is it what comes over us when beautiful memories shatter in hindsight because the remembered happiness fed not just on actual circumstances but on a promise that was not kept?

She – I should start calling her Hanna, just as I started calling her Hanna back then – she certainly didn't nourish herself on promises, but was rooted in the here and now.

I asked her about her life, and it was as if she rummaged around in a dusty chest to get me the answers. She had grown up in a German community in Rumania, then came to Berlin at the age of sixteen, taken a job at the Siemens factory, and ended up in the army at twenty-one. Since the end of the war, she had done all manner of jobs to get by. She had been a tram conductor for several years; what she liked about the job was the uniform and the constant motion, the changing scenery and the wheels rolling under her feet. But that was all she liked about it. She had no family. She was thirty-six. She told me all this as if it were not her life but somebody else's, someone she didn't know well and who wasn't important to her. Things I wanted to know more about had vanished completely from her mind, and she didn't understand why I was interested in what had happened to her parents, whether she had had brothers and sisters, how she had lived in Berlin, and what she'd done in the army. 'The things you ask, kid!'

It was the same with the future – of course I wasn't hammering out plans for marriage and future. But I identified more with Julien Sorel's relationship with Madame de Renal than with his one with Mathilde de la Mole. I was glad to see Felix Krull end up in the arms of the mother rather than the daughter. My sister, who was studying German literature, delivered a report at the dinner table about the controversy as to whether Mr von Goethe and Madame von Stein had had a relationship, and I vigorously defended the idea, to the bafflement of my family. I imagined how our relationship might be in five or ten years. I asked Hanna how she imagined it. She didn't even want to think ahead to Easter, when I wanted to take a bicycle trip with her over the holiday. We could get a room together as mother and son, and spend the whole night together.

Strange that this idea and suggesting it were not embarrassing to me. On a trip with my mother I would have fought to get a room of my own. Having my mother with me when I went to the doctor or to buy a new coat or to be picked up by her after a trip seemed to me to be something I had outgrown. If we went somewhere together and we ran into my schoolfriends, I was afraid they would think I was a mother's boy. But to be seen with Hanna, who was ten years younger than my mother but could have been my mother, didn't bother me. It made me proud.

When I see a woman of thirty-six today, I find her young. But when I see a boy of fifteen, I see a child. I am amazed at how much confidence Hanna gave me. My success at school got my teachers' attention and assured me of their respect. The girls I met noticed and liked it that I wasn't afraid of them. I felt at ease in my own body.

The memory that illuminates and fixes my first meetings with Hanna makes a single blur of the weeks between our first conversation and the end of the academic year. One reason for that is we saw each other so regularly and our meetings always followed the same course. Another is that my days had never been so full and my life had never been so swift and so dense. When I think about the work I did in those weeks, it's as if I had sat down at my desk and stayed there until I had caught up with everything I'd missed during my hepatitis, learned all the vocabulary, read all the texts, worked through all the theorems and linked all the chemical formulas. I had already done the reading about the Weimar Republic and the Third Reich while I was in my sickbed. And I remember our meetings in those weeks as one single long meeting. After our conversation, they were always in the afternoon: if she was on the late shift, then from three to four-thirty, otherwise until five-thirty. Dinner was at seven, and at first Hanna forced me to be home on time. But after a while it lasted beyond the hour and a half, and I began to think up excuses to miss dinner.

It all happened because of reading aloud. The day after our conversation, Hanna wanted to know what I was learning in school. I told her about Homer, Cicero, and Hemingway's story about the old man and his battle with the fish and the sea. She wanted to hear what Greek and Latin sounded like, and I read to her from the *Odyssey* and the speeches against Cataline.

'Are you also learning German?'

'How do you mean?'

'Do you only learn foreign languages, or is there still stuff you have to learn in your own?'

'We read texts.' While I was sick, the class had read *Emilia Galotti* and *Intrigues and Love*, and there was an essay due on them. So I had to read both, which I did after finishing everything else. By then it was late, and I was tired, and the next day I'd forgotten it all and had to start all over again.

'So read it to me!'

'Read it yourself. I'll bring it for you.'

'You have such a nice voice, kid, I'd rather listen to you than read it myself.'

'Oh, come on.'

But next day when I arrived and wanted to kiss her, she pulled back. 'First you have to read.'

She was serious. I had to read *Emilia Galotti* to her for half an hour before she took me into the shower and then to bed. Now I enjoyed showering too – the desire I felt when I arrived had got lost as I read aloud to her. Reading a play out loud so that the various characters are more or less recognizable and come to life takes a certain concentration. Lust reasserted itself under the shower. So reading to her, showering with her, making love to her, and lying next to her for a while afterwards — that became the ritual in our meetings.

She was an attentive listener. Her laugh, her sniffs of contempt, and her angry or enthusiastic remarks left no doubt that she was following the action intently, and she found both Emilia and Luise to be silly little girls. Her impatience when she sometimes asked me to go on reading seemed to come from the hope that all this imbecility would eventually play itself out. 'Unbelievable!' Sometimes this made even me eager to keep reading. As the days grew longer, I read longer, so that I could be in bed with her in the twilight. When she had fallen asleep lying on top of me, and the saw in the yard was quiet, and a blackbird was singing as the colours of things in the kitchen dimmed until nothing remained of them but lighter and darker shades of grey, I was completely happy.

CHAPTER TEN

ON THE FIRST DAY OF THE EASTER holidays, I got up at four. Hanna was working the early shift. She rode her bicycle to the tram depot at a quarter past four and was on the tram to Schwetzingen at four-thirty. On the way out, she'd told me, the tram was often empty. It only filled up on the return journey.

I got on at the second stop. The second carriage was empty; Hanna was standing in the first carriage close to the driver. I debated whether I should sit in the first or the second carriage, and decided on the second. It promised privacy, a hug, a kiss. But Hanna didn't come.

She must have seen that I had been waiting at the stop and had got on. That's why the tram had stopped. But she stayed up with the driver, talking and joking. I could see them.

The tram passed one stop after another. No one was waiting to get on. The streets were empty. It was not yet sunrise, and under a colourless sky everything lay pale in the pale light: buildings, parked cars, the new leaves on the trees and first flowers on the shrubs, the gas tank, and the mountains in the distance. The tram was moving slowly; presumably the schedule was based both on stopping times and on the time between each stop, and so the speed of travel had to be slowed down when there were no actual stops. I was imprisoned in the slow-moving tram. At first I sat, then I went and stood on the front platform and tried to impale Hanna with my stare; I wanted her to feel my eyes in her back. After some time she turned around and glanced at me. Then she went on talking to the driver. The journey continued. Once we'd passed Eppelheim the rails were no longer in the surface of the road, but laid alongside on a gravelled embankment. The tram accelerated, with the regular *clackety-clack* of a train. I knew that this stretch continued through various places and ended up in Schwetzingen. But I felt rejected, exiled from the real world in which people lived and worked and loved. It was as if I were condemned to ride forever in an empty tram to nowhere.

Then I saw another stop, a shelter in the middle of

open country. I pulled the cord the conductors used to signal the driver to stop or start. The tram stopped. Neither Hanna nor the driver looked back at me when they heard the bell. As I got off, I thought they were looking at me and laughing. But I wasn't sure. Then the tram moved on, and I looked after it until it headed down into a dip and disappeared behind a hill. I was standing between the embankment and the road, there were fields around me, and fruit trees, and further on a nursery with greenhouses. The air was cool, and filled with the twittering of birds. Above the mountains the pale sky shone pink.

The trip on the tram had been like a bad dream. If I didn't remember its epilogue so vividly, I would actually be tempted to think of it as a bad dream. Standing at the tram stop, hearing the birds and watching the sun come up was like an awakening. But waking from a bad dream does not necessarily console you. It can also make you fully aware of the horror you just dreamed, and even of the truth residing in that horror. I set off towards home in tears, and couldn't stop crying until I reached Eppelheim.

I walked all the way back. I tried more than once to hitch a lift. When I was halfway there, the tram passed me. It was full. I didn't see Hanna.

I was waiting for her on the landing outside her flat at noon, miserable, anxious, and furious.

'Are you missing lessons again?'

'I'm on holiday. What was going on this morning?'

She unlocked the door and I followed her into the apartment and into the kitchen.

'What do you mean, what was wrong this morning?'

'Why did you behave as if you didn't know me? I wanted . . .'

'I behaved as if I didn't know you?' She turned around and stared at me coldly. 'You didn't want to know me. Getting into the second carriage when you could see I was in the first.'

'Why would I get up at four-thirty on my first day of holiday to ride to Schwetzingen? Just to surprise you, because I thought you'd be happy. I got into the second carriage . . .'

'You poor baby. Up at four-thirty, and on your holiday too.'

I had never seen her sarcastic before. She shook her head.

'How should I know why you're going to Schwetzingen. How should I know why you choose not to know me. It's your business, not mine. Would you leave now?'

I can't describe how furious I was. 'That's not fair, Hanna. You knew, you had to know that I only got on the tram to be with you. How can you believe I didn't want to know you? If I didn't, I would not have got on at all.'

'Oh, leave me alone. I already told you, what you do is your business, not mine.' She had moved so that the kitchen table was between us; everything in her look, her voice, and her gestures told me I was an intruder and should leave.

I sat down on the sofa. She had treated me badly and I had wanted to challenge her on it. But I hadn't got through to her. Instead, she was the one who'd attacked me. And I became uncertain. Could she be right, not objectively, but subjectively? Could she have, must she have misunderstood me? Had I hurt her, unintentionally, against my will, but hurt her anyway?

'I'm sorry, Hanna. Everything went wrong. I didn't mean to upset you, but it looks . . .'

'It looks? You think it looks like you upset me? *You* don't have the power to upset me. And will you please go, finally? I've been working, I want to take a bath, and I want a little peace.' She looked at me commandingly. When I didn't get up, she shrugged, turned around, ran water into the bath, and took off her clothes.

Then I stood up and left. I thought I was leaving for good. But half an hour later I was back at her door. She let me in, and I said the whole thing was my fault. I had behaved thoughtlessly, inconsiderately, unlovingly. I understood that she was upset. I understood that she wasn't upset because I couldn't upset her. I understood that I couldn't upset her, but that she simply couldn't allow me to behave that way to her. In the end, I was happy that she admitted I'd hurt her.

So she wasn't as unmoved and uninvolved as she'd been making out, after all.

'Do you forgive me?'

She nodded.

'Do you love me?'

She nodded again. 'The bath is still full. Come, I'll bathe you.'

Later I wondered if she had left the water in the bath because she knew I would come back. If she had taken her clothes off because she knew I wouldn't be able to get that out of my head and that it would bring me back. If she had just wanted to win a power game.

After we'd made love and were lying next to each other and I told her why I'd got into the second carriage and not the first, she teased me. 'You want to do it with me in the tram too? Kid, kid!' It was as if the actual cause of our fight had been meaningless.

But its results had meaning. I had not only lost this fight. I had caved in after a short struggle when she threatened to send me away and withhold herself. In the weeks that followed I didn't fight at all. If she threatened, I instantly and unconditionally surrendered. I took all the blame. I admitted mistakes I hadn't made, intentions I'd never had. Whenever she turned cold and hard, I begged her to be good to me again, to forgive me and love me. Sometimes I had the feeling that she hurt herself when she turned cold and rigid. As if what she was yearning for was the warmth of my apologies, protestations, and entreaties. Sometimes I thought she just bullied me. But either way, I had no choice.

I couldn't talk to her about it. Talking about our fights only led to more fighting. Once or twice I wrote her letters. But she didn't react, and when I asked her about them, she said, 'Are you starting that again?'

CHAPTER ELEVEN

*N*OT THAT HANNA AND I WERE never happy again after the first day of the Easter holiday. We were never happier than in those weeks of April. As sham as our first fight and indeed all our fights were, everything that enlarged our ritual of reading, showering, making love, and lying beside each other did us good. Besides which, she had trumped herself with her accusation that I hadn't wanted to know her. When I wanted to be seen with her, she couldn't raise any fundamental objections. 'So it was you who didn't want to be seen with me' – she didn't want to have to listen to that. So the week after Easter we set off by bike on a four-day trip to Wimpfen, Amorbach, and Miltenberg.

I don't remember what I told my parents. That I was doing the trip with my friend Matthias? With a group? That I was going to visit a former classmate? My mother was probably worried, as usual, and my father probably thought, as usual, that she should stop worrying. Hadn't I just passed the class, when nobody thought I could do it?

While I was sick, I hadn't spent any of my pocket money. But that wouldn't be enough if I wanted to pay for Hanna as well. So I offered to sell my stamp collection to the stamp dealer next to the Church of the Holy Spirit. It was the only shop that said on the door that it purchased collections. The salesman looked through my album and offered me sixty marks. I made him look at my showpiece, a straight-edged Egyptian stamp with a pyramid that was listed in the catalogue for four hundred marks. He shrugged. If I cared that much about my collection, maybe I should hang on to it. Was I even allowed to be selling it? What did my parents say about it? I tried to bargain. If the stamp with the pyramid wasn't that valuable, I would just keep it. Then he could only give me thirty marks. So the stamp with the pyramid was valuable after all? In the end I got seventy marks. I felt cheated, but I didn't care.

I was not the only one with itchy feet. To my amazement, Hanna started getting restless days before we left. She went this way and that over what to take, and packed and repacked the saddlebag and rucksack I had got hold of for her. When I wanted to show her the route I had worked out on the map, she didn't want to look, or even hear about it. 'I'm too excited already. You'll have worked it out right anyway, kid.'

We set off on Easter Monday. The sun was shining and went on shining for four days. The mornings were cool and then the days warmed up, not too warm for cycling, but warm enough to have picnics. The woods were carpets of green, with yellow green, bright green, bottle green, blue green, and black green daubs, flecks, and patches. In the flatlands along the Rhine, the first fruit trees were already in bloom. In Odenwald the first forsythias were out.

Often we could ride side by side. Then we pointed out to each other the things we saw: the castle, the fisherman, the boat on the river, the tent, the family walking single file along the bank, the enormous American convertible with the top down. When we changed directions or roads, I had to ride ahead; she didn't want to have to bother with such things. Otherwise, when the traffic was too heavy, she sometimes rode behind me and sometimes vice versa. Her bike had covered spokes, pedals, and gears, and she wore a blue dress with a big skirt that fluttered in her wake. It took me some time to stop worrying that the skirt would get caught in the spokes or the gears and she would fall off. After that, I liked watching her ride ahead of me.

How I had looked forward to the nights. I had imagined that we would make love, go to sleep, wake up, make love again, go to sleep again, wake up again and so on, night after night. But the only time I woke up again was the first night. She lay with her back to me, I leaned over her and kissed her, and she turned on her back, took me into her and held me in her arms. 'Kid, kid.' Then I fell asleep on top of her. The other nights we slept right through, worn out by the cycling, the sun, and the wind. We made love in the mornings.

Hanna didn't just let me be in charge of choosing our direction and the roads to take. I was the one who picked out the inns where we spent the nights, registered us as mother and son while she just signed her name, and selected our food from the menu for both of us. 'I like not having to worry about a thing for a change.'

The only fight we had took place in Amorbach. I had woken up early, dressed quietly, and crept out of the room. I wanted to bring up breakfast and also see if I could find a flower shop open where I could get a rose for Hanna. I had left a note on the night table. 'Good morning! Bringing breakfast, be right back,' or words to that effect. When I returned, she was standing in the room, trembling with rage and white-faced.

'How could you go just like that?'

I put down the breakfast tray with the rose on it and wanted to take her in my arms. 'Hanna.'

'Don't touch me.' She was holding the narrow leather

belt that she wore around her dress; she took a step backwards and hit me across the face with it. My lip split and I tasted blood. It didn't hurt. I was horrorstruck. She swung again.

But she didn't hit me. She let her arm fall, dropped the belt, and burst into tears. I had never seen her cry. Her face lost all its shape. Wide-open eyes, wide-open mouth, eyelids swollen after the first tears, red blotches on her cheeks and neck. Her mouth was making croaking, throaty sounds like the toneless cry when we made love. She stood there looking at me through her tears.

I should have taken her in my arms. But I couldn't. I didn't know what to do. At home none of us cried like that. We didn't hit, not even with our hands, let alone a leather belt. We talked. But what was I supposed to say now?

She took two steps towards me, beat her fists against me, then clung to me. Now I could hold her. Her shoulders trembled, she knocked her forehead against my chest. Then she gave a deep sigh and snuggled into my arms.

'Shall we have breakfast?' She let go of me. 'My God, kid, look at you.' She fetched a wet towel and cleaned my mouth and chin. 'And your shirt is covered with blood.' She took off the shirt and trousers, and we made love.

'What was the matter? Why did you get so angry?' We were lying side by side, so satiated and content that I thought everything would be cleared up now.

'What was the matter, what was the matter – you always ask such silly questions. You can't just leave like that.'

'But I left you a note . . .'

'Note?'

I sat up. The note was no longer on the night table where I had left it. I got to my feet, and searched next to the night table, and underneath, and under the bed and in it. I couldn't find it. 'I don't understand. I wrote you a note saying I was going to get breakfast and I'd be right back.'

'You did? I don't see any note.'

'You don't believe me?'

'I'd love to believe you. But I don't see any note.'

We didn't go on fighting. Had a gust of wind come and taken the note and carried it away to God knows where? Had it all been a misunderstanding, her fury, my split lip, her wounded face, my helplessness?

Should I have gone on searching, for the note, for the cause of Hanna's fury, for the source of my helplessness? 'Read me something, kid!' She cuddled up to me and I picked up Eichendorff's *Memoirs of a Good-for-Nothing* and continued from where I had left off. *Memoirs of a Good-for-Nothing* was easy to read aloud, easier than *Emilia Galotti* and *Intrigues and Love*. Again, Hanna followed everything eagerly. She liked the scattering of poems. She liked the disguises, the mix-ups, the complications and pursuits which the hero gets tangled up in in Italy. At the same time, she held it against him that he's a good-for-nothing who doesn't achieve anything, can't do anything, and doesn't want to besides. She was torn in all directions; hours after I stopped reading, she was still coming up with questions. 'Customs collector – wasn't much of a job?'

Once again the report on our fight has become so detailed that I would like to report on our happiness. The fight made our relationship more intimate. I had seen her crying. The Hanna who could cry was closer to me than the Hanna who was only strong. She began to show a soft side that I had never seen before. She kept looking at my split lip, until it healed, and stroking it gently.

We made love a different way. For a long time I had abandoned myself to her and her power of possession. Then I had also learned to take possession of her. On this trip and afterwards, we no longer merely took possession of each other.

I have a poem that I wrote back then. As poetry, it's worthless. At the time I was in love with Rilke and Benn, and I can see that I wanted to imitate them both. But I can also see how close we were at that time. Here is the poem:

> *When we open ourselves*
> *you yourself to me and I myself to you,*
> *when we submerge*
> *you into me and I into you*

T042728

when we vanish
you into me, and into you I

Then
am I me
and you are you

CHAPTER TWELVE

WHILE I HAVE NO MEMORY OF THE lies I told my parents about the trip with Hanna, I do remember the price I had to pay to stay alone at home the last week of the holidays. I can't recall where my parents and my older brother and sister were going. The problem was my little sister. She was supposed to go and stay with a friend's family. But if I was going to be at home, she wanted to be at home as well. My parents didn't want that. So I was supposed to go and stay with a friend too.

As I look back, I find it remarkable that my parents were willing to leave me, a fifteen-year-old, at home alone for a week. Had they noticed the independence that had been growing in me since I met Hanna? Or had they simply registered that fact that I had passed the class despite the months of illness and decided that I was more responsible and trustworthy than I had shown myself to be until then? Nor do I remember being called on to explain the many hours I spent at Hanna's. My parents apparently believed that, now that I was healthy again, I wanted to be with my friends as much as possible, whether studying or just enjoying our free time. Besides, when parents have a pack of four children, their attention cannot cover everything, and tends to focus on whichever one is causing the most problems at the moment. I had caused problems for long enough; my parents were relieved that I was healthy and would be moving up into the next class.

When I asked my little sister what her price was for going to stay with her friend while I stayed at home, she demanded jeans — we called them blue jeans back then, or studded pants — and a Nicki, which was a velour jumper. That made sense. Jeans were still something special at that time, they were chic, and they promised liberation from herringbone suits and big-flowered dresses. Just as I had to wear my brother's things, my little sister had to wear her big sister's. But I had no money.

'Then steal them!' said my little sister with perfect equanimity.

It was astonishingly easy. I tried on various jeans, took a pair her size with me into the fitting room, and carried them out of the store against my stomach under my wide suit trousers. The jumper I stole from the big main department store. My little sister and I went in one day and strolled from stand to stand in the fashion department until we found the right stand and the right jumper. Next day I marched quickly through the department, seized the jumper, hid it under my suit jacket, and was outside again. The day after that I stole a silk nightdress for Hanna, was spotted by the store detective, ran for my life, and escaped by a hair. I didn't go back to the department store for years after that.

Since our nights together on the trip, I had longed every night to feel her next to me, to curl up against her, my stomach against her behind and my chest against her back, to rest my hand on her breasts, to reach out for her when I woke up in the night, find her, push my leg over her legs, and press my face against her shoulder. A week alone at home meant seven nights with Hanna.

One evening I invited her to the house and cooked for her. She stood in the kitchen as I put the finishing touches on the food. She stood in the open double doors between the dining room and sitting room as I served. She sat at the round dining table where my father usually sat. She looked around.

Her eyes explored everything – the Biedermeier furniture, the piano, the old grandfather clock, the pictures, the bookcases, the plates and cutlery on the table. When I left her alone to prepare pudding, she was not at the table when I came back. She had gone from room to room and was standing in my father's study. I leaned quietly against the doorpost and watched her. She let her eyes drift over the bookshelves that filled the walls, as if she were reading a text. Then she went to a shelf, raised her right index finger chest high and ran it slowly along the backs of the books, moved to the next shelf, ran her finger further along, from one spine to the next, pacing off the whole room. She stopped at the window, looked out into the darkness, at the reflection of the bookshelves, and at her own.

It is one of the pictures of Hanna that has stayed with me. I have them stored away, I can project them on a mental screen and watch them, unchanged, unconsumed. There are long periods when I don't think about them at all. But they always come back into my head, and then I sometimes have to run them repeatedly through my mental projector and watch them. One is Hanna putting on her stockings in the kitchen. Another is Hanna standing in front of the bath holding the towel in her outstretched arms. Another is Hanna riding her bike with her skirt blowing in her slipstream. Then there is the picture of Hanna in my father's study. She's wearing a blue-and-white striped dress, what they called a shirt-waister back then. She looks young in it. She has run her finger along the backs of the books and looked into the darkness of the window. She turns to me, quickly enough that the skirt swings out around her legs for a moment before it hangs smooth again. Her eyes are tired.

'Are these books your father has just read, or did he write them too?'

I knew there was a book on Kant and another on Hegel that my father had written, and I searched for them and showed them to her.

'Read me something from them. Please, kid?'

'I . . .' I didn't want to, but didn't like to refuse her either. I took my father's Kant book and read her a passage on analysis and dialectics that neither of us understood. 'Is that enough?'

She looked at me as though she had understood it all, or as if it didn't matter whether anything was understandable or not. 'Will you write books like that some day?'

I shook my head.

'Will you write other books?'

'I don't know.'

'Will you write plays?'

'I don't know, Hanna.'

She nodded. Then we ate pudding and went to her flat. I would have liked to sleep with her in my bed, but she didn't want to. She felt like an intruder in our house. She didn't say it in so many words, but in the way she stood in the kitchen or in the open double doors, or walked from room to room, inspected my father's books and sat with me at dinner.

I gave her the silk nightdress. It was aubergine-coloured with narrow straps that left her shoulders and arms bare, and came down to her ankles. It shone and shimmered. Hanna was delighted; she laughed and beamed. She looked down at herself, turned around, danced a few steps, looked at herself in the mirror, checked her reflection, and danced some more. That too is a picture of Hanna that has stayed with me.

CHAPTER THIRTEEN

*I*ALWAYS EXPERIENCED THE BEGIN-
ning of a new school year as a watershed.
Moving up into the sixth form was a major one.
My class was disbanded and divided into three parallel
classes. Quite a few students had failed to make the grade,
so four small classes were combined into three larger
ones.

My school traditionally had taken only boys. When
girls began to be accepted, there were so few of them to
begin with that they were not divided equally among the
parallel classes, but were assigned to a single class, then
later to a second and a third, until they made up a third

of each class. There were not enough girls in my year for any to be assigned to my former class. We were the fourth parallel class, and all boys, which is why we were the ones to be disbanded and reassigned, and not one of the other classes.

We didn't find out about it until school began. The headmaster summoned us into a classroom and informed us about the why and how of our reassignment. Along with six others, I crossed the empty halls to the new classroom. We got the seats that were left over; mine was in the second row. They were individual seats, but in pairs, divided into three rows. I was in the middle row. On my left I had a classmate from my old class, Rudolf Bargen, a heavy-set, calm, dependable chess and hockey player with whom I hadn't ever spent any time in my old class, but who soon became a good friend. On my right, across the aisle, were the girls.

My neighbour was Sophie. Brown hair, brown eyes, brown summer skin, with tiny golden hairs on her bare arms. After I'd sat down and looked around, she smiled at me.

I smiled back. I felt good, I was excited about a new start in a new class, and the girls. I had observed my year in the fifth form: whether they had girls in their class or not, they were afraid of them, or kept out of their way, or showed off to them, or worshipped them. I knew my way around women, and could be comfortable and open in a friendly way. The girls liked that. I would get along with them well in the new class, which meant I'd get along with the boys too.

Does everyone feel this way? When I was young, I was perpetually overconfident or insecure. Either I felt completely useless, unattractive, and worthless, or that I was pretty much a success, and everything I did was bound to succeed. When I was confident, I could overcome the hardest challenges. But all it took was the smallest setback, for me to be sure that I was utterly worthless. Regaining my self-confidence had nothing to do with success; every goal I set myself, every recognition I craved made anything I actually did seem paltry by comparison, and whether I experienced it as a failure or triumph was utterly dependent on my mood. With Hanna things felt good for weeks – in spite of our fights, in spite of the fact that she pushed me away again and again, and again and again I crawled to her. And so summer in the new class began well.

I can still see the classroom: right front, the door; along the right-hand wall the board with the clothes hooks; on the left a row of windows looking onto the Heiligenberg and – when we stood next to the glass at break – down at the streets, the river and the meadows on the opposite bank; in front, the blackboard, the stands for maps and diagrams, and the reader's desk and chair on a foot-high platform. The walls had yellow oil paint on them to about head height, and above that, white; and from the ceiling hung two milky glass globes. There was not one superfluous thing in the room: no pictures, no plants, no extra chair, no cupboard with forgotten books and notebooks and coloured chalk. When your eyes wandered, they wandered to what was outside the window, or to whoever was sitting next to you. When Sophie saw me looking at her, she turned and smiled at me.

'Berg, Sophia may be a Greek name, but that is no reason for you to study your neighbour in a Greek lesson. Translate!'

We were translating the *Odyssey*. I had read it in German, loved it, and love it to this day. When it was my turn, it took me only seconds to find my place and translate. After the teacher had stopped teasing me about Sophie and the class had stopped laughing, it was something else that made me stutter. Nausicaa, white-armed and virginal, who in body and features resembled the immortals – should I imagine her as Hanna or as Sophie? It had to be one of the two.

CHAPTER FOURTEEN

WHEN AN AEROPLANE'S ENGINES fail, it is not the end of the flight. Aeroplanes don't fall out of the sky like stones. They glide on, the enormous multi-engined passenger jets, for thirty, forty-five minutes, only to smash themselves up when they attempt a landing. The passengers don't notice a thing. Flying feels the same whether the engines are working or not. It's quieter, but only slightly: the wind drowns out the engines as it buffets the tail and wings. At some point, the earth or sea look dangerously close through the window. But perhaps the film is on, and the stewards and air hostesses have closed the blinds. Maybe the very quietness of the flight strikes the passengers as an improvement.

That summer was the glide path of our love. Or rather, of my love for Hanna. I don't know about her love for me.

We kept up our ritual of reading aloud, showering, making love, and then lying together. I read her *War and Peace* with all of Tolstoy's disquisitions on history, great men, Russia, love and marriage; it must have lasted forty or fifty hours. Again, Hanna became absorbed in the unfolding of the story. But it was different this time; she withheld her own opinions; she didn't make Natasha, Andrei, and Pierre part of her world, as she had Luise and Emilia, but entered their world the way one sets out on a long and dazzling journey, or enters a castle which one is allowed to visit, even stay in until one feels at home, but without ever really shedding one's inhibitions. All the things I had read to her before were already familiar to me. *War and Peace* was new for me, too. We took the long journey together.

We thought up pet names for each other. She began not just to call me Kid, but gave me other attributes and diminutives, such as Frog or Toad, Puppy, Toy, and Rose. I stuck to Hanna, until she asked me, 'Which animal do you see when you hold me and close your eyes and think of animals?' I closed my eyes and thought of animals. We were lying snuggled close together, my head on her neck, my neck on her breasts, my right arm underneath her against her back and my left hand on her bottom. I ran my arms and hands over her broad back, her hard thighs, her firm bottom, and also felt the solidity of her breasts and stomach against my neck and chest. Her skin was smooth and soft to the touch, the body beneath it strong and reliable. When my hand lay on her calf, I felt the constant twitching play of muscles. It reminded me of the way a horse twitches its hide to repel flies. 'A horse.'

'A horse?' She disentangled herself, sat up and stared at me, stared in shock.

'You don't like it? It came to me because you feel so good, smooth and soft and all firm and strong underneath. And because your calf twitches.' I explained my association.

She looked at the ripple of the muscles in her calf. 'Horse.' She shook her head. 'I don't know . . .'

That wasn't how she usually was. Usually she was absolutely single-minded, whether in agreement or disagreement. Faced with her look of shock, I had been ready to take it all back if necessary, blame myself, and apologize. But now I tried to reconcile her to the horse. 'I could call you Cheval or Pony or Little Equus. When I think of horses, I don't think horse's teeth or horse face or whatever it is that worries you, I think of something good, warm, soft, strong. You're not a bunny or a kitten, and whatever there is in a tiger – that evil something – that's not you either.'

She lay down on her back, arms behind her head. Now

it was me who sat up to look at her. She was staring into space. After a while she turned her face to me. Her expression was curiously naked. 'Yes, I like it when you call me Horse or those other horse names – can you explain them to me?'

Once we went to the theatre in the next town to see Schiller's *Intrigues and Love*. It was the first time Hanna had been to the theatre and she loved all of it, from the performance to the champagne at the interval. I put my arm around her waist, and didn't care what people might think of us as a couple, and I was proud that I didn't care. At the same time, I knew that in the theatre in our home town I would care. Did she know that too?

She knew that my life that summer no longer revolved around her, and school, and my studies. More and more, when I came to her in the late afternoon, I came from the swimming pool. That was where our class got together, did our homework, played football and volleyball and skat, and flirted. That was where our class socialized, and it meant a lot to me to be part of it and to belong. The fact that I came later than the others or left earlier, depending on Hanna's shifts, didn't hurt my reputation, but made me interesting. I knew that. I also knew that I wasn't missing anything, and yet I often had the feeling that absolutely everything could be happening while I wasn't there. There was a long stretch when I did not dare ask myself whether I would rather be at the swimming pool or with Hanna. But on my birthday in

July, there was a party for me at the pool, and it was hard to tear myself away from it when they didn't want me to go, and then an exhausted Hanna received me in a bad mood. She didn't know it was my birthday. When I had asked her about hers, and she had told me it was the twenty-first of October, she hadn't asked me when mine was. She was also no more bad-tempered than she always was when she was exhausted. But I was annoyed by her bad temper, and I wanted to be somewhere else, at the pool, away with my classmates, swept up in the exuberance of our talk, our banter, our games, and our flirtations. Then when I proceeded to get bad-tempered myself and we started a fight and Hanna treated me like a nonentity, the fear of losing her returned and I humbled myself and begged her pardon until she took me back. But I was filled with resentment.

CHAPTER FIFTEEN

*T*HEN I BEGAN TO BETRAY HER.

Not that I gave away any secrets or exposed Hanna. I didn't reveal anything that I should have kèpt to myself. I kept something to myself that I should have revealed. I didn't acknowledge her. I know that disavowal is an unusual form of betrayal. From the outside it is impossible to tell if you are disowning someone or simply exercising discretion, being considerate, avoiding embarrassments and sources of irritation. But you, who are doing the disowning, you know what you're doing. And disavowal pulls the underpinnings away from a relationship just as surely as other more flamboyant types of betrayal.

I no longer remember when I first denied Hanna. Friendships coalesced out of the casual ease of those summer afternoons at the swimming pool. Aside from the boy who sat next to me in school, whom I knew from the old class, the person I liked especially in the new class was Holger Schlüter, who like me was interested in history and literature, and with whom I quickly felt at ease. He also got along with Sophie, who lived a few streets away from me, which meant that we went to and from the swimming pool together. At first I told myself that I wasn't yet close enough to my friends to tell them about Hanna. Then I didn't find the right opportunity, the right moment, the right words. And finally it was too late to tell them about Hanna, to present her along with all my other youthful secrets. I told myself that talking about her so belatedly would misrepresent things, make it seem as if I had kept silent about Hanna for so long because our relationship wasn't right and I felt guilty about it. But no matter what I pretended to myself, I knew that I was betraying Hanna when I acted as if I was letting my friends in on everything important in my life but said nothing about Hanna.

The fact that they knew I wasn't being completely open only made things worse. One evening Sophie and I got caught in a thunderstorm on our way home and took shelter under the overhang of a garden shed in

Neuenheimer Feld, which had no university buildings on it then, just fields and gardens. It thundered, the lightning crackled, the wind came in gusts, and rain fell in big heavy drops. At the same time the temperature dropped a good ten degrees. We were freezing, and I put my arm around her.

'You know . . .' She wasn't looking at me, but out at the rain.

'What?'

'You were sick with hepatitis for a long time. Is that what's on your mind? Are you afraid you won't really get well again? Did the doctors say something? And do you have to go to the clinic every day to give blood or get transfusions?'

Hanna as illness. I was ashamed. But I really couldn't start talking about Hanna at this point. 'No, Sophie, I'm not sick any more. My liver is normal, and in a year I'll even be able to drink alcohol if I want, but I don't. What's . . .' Talking about Hanna, I didn't want to say 'what's bothering me.' 'There's another reason I arrive later or leave earlier.'

'Do you not want to talk about it, or is it that you want to but you don't know how?'

Did I not want to, or didn't I know how? I didn't know the answer. But as we stood there under the lightning, with the explosions of thunder rumbling almost overhead and the pounding of the rain, both freezing, warming each other a little, I had the feeling that I had to tell her, of all people, about Hanna. 'Maybe I can tell you some other time.'

But there never was another time.

CHAPTER SIXTEEN

I NEVER FOUND OUT WHAT HANNA DID when she wasn't working and we weren't together. When I asked, she turned away my questions. We did not have a world that we shared; she gave me the space in her life that she wanted me to have. I had to be content with that. Wanting more, even wanting to know more, was presumption on my part. If we were particularly happy with each other and I asked her something because at that moment it felt as if everything was possible and allowed, then she sometimes ducked my questions, instead of refusing outright to answer them. 'The things you ask, kid!' Or she would take my hand and lay it on her stomach. 'Are you trying to make holes in me?' Or she would count on her fingers. 'Laundry, ironing, sweeping, dusting, shopping, cooking, shake plums out of tree, pick up plums, bring plums home and cook them quick before the little one' – and here she would take hold of the fifth finger of her left hand between her right thumb and forefinger – 'eats them all himself.'

I never met her unexpectedly on the street or in a store or a cinema, although she told me she loved going to the movies, and in our first months together I always wanted to go with her, but she wouldn't let me. Sometimes we talked about films we had both seen. She went no matter what was showing, and saw everything, from German war and folk movies to Westerns and New Wave films, and I liked what came out of Hollywood, whether it was set in ancient Rome or the Wild West. There was one Western in particular that we both loved: the one with Richard Widmark playing a sheriff who has to fight a duel next morning that he's bound to lose, and in the evening he knocks on Dorothy Malone's door – she's been trying, but failing, to get him to make a break for it. She opens up. 'What do you want now? Your whole life in one night?' Sometimes Hanna teased me when I came to her full of desire, with 'What do you want now? Your whole life in one hour?'

Only once did I ever see Hanna by chance. It was the end of July or the beginning of August, in the last few days before the summer holidays.

Hanna had been behaving oddly for days, moody and peremptory, and at the same time palpably under some kind of pressure that was absolutely tormenting her and left her acutely sensitive and vulnerable. She pulled herself together and held herself tight as if to stop herself from exploding. When I asked what was upsetting her so, she snapped at me. That was hard for me to take. I felt rejected, but I also felt her helplessness, and I tried to be there for her and at the same time to leave her in peace. One day the pressure was gone. At first I thought Hanna was her usual self again. We had not started a new book after the end of *War and Peace*, but I had promised I'd see to it, and had brought several books to choose from.

But she didn't want that. 'Let me bathe you, kid.'

It wasn't summer's humidity that had settled on me like a heavy net when I came into the kitchen. Hanna had turned on the boiler for the bathwater. She filled the bath, put in a few drops of lavender oil, and washed me. She wore her pale blue flowered smock with no underwear underneath; the smock stuck to her sweating body in the hot, damp air. She excited me very much. When we made love, I sensed that she wanted to push me to the point of feeling things I had never felt before, to the point where I could no longer stand it. She also gave herself in a way she had never done before. She didn't abandon all reserve, she never did that. But it was as if she wanted us to drown together.

'Now go to your friends.' She dismissed me, and I went. The heat stood solidly between the buildings, lay over the fields and gardens, and shimmered above the tarmac. I was numb. At the swimming pool the shrieks of playing, splashing children reached me as if from far, far away. I moved through the world as if it had nothing to do with me nor I with it. I dived into the milky chlorinated water and felt no compulsion to surface again. I lay near the others, listening to them, and found what they said silly and pointless.

Eventually the feeling passed. Eventually it turned into an ordinary afternoon at the swimming pool with homework and volleyball and gossip and flirting. I can't remember what it was I was doing when I looked up and saw her.

She was standing twenty or thirty metres away, in shorts and an open blouse knotted at the waist, looking at me. I looked back at her. She was too far away for me to read her expression. I didn't jump to my feet and run to her. Questions raced through my head: why was she at the pool, did she want to be seen with me, did I want to be seen with her, why had we never met each other by accident, what should I do? Then I stood up. And in that briefest of moments in which I took my eyes off her, she was gone.

Hanna in shorts, with the tails of her blouse knotted, her face turned towards me but with an expression I cannot read at all – that is another picture I have of her.

CHAPTER SEVENTEEN

*N*EXT DAY, SHE WAS GONE. I CAME at the usual time and rang the bell. I looked through the door, everything looked the way it always did. I could hear the clock ticking.

I sat down on the stairs once again. During our first few months, I had always known what line she was working on, even though I had never repeated my attempt to accompany her or even pick her up afterwards. At some point I had stopped asking, stopped even wondering. It hadn't even occurred to me until now.

I used the telephone booth at the Wilhelmsplatz to call the tram company, was transferred from one person to the next, and finally was told that Hanna Schmitz had not come to work. I went back to Bahnhofstrasse, asked at the carpenter's shop in the yard for the name of the owner of the building, and got a name and address in Kirchheim. I rode over there.

'Frau Schmitz? She moved out this morning.'

'And her furniture?'

'It's not her furniture.'

'How long did she live in the flat?'

'What's it to you?' The woman who had been talking to me through a window in the door slammed it shut.

In the administration building of the tram company, I talked my way through to the personnel department. The man in charge was friendly and concerned.

'She called this morning early enough for us to arrange for a substitute, and said that she wouldn't be coming back, full stop.' He shook his head. 'Two weeks ago she was sitting there in your chair and I offered to have her trained as a driver, and she throws it all away.'

It took me some days to think of going to the citizen's registration office. She had informed them she was moving to Hamburg, but without giving an address.

The days went by and I felt sick. I took pains to make sure my parents and my brother and sisters noticed nothing. I joined in the conversation at table a little, ate a little, and when I had to throw up, I managed to make it to the toilet. I went to school and to the swimming pool. I spent my afternoons there in an out-of-the-way place where no one would look for me. My body yearned for Hanna. But even worse than my physical desire was my sense of guilt. Why hadn't I jumped up immediately when she stood there and run to her! It was a microcosm of all my half-heartedness of the past months, which had produced my denial of her, and my betrayal. Leaving was her punishment.

Sometimes I tried to tell myself that it wasn't her I had seen. How could I be sure it was her when I hadn't been able to make out the face? If it had been her, wouldn't I have had to recognize her face? So couldn't I be sure it wasn't her at all?

But I knew it was her. She stood and looked – and it was too late.

Part Two

CHAPTER ONE

*A*FTER HANNA LEFT THE CITY, IT TOOK a while before I stopped expecting to see her everywhere, before I got used to the fact that afternoons had lost their shape, and before I could look at books and open them without asking myself whether they were suitable for reading aloud. It took a while before my body stopped yearning for hers; sometimes I myself was aware of my arms and legs groping for her in my sleep, and my brother reported more than once at table that I had called out 'Hanna' in the night. I can also remember classes at school when I did nothing but dream of her, think of her. The feeling of guilt that had tortured me in the first weeks gradually faded. I avoided her building, took other routes, and six months later my family moved to another part of town. It wasn't that I forgot Hanna. But at a certain point the memory of her stopped accompanying me wherever I went. She stayed behind, the way a city stays behind as a train pulls out of the station. It's there, somewhere behind you, and you could go back and make sure of it. But why should you?

I remember my last years of school and my first years at university as happy. Yet I can't say very much about them. They were effortless; I had no difficulty with my final exams at school or with the legal studies that I chose because I couldn't think of anything else I really wanted to do; I had no difficulty with friendships, with relationships or the end of relationships – I had no difficulty with anything. Everything was easy; nothing weighed heavily. Perhaps that is why my bundle of memories is so small. Or do I keep it small? I wonder if my memory of happiness is even true. If I think about it more, plenty of embarrassing and painful situations come to mind, and I know that even if I had said goodbye to my memory of Hanna, I had not overcome it. Never to let myself be humiliated or humiliate myself after Hanna, never to take guilt upon myself or feel guilty, never again to love anyone whom it would hurt to lose – I didn't formulate any of this as I thought back then, but I know that's how I felt.

I adopted a posture of arrogant superiority. I behaved as if nothing could touch or shake or confuse me. I got involved in nothing, and I remember a teacher who saw through this and spoke to me about it; I was arrogantly dismissive. I also remember Sophie. Not long after Hanna left the city, Sophie was diagnosed with tuberculosis. She spent three years in a sanatorium, returning just as I went to university. She felt lonely, and sought out contact with her old friends. It wasn't hard for me to find a way into her heart. After we slept together, she realized I wasn't interested in her; in tears, she asked, 'What's happened to you, what's happened to you?' I remember my grandfather during one of my last visits before his death; he wanted to bless me, and I told him I didn't believe in any of that and didn't want it. It is hard for me to imagine that I felt good about behaving like that. I also remember that the smallest gesture of affection would bring a lump to my throat, whether it was directed at me or at someone else. Somehow all it took was a scene in a film. This juxtaposition of callousness and extreme sensitivity seemed suspicious even to me.

CHAPTER TWO

*W*HEN I SAW HANNA AGAIN, IT WAS in a courtroom.

It wasn't the first trial dealing with the camps, nor was it one of the major ones. Our professor, one of the few at that time who were working on the Nazi past and the related trials, made it the subject of a seminar, in the hope of being able to follow the entire trial with the help of his students, and evaluate it. I can no longer remember what it was he wanted to examine, confirm, or disprove. I do remember that we argued the prohibition of retroactive justice in the seminar. Was it sufficient that the ordinances under which the camp guards and enforcers were convicted were already on the statute books at the time they committed their crimes? Or was it a question of how the laws were actually interpreted and enforced at the time they committed their crimes, and that they were not applied to them? What is law? Is it what is on the books, or what is actually enacted and obeyed in a society? Or is law what must be enacted and obeyed, whether or not it is on the books, if things are to go right? The professor, an old gentleman who had returned from exile but remained an outsider among German legal scholars, participated in these debates with all the force of his scholarship, and yet at the same time with a detachment that no longer relied on pure scholarship to provide the solution to a problem. 'Look at the defendants – you won't find a single one who really believes he had the dispensation to murder back then.'

The seminar began in winter, the trial in spring. It lasted for weeks. The court was in session Monday to Thursday, and the professor assigned a group of students to keep a word-for-word record for each day. The seminar was held on Fridays, and explored the data gathered during the preceding week.

Exploration! Exploring the past! We students in the camps seminar considered ourselves radical explorers. We tore open the windows and let in the air, the wind that finally whirled away the dust that society had permitted to settle over the horrors of the past. We made sure people could breathe and see. And we placed no reliance on legal scholarship. It was evident to us that there had to be convictions. It was just as evident that conviction of this or that camp guard or enforcer was only the prelude. The generation that had been served by the guards and enforcers, or had done nothing to stop them, or had not banished them from its midst as it could have done after 1945, was in the dock, and we explored it, subjected it to trial by daylight, and condemned it to shame.

Our parents had played a variety of roles in the Third Reich. Several among our fathers had been in the war, two or three of them as officers of the Wehrmacht and one as an officer of the Waffen SS. Some of them had held positions in the judiciary or local government. Our parents also included teachers and doctors, and one of us had an uncle who had been a high official in the Ministry of the Interior. I am sure that to the extent that we asked and to the extent that they answered us, they had very different stories to tell. My father did not want to talk about himself, but I knew that he had lost his job as a university lecturer in philosophy for scheduling a lecture on Spinoza, and had got himself and us through the war as an editor for a house that published hiking maps and books. How did I decide that he too was under sentence of shame? But I did. We all condemned our parents to shame, even if the only charge we could bring was that after 1945 they had tolerated the perpetrators in their midst.

We students in the seminar developed a strong group

identity. We were the students of the camps – that's what the other students called us, and how we soon came to describe ourselves. What we were doing didn't interest the others; it alienated many of them, literally repelled some. When I think about it now, I think that our eagerness to assimilate the horrors and our desire to make everyone else aware of them was in fact repulsive. The more horrible the events about which we read and heard, the more certain we became of our responsibility to enlighten and accuse. Even when the facts took our breath away, we held them up triumphantly. Look at this!

I had enrolled in the seminar out of sheer curiosity. It was finally something new, not buyer's rights and not ordinary criminal activity or conspiracy thereto, not Saxon precedents or ancient bits of philosophical jurisprudence. I brought to the seminar my arrogant, superior airs. But as the winter went on, I found it harder and harder to withdraw – either from the events we read and heard about, or from the zeal that seized the students in the seminar. At first, I pretended to myself that I only wanted to participate in the scholarly debate, or the political and moral fervour. But I wanted more; I wanted to share in the general passion. The others may have found me distant and arrogant; for my part, I had the good feeling all that winter that I belonged, and that I was at peace with myself about what I was doing and the people with whom I was doing it.

CHAPTER THREE

*T*HE TRIAL WAS IN ANOTHER TOWN, about an hour's drive away. I had no other reason ever to go there. Another student drove. He had grown up there and knew the place.

It was a Thursday. The trial had begun on Monday. The first three days of proceedings had been taken up with defence motions to recuse. Our group was the fourth, and so would witness the examination of the defendants at the actual start of proceedings.

We drove along Bergstrasse under blossoming fruit trees. We were bubbling over with exhilaration: finally we could put all our training into practice. We did not feel like mere spectators, or listeners, or recorders. Watching and listening and recording were our contributions to the exploration of history.

The court was in a turn-of-the-century building, but devoid of the gloomy pomposity so characteristic of court buildings of the time. The room that housed the assize court had a row of large windows down the left-hand side, with milky glass that blocked the view of the outdoors but let in a great deal of light. The prosecutors sat in front of the windows, and against the bright spring and summer daylight they were no more than black silhouettes. The court, three judges in black robes and six selected citizens, was in place at the head of the courtroom and on the right-hand side was the bench of defendants and their lawyers: there were so many of them that the extra chairs and tables stretched into the middle of the room in front of the public seats. Some of the defendants and their lawyers were sitting with their backs to us. One of them was Hanna. I did not recognize her until she was called, and she stood up and stepped forward. Of course I recognized the name as soon as I heard it: Hanna Schmitz. Then I also recognized the body, the head with the hair gathered in an unfamiliar knot, the neck, the broad back, and the strong arms. She held herself very straight, balanced on both feet. Her arms were relaxed at her sides. She wore a grey dress with short sleeves. I recognized her, but I felt nothing. Nothing at all.

Yes, she wished to stand. Yes, she was born on 21 October 1922, near Hermannstadt and was now forty-three years old. Yes, she had worked at Siemens in Berlin and had joined the SS in the autumn of 1943.

'You enrolled voluntarily?'

'Yes.'

'Why?'

Hanna did not answer.

'Is it true that you joined the SS even though Siemens had offered you a job as a foreman?'

Hanna's lawyer was on his feet. 'What do you mean by "even though"? Do you mean to suggest that a woman should prefer to become a foreman at Siemens than join the SS? There are no grounds for making my client's decision the object of such a question.'

He sat down. He was the only young defence attorney; the others were old – some of them, as became apparent, old Nazis. Hanna's lawyer avoided both their jargon and their lines of reasoning. But he was too hasty and too zealous in ways that were as damaging to his client as his colleagues' Nazi tirades were to theirs. He did succeed in making the judge grimace and stop pursuing the question of why Hanna had joined the SS. But the impression remained that she had done it of her own accord and not under pressure. When one of the lay members of the court asked Hanna what kind of work she expected to do for the SS and she said that the SS was recruiting women at Siemens and other factories for guard duties and she had applied and was hired, the negative impression was reinforced.

To the judge's questions, Hanna testified in mono-syllables that yes, she had served in Auschwitz until early 1944 and then in a small camp near Cracow until the winter of 1944–5, that yes, when the prisoners were moved to the west she went with them all the way, that she was in Kassel at the end of the war and since then had lived in one place and another. She had been in my city for eight years; it was the longest time she had spent in any one place.

'Is her frequent change of residence supposed to be grounds for viewing her as a flight risk?' The lawyer was openly sarcastic. 'My client registered with the police each time she arrived at a new address and each time she left. There is no reason to assume she would run away, and there is nothing for her to hide. Did the judge feel it impossible to release my client on her own recognizance because of the gravity of the charges and the risk of public agitation? That, members of the court, is a Nazi rationale for custody; it was introduced by the Nazis and abolished after the Nazis. It no longer exists.' The lawyer's malicious emphasis underlined the irony in this truth.

I was jolted. I realized that I had assumed it was both natural and right that Hanna should be in custody. Not because of the charges, the gravity of the allegations, or the force of the evidence, of which I had no real knowl-edge, but because in a cell she was out of my world, out of my life. I wanted her far away from me, so unattainable that she could continue as the mere memory she had become and remained all these years. If the lawyer was successful, I would have to prepare myself to meet her again, and I would have to work out how I wanted to do that, and how it should be. And I could see no reason why he should fail. If Hanna had not tried to escape the law so far, why should she try now? And what evidence could she suppress? There were no other reasons at that time to hold someone in custody.

The judge seemed irritated again, and I began to realize that this was his particular trick. Whenever he found a statement either obstructive or annoying, he took off his glasses, stared at the speaker with a blank, short-sighted gaze, frowned, and either ignored the statement altogether or began with 'So you mean' or 'So what you're trying to say is' and then repeated what had been said in a way as to leave no doubt that he had no desire to deal with it and that trying to compel him to do so would be pointless.

'So you're saying that the arresting judge misinterpreted the fact that the defendant ignored all letters and summonses, and did not present herself either to the police, or the prosecutor, or the judge? You wish to make a motion to lift the order of detention?'

The lawyer made the motion and the court denied it.

CHAPTER FOUR

I DID NOT MISS A SINGLE DAY OF THE trial. The other students were surprised. The professor was pleased that one of us was making sure that the next group found out what the last one had heard and seen.

Only once did Hanna look at the spectators and over at me. Usually she was brought in by a guard and took her place and then kept her eyes fixed on the bench throughout the day's proceedings. It appeared arrogant, as did the fact that she didn't talk to the other defendants and almost never with her lawyer either. However, as the trial went on, the other defendants talked less among themselves too. When there were breaks in the proceedings, they stood with relatives and friends, and in the mornings they waved and called hello to them when they saw them in the public benches. During the breaks Hanna remained in her seat.

So I watched her from behind. I saw her head, her neck, her shoulders. I decoded her head, her neck, her shoulders. When she was being discussed, she held her head very erect. When she felt she was being unjustly treated, slandered, or attacked and she was struggling to respond, she rolled her shoulders forward and her neck swelled, showing the play of muscles. The objections were regularly overruled, and her shoulders regularly sank. She never shrugged, and she never shook her head. She was too wound up to allow herself anything as casual as a shrug or a shake of the head. Nor did she allow herself to hold her head at an angle, or to let it fall, or to lean her chin on her hand. She sat as if frozen. It must have hurt to sit that way.

Sometimes strands of hair slipped out of the tight knot, began to curl, lay on the back of her neck, and moved gently against it in the draught. Sometimes Hanna wore a dress with a neckline low enough to reveal the birthmark high on her left shoulder. Then I remembered how I had blown the hair away from that neck and how I had kissed that birthmark and that neck. But the memory was like a retrieved file. I felt nothing.

During the weeks of the trial, I felt nothing: my feelings were numbed. Sometimes I poked at them, and imagined Hanna doing what she was accused of doing as clearly as I could, and also doing what the hair on her neck and the birthmark on her shoulder recalled to my mind. It was like a hand pinching an arm numbed by an injection. The arm doesn't register that it is being pinched by the hand, the hand registers that it is pinching the arm, and at first the mind cannot tell the two of them apart. But a moment later it distinguishes them quite clearly. Perhaps the hand has pinched so hard that the flesh stays white for a while. Then the blood flows back and the spot regains its colour. But that does not bring back sensation.

Who had given me the injection? Had I done it myself, because I couldn't manage without anaesthesia? The anaesthetic functioned not only in the courtroom, and not only to allow me to see Hanna as if it was someone else who had loved and desired her, someone I knew well but who wasn't me. In every part of my life, too, I stood outside myself and watched; I saw myself functioning at the university, with my parents and brother and sisters and my friends, but inwardly I felt no involvement.

After a time I thought I could detect a similar numbness in other people. Not in the lawyers, who carried on throughout the trial with the same rhetorical legalistic pugnacity, jabbing pedantry, or loud, calculated truculence, depending on their personalities and their political standpoint. Admittedly the trial proceedings exhausted them; in the evenings they were tired and grew more shrill. But overnight they recharged or reinflated themselves and droned and hissed away the next morning just as they had twenty-four hours before. The prosecutors made an effort to keep up and display the same level of attack day after day. But they didn't succeed, at first because the facts and their outcome as laid out at the trial horrified them so much, and later because the numbness began to take hold. The effect was strongest on the judges and the lay members of the court. During the first weeks of the trial they took in the horrors – sometimes recounted in tears, sometimes in choking voices, sometimes in agitated or broken sentences – with visible shock or obvious efforts at self-control. Later their faces returned to normal; they could smile and whisper to one another or even show traces of impatience when a witness lost the thread while testifying. When going to Israel to question a witness was discussed, they were evidently itching to travel. The other students kept being horrified all over again. They only came to the trial once a week, and each time the same thing happened: the intrusion of horror into daily life. I, who was in court every day, observed their reactions with detachment.

It was like being a prisoner on death row who survives month after month and becomes accustomed to the life, while he registers with an objective eye the horror of the new arrivals: registers it with the same numbness that he brings to the murders and deaths themselves. All survivor literature talks about this numbness, in which life's functions are reduced to a minimum, behaviour becomes completely selfish and indifferent to others, and gassing and burning are everyday occurrences. In the rare accounts by perpetrators, too, the gas chambers and ovens become ordinary scenery, the perpetrators reduced to their few functions and exhibiting a mental paralysis and indifference, a dullness that makes them seem drugged or drunk. The defendants seemed to me to be trapped still, and forever, in this drugged state, in a sense petrified in it.

Even then, when I was preoccupied by this general numbness, and by the fact that it had taken hold not only of the perpetrators and victims, but of all of us, judges and lay members of the court, prosecutors and recorders, who had to deal with these events now; when I likened perpetrators, victims, the dead, the living, survivors, and their descendants to each other, I didn't feel good about it and I still don't.

Can one see them all as linked in this way? When I began to make such comparisons in discussions, I always emphasized that the linkage was not meant to relativize the difference between being forced into the world of the death camps and entering it voluntarily, between enduring suffering and imposing it on others, and that this difference was of the greatest, most critical import-ance. But I met with shock and indignation when I said this not in reaction to the others' objections, but before they had even had the chance to demur.

At the same time I ask myself, as I had already begun to ask myself back then: What should our second generation have done, what should it do with the knowledge of the horrors of the extermination of the Jews? We should not believe we can comprehend the incomprehensible, we may not compare the incomparable, we may not inquire because to inquire is to make the horrors an object of discussion, even if the horrors themselves are not questioned, instead of accepting them as something in the face of which we can only fall silent in revulsion, shame, and guilt. Should we only fall silent in revulsion, shame, and guilt? To what purpose? It was not that I had lost my eagerness to explore and cast light on things which had filled the seminar, once the trial got under way. But that some few would be convicted and punished while we of the second generation were silenced by revulsion, shame, and guilt – was that all there was to it now?

CHAPTER FIVE

*I*N THE SECOND WEEK, THE INDICT-
ment was read out. It took a day and a half to
read – a day and a half in the subjunctive. The
first defendant is alleged to have . . . Furthermore she is
alleged . . . In addition, she is alleged . . . Thus she comes
under the necessary conditions of paragraph so-and-so,
furthermore she is alleged to have committed this and
that act . . . She is alleged to have acted illegally and
culpably. Hanna was the fourth defendant.

The five accused women had been guards in a small
camp near Cracow, a satellite camp for Auschwitz. They
had been transferred there from Auschwitz in early 1944

to replace guards killed or injured in an explosion in the factory where the women in the camp worked. One count of the indictment involved their conduct at Auschwitz, but that was of minor significance compared with the other charges. I no longer remember it. Was it because it didn't involve Hanna, but only the other women? Was it of minor importance in relation to the other counts, or minor, period? Did it simply seem inexcusable to have someone on trial who had been in Auschwitz and not charge them about their conduct in Auschwitz?

Of course the five defendants had not been in charge of the camp. There was a commandant, special troops, and other female guards. Most of the troops and guards had not survived the bombing raid that put an end one night to the prisoners' westward march. Some fled the same night, and vanished as surely as the commandant, who had made himself scarce as soon as the column of prisoners set off on the forced march to the west.

None of the prisoners should, by rights, have survived the night of the bombing. But two did survive, a mother and her daughter, and the daughter had written a book about the camp and the march west and published it in America. The police and prosecutors had tracked down not only the five defendants but several witnesses who had lived in the village which had taken the bombing hits that ended the death march. The most important witnesses were the daughter, who had come to Germany, and the mother, who had remained in Israel. To take the mother's deposition the court, prosecutors, and defence lawyers were going to go to Israel – the only part of the trial I did not attend.

One main charge concerned selections in the camp. Each month around sixty new women were sent out from Auschwitz and the same number were sent back, minus those who had died in the meantime. It was clear to everyone that the women would be killed in Auschwitz; it was those who could no longer perform useful work in the factory who were sent back. The factory made munitions; the actual work was not difficult, but the women hardly ever got to do the actual work, because they had to do raw construction to repair the devastating damage caused by the explosion early in the year.

The other main charge involved the night of the bombing that ended everything. The troops and guards had locked the prisoners, several hundred women, in a church in a village that had been abandoned by most of its inhabitants. Only a few bombs fell, possibly intended for the nearby railway or a factory, or maybe simply released because they were left over from a raid on a larger town. One of them hit the priest's house in which the troops and guards were sleeping. Another landed on the church steeple. First the steeple burned, then the roof; then the blazing rafters collapsed into the nave, and the pews caught fire. The heavy doors could not be budged. The defendants could have unlocked them. They did not, and the women locked in the church burned to death.

CHAPTER SIX

HE TRIAL COULD NOT HAVE GONE any worse for Hanna. She had already made a bad impression on the court during the preliminary questioning. After the indictment had been read out, she spoke up to say that something was incorrect; the presiding judge rebuked her irritably, telling her that she had had plenty of time before the trial to study the charges and register objections; now the trial was in progress and the evidence would show what was correct and incorrect. When the presiding judge proposed at the beginning of the actual testimony that the German version of the daughter's book not be read into the record, as it had been prepared for publication by a German publisher and the manuscript made available to all participants in the trial, Hanna had to be argued into it by her lawyer under the exasperated eyes of the judge. She did not willingly agree. She also did not want to acknowledge that she had admitted, in an earlier deposition, to having had the key to the church. She had not had the key, no one had had the key, there had not been any one key to the church, but several keys to several different doors, and they had all only worked from outside. But the court record of her examination by the judge, approved and signed by her, read differently, and the fact that she asked why they were trying to pin something on her did not make matters any better. She didn't ask loudly or arrogantly, but with determination, and, I think, in visible and audible confusion and helplessness, and the fact that she spoke of others trying to pin something on her did not mean she was claiming any miscarriage of justice by the court. But the presiding judge interpreted it that way and responded sharply. Hanna's lawyer leapt to his feet and let loose, overeagerly; he was asked whether he was agreeing with his client's accusations, and sat down again.

Hanna wanted to do the right thing. When she thought she was being done an injustice, she contradicted it, and when something was rightly claimed or alleged, she acknowledged it. She contradicted vigorously and admitted willingly, as though her admissions gave her the right

to her contradictions or as though, along with her contradictions, she took on a responsibility to admit what she
could not deny. But she did not notice that her insistence
annoyed the presiding judge. She had no sense of context,
of the rules of the game, of the formulae by which her
statements and those of the others were totted up into
guilt and innocence, conviction and acquittal. To compensate for her defective grasp of the situation, her lawyer
would have had to have more experience and self-confidence, or simply to have been a better lawyer. But Hanna
should not have made things so hard for him; she was
obviously withholding her trust from him, but had not
chosen another lawyer she trusted more. Her lawyer was
a public defender appointed by the court.

Sometimes Hanna achieved her own kind of success. I
remember her examination on the selections in the camp.
The other defendants denied ever having had anything to
do with them. Hanna admitted so readily that she had
participated – not alone, but just like the others and along
with them – that the judge felt he had to probe further.

'What happened at the selections?'

Hanna described how the guards had agreed among
themselves to tally the same number of prisoners from
their six equal areas of responsibility, ten each and sixty
in all, but that the figures could fluctuate when the
number of sick was low in one person's area of responsibility and high in another's, and that all the guards on
duty had decided together who was to be sent back.

'None of you held back, you all acted together?'

'Yes.'

'Did you not know that you were sending the prisoners to their death?'

'Yes, but the new ones came, and the old ones had to make room for the new ones.'

'So because you wanted to make room, you said you and you and you have to be sent back to be killed?'

Hanna didn't understand what the presiding judge was getting at.

'I . . . I mean . . . so what would you have done?' Hanna meant it as a serious question. She did not know what she should or could have done differently, and therefore wanted to hear from the judge, who seemed to know everything, what he would have done.

Everything was quiet for a moment. It is not the custom at German trials for defendants to question the judges. But now the question had been asked, and everyone was waiting for the judge's answer. He had to answer; he could not ignore the question or brush it away with a reprimand or a dismissive counterquestion. It was clear to everyone, it was clear to him too, and I understood why he had adopted an expression of irritation as his defining feature. It was his mask. Behind it, he could take a little time to find an answer. But not too long; the longer he took, the greater the tension and expectation, and the better his answer had to be.

'There are matters one simply cannot get drawn into,

that one must distance oneself from, if the price is not life and limb.'

Perhaps this would have been all right if he had said the same thing, but referred directly to Hanna or himself. Talking about what 'one' must and must not do and what it costs did not do justice to the seriousness of Hanna's question. She had wanted to know what she should have done in her particular situation, not that there are things that are not done. The judge's answer came across as hapless and pathetic. Everyone felt it. They reacted with sighs of disappointment and stared in amazement at Hanna, who had more or less won the exchange. But she herself was lost in thought.

'So should I have . . . should I have not . . . should I not have signed up at Siemens?'

It was not a question directed at the judge. She was talking out loud to herself, hesitantly, because she had not yet asked herself that question and did not know whether it was the right one, or what the answer was.

CHAPTER SEVEN

*J*UST AS HANNA'S INSISTENT CONTRA-
dictions annoyed the judge, her willing-
ness to admit things annoyed the other
defendants. It was damaging for their defence,
but also her own.

In fact the evidence itself was favourable to the defendants. The only evidence for the main count of the indictment was the testimony of the mother who had survived,
her daughter, and the daughter's book. A competent
defence would have been able, without attacking the
substance of the mother's and daughter's testimony, to
cast reasonable doubt on whether these defendants were

the actual ones who had done the selections. Witnesses' testimony on this point was not precise, nor could it be; there had, after all, been a commandant, uniformed men, other female guards, and a whole hierarchy of responsibilities and order with which the prisoners had only been partially confronted and which, consequently, they could only partially understand. The same was true of the second count. Mother and daughter had both been locked inside the church, and could not testify as to what had happened outside. Certainly the defendants could not claim not to have been there. The other witnesses who had been living in the village then had spoken with them and remembered them. But these other witnesses had to be careful to avoid the charge that they themselves could have rescued the prisoners. If the defendants had been the only ones there – could the villagers not have overpowered the few women and unlocked the church doors themselves? Would they not have to fall in line with the defence, that the defendants had acted under a power of compulsion that also extended to them, the witnesses? That they had been forced by, or acted on the orders of, the soldiers who had either not yet fled or who, in the reasonable assumption of the guards, had left for a brief interval, perhaps to bring the wounded to the field hospital, and would be returning soon?

When the other defendants' lawyers realized that such strategies were being undone by Hanna's voluntary concessions, they switched to another strategy, which used her concessions to incriminate Hanna and exonerate the other defendants. The defence lawyers did this with professional objectivity. The other defendants backed them up with impassioned interjections.

'You stated that you knew you were sending the prisoners to their deaths – that was only true of you, wasn't it? You cannot know what your colleagues knew. Perhaps you can guess at it, but in the final analysis you cannot judge, is that not so?' Hanna was asked by one of the other defendants' lawyers.

'But we all knew . . .'

'Saying "we," "we all" is easier than saying "I," "I alone," isn't it? Isn't it true that you and only you had special prisoners in the camp, young girls, first one for a period, and then another one?'

Hanna hesitated. 'I don't think I was the only one who . . .'

'You dirty liar! Your favourites – all that was just you, no one else!' Another of the accused, a coarse woman, not unlike a fat broody hen but with a spiteful tongue, was visibly worked up.

'Is it possible that when you say "knew," the most you can actually do is assume, and that when you say "believe," you are actually just making things up?' The lawyer shook his head, as if disturbed by her acknowledgment of this. 'And is it also true that once you were tired of your special prisoners, they all went back to Auschwitz with the next transport?'

Hanna did not answer.

'That was your special, your personal selection, wasn't it? You don't want to remember, you want to hide behind something that everyone did, but . . .'

'Oh God!' The daughter, who had taken a seat in the public benches after being examined, covered her face with her hands. 'How could I have forgotten?' The presiding judge asked if she wished to add anything to her testimony. She did not wait to be called to the front. She stood up and spoke from her seat among the spectators.

'Yes, she had favourites, always one of the young ones who was weak and delicate, and she took them under her wing and made sure that they didn't have to work, got them better barracks space and took care of them and fed them better, and in the evenings she had them brought to her. And the girls were never allowed to say what she did with them in the evening, and we assumed she was . . . also because they all ended up on the transports, as if she had had her fun with them and then had got bored. But it wasn't like that at all, and one day one of them finally talked, and we learned that the girls read aloud to her, evening after evening after evening. That was better than if they . . . and better than working themselves to death on the building site. I must have thought it was better, or I couldn't have forgotten it. But was it better?' She sat down.

Hanna turned around and looked at me. Her eyes found me at once, and I realized that she had known the whole time I was there. She just looked at me. Her face didn't ask for anything, beg for anything, assure me of anything or promise anything. It simply presented itself. I saw how tense and exhausted she was. She had circles under her eyes, and there were lines on each cheek that ran from top to bottom that I'd never seen before, that weren't yet deep, but already marked her like scars. When I turned red under her gaze, she turned away and back to the judges' bench.

The presiding judge asked the lawyer who had cross-examined Hanna if he had any further questions for the defendant. He also asked Hanna's lawyer. Ask her, I thought. Ask her if she chose the weak and delicate girls, because they could never have stood up to the work on the building site anyway, because they would have been sent on the next transport to Auschwitz in any case, and because she wanted to make that final month bearable. Say it, Hanna. Say you wanted to make their last month bearable. That that was the reason for choosing the delicate and the weak. That there was no other reason, and could not be.

But the lawyer did not ask Hanna, and she did not speak of her own accord.

CHAPTER EIGHT

THE GERMAN VERSION OF THE BOOK that the daughter had written about her time in the camps did not appear until after the trial. During the trial the manuscript was available, but only to those directly involved. I had to read the book in English, an unfamiliar and laborious exercise at the time. And as always, the alien language, unmastered and struggled over, created a strange combination of distance and immediacy. One worked through the book with particular thoroughness and yet did not make it one's own. It remained alien, in the way that language is alien.

Years later I reread it and discovered that it is the book

that creates distance. It does not invite one to identify with it and makes no one sympathetic, neither the mother nor the daughter, nor those who shared their fate in various camps and finally in Auschwitz and the satellite camp near Cracow. It never gives the barracks leaders, the female guards, or the uniformed security force clear enough faces or shapes for the reader to be able to relate to them, to judge their acts for better or worse. It exudes the very numbness I have tried to describe before. But even in her numbness the daughter did not lose the ability to observe and analyze. And she had not allowed herself to be corrupted either by self-pity or by the self-confidence she had obviously drawn from the fact that she had survived and not only come through the years in the camps but given literary form to them. She writes about herself and her pubescent, precocious, and, when necessary, cunning behaviour with the same sober tone she uses to describe everything else.

Hanna is neither named in the book, nor is she recognizable or identifiable in any way. Sometimes I thought I recognized her in one of the guards, who was described as young, pretty, and obliviously conscientious in the fulfilment of her duties, but I wasn't sure. When I considered the other defendants, only Hanna could be the guard described. But there had been other guards. In one camp the daughter had known a guard who was called 'Mare', also young, beautiful, and diligent, but cruel and uncontrolled. The guard in the camp reminded her of that one. Had others drawn the same comparison? Did Hanna know about it? Did she remember it? Was that why she was upset when I compared her to a horse?

The camp near Cracow was the last stop for mother and daughter after Auschwitz. It was a step forward; the work was hard, but easier, the food was better, and it was better to sleep six women to a room than a hundred to a barracks. And it was warmer; the women could forage for wood on the way from the factory to the camp, and bring it back with them. There was the fear of selections, but it wasn't as bad as at Auschwitz. Sixty women were sent back each month, sixty out of around twelve hundred; that meant each prisoner had a life expectancy of twenty months, even if she only possessed average strength, and there was always the hope of being stronger than the average. Moreover, there was also the hope that the war would be over in less than twenty months.

The misery began when the camp was closed and the prisoners set off towards the west. It was winter, it was snowing, and the clothing in which the women had frozen in the factory and just managed to hold out in the camp was completely inadequate, but not as inadequate as what was on their feet, often rags and sheets of newspaper tied so as to stay on when they stood or walked around, but impossible to make withstand long marches in snow and ice. And the women did not just march; they were driven, and forced to run. 'Death march?' asks the daughter in the book, and answers, 'No, death trot, death gallop.'

Many collapsed along the way; others never got to their feet again after nights spent in barns or leaning against a wall. After a week, almost half the women were dead.

The church made a better shelter than the barns and walls the women had had before. When they had passed abandoned farms and stayed overnight, the uniformed security force and the female guards had taken the living quarters for themselves. Here, in the almost deserted village, they could commandeer the priest's house and still leave the prisoners something more than a barn or a wall. That they did it, and that the prisoners even got something warm to eat in the village seemed to promise an end to the misery. The women went to sleep. Shortly afterwards the bombs fell. As long as the steeple was the only thing burning, the fire could be heard in the church, but not seen. When the tip of the steeple collapsed and crashed down onto the rafters, it took several minutes for the glow of the fire to become visible. By then the flames were already licking downwards and setting clothes alight, collapsing burning beams set fire to the pews and pulpit, and soon the whole roof crashed into the nave and started a general conflagration.

The daughter thinks the women could have saved themselves if they had immediately got together to break down one of the doors. But by the time they realized what had happened and what was going to happen, and that no one was coming to open the doors, it was too late. It was completely dark when the sound of the falling bombs woke them. For a while they heard nothing but an eerie, frightening noise in the steeple, and kept absolutely quiet, so as to hear the noise better and work out what it was. That it was the crackling and snapping of a fire, that it was the glow of flames that flared up now and again behind the windows, that the crash above their heads signalled the spread of the fire from the steeple to the roof – all this the women realized only once the rafters began to burn. They realized, they screamed in horror, screamed for help, threw themselves at the doors, shook them, beat at them, screamed.

When the burning roof crashed into the nave, the shell of the walls acted like a chimney. Most of the women did not suffocate, but burned to death in the brilliant roar of the flames. In the end, the fire even burned its glowing way through the ironclad church doors. But that was hours later.

Mother and daughter survived because the mother did the right thing for the wrong reasons. When the women began to panic, she couldn't bear to be among them any more. She fled to the gallery. She didn't care that she was closer to the flames, she just wanted to be alone, away from the screaming, thrashing, burning women. The gallery was narrow, so narrow that it was barely touched by the burning beams. Mother and daughter stood pressed against the wall and saw and heard the raging of the fire. Next day they didn't dare come down and out of the church. In the darkness of the following night, they were afraid of not finding the stairs and the way out. When they left the church in the dawn of the day after that, they met some of the villagers, who gaped at them in silent astonishment, but gave them clothing and food and let them walk on.

CHAPTER NINE

'WHY DID YOU NOT UNLOCK THE doors?'

The presiding judge put the question to one defendant after another. One after the other, they gave the same answer. They couldn't unlock the doors. Why? They had been wounded when the bombs hit the priest's house. Or they had been in shock as a result of the bombardment. Or they had been busy after the bombs hit, with the wounded guard contingent, pulling them out of the rubble, bandaging them, taking care of them. They had not thought about the church, had not seen the fire in the church, had not heard the screams from the church.

The judge made the same statement to one defendant after another. The record indicated otherwise. This was deliberately cautiously phrased. To say that the record found in the SS archives said otherwise would be wrong. But it was true that it suggested something different. It listed the names of those who had been killed in the priest's house and those who had been wounded, those who had brought the wounded to a field hospital in a truck, and those who had accompanied the truck in a jeep. It indicated that the women guards had stayed behind to wait out the end of the fires, to prevent any of them from spreading and to prevent any attempts to escape under the cover of the flames. It referred to the deaths of the prisoners.

The fact that the names of the defendants appeared nowhere in the report suggested that the defendants were among the female guards who had remained behind. That these guards had remained behind to prevent attempts at escape indicated that the affair didn't end with the rescue of the wounded from the priest's house and the departure of the transport to the field hospital. The guards who remained behind, the report indicated, had allowed the fire to rage in the church and had kept the church doors locked. Among the guards who remained behind, the report indicated, were the defendants.

No, said one defendant after the other, that is not the way it was. The report was wrong. That much was evident from the fact that it mentioned the obligation of the guards to prevent the fires from spreading. How could they have carried out that responsibility? It was ridiculous, as was the other responsibility of preventing attempted escapes under the cover of the fires. Attempted escapes? By the time they no longer had to worry about their own people and could worry about the others, the prisoners, there was no one left to escape. No, the report completely ignored what they had done and achieved and suffered that night. How could such a false report have been filed? They didn't know.

Until it was the turn of the plump and vicious defendant. She knew. 'Ask that one there!' She pointed at Hanna. 'She wrote the report. She's the guilty one, she did it all, and she wanted to use the report to cover it up and drag us into it.'

The judge asked Hanna. But it was his last question. His first was 'Why did you not unlock the doors?'

'We were . . . we had . . .' Hanna was groping for the answer. 'We didn't have any alternative.'

'You had no alternative?'

'Some of us were dead, and the others had left. They said they were taking the wounded to the field hospital and would come back, but they knew they weren't coming back and so did we. Perhaps they didn't even go to the hospital, the wounded were not that badly hurt. We would have gone with them, but they said they needed the room for the wounded, and anyway they didn't ... they weren't keen to have so many women along. I don't know where they went.'

'What did you do?'

'We didn't know what to do. It all happened so fast, with the priest's house burning and the church spire, and the men and the cart were there one minute and gone the next, and suddenly we were alone with the women in the church. They left behind some weapons, but we didn't know how to use them, and even if we had, what good would it have done, since we were only a handful of women? How could we have guarded all those women? A line like that is very long, even if you keep it as tight together as possible, and to guard such a long column, you need far more people than we had.' Hanna paused. 'Then the screaming began and got worse and worse. If we had opened the doors and they had all come rushing out...'

The judge waited a moment. 'Were you afraid? Were you afraid the prisoners would overpower you?'

'That they would ... no, but how could we have restored order? There would have been chaos, and we had no way to handle that. And if they'd tried to escape...'

Once again the judge waited, but Hanna didn't finish the sentence. 'Were you afraid that if they escaped, you would be arrested, convicted, shot?'

'We couldn't just let them escape! We were responsible for them ... I mean, we had guarded them the whole time, in the camp and on the march, that was the point, that we had to guard them and not let them escape. That's why we didn't know what to do. We also had no idea how many of the women would survive the next few days. So many had died already, and the ones who were still alive were so weak . . .'

Hanna realized that what she was saying wasn't doing her case any good. But she couldn't say anything else. She could only try to say what she was saying better, to describe it better and explain it. But the more she said, the worse it looked for her. Because she was at her wit's end, she turned to the judge again.

'What would you have done?'

But this time she knew she would get no answer. She wasn't expecting one. Nobody was. The judge shook his head silently.

Not that it was impossible to imagine the confusion and helplessness Hanna described. The night, the cold, the snow, the fire, the screaming of the women in the church, the sudden departure of the people who had commanded and escorted the female guards – how could the situation have been easy? But could an acknowledgment that the situation had been hard be any mitigation for what the defendants had done or not done? As if it had been a car accident on a lonely road on a cold winter night, with injuries and vehicles written off, and no one knowing what to do? Or as if it had been a conflict between two equally compelling duties that required action? That is how one could imagine what Hanna was describing, but nobody was willing to look at it in such terms.

'Did you write the report?'

'We all discussed what we should write. We didn't want to hang any of the blame on the ones who had left. But we didn't want to attract charges that we had done anything wrong either.'

'So you're saying you talked it through together. Who wrote it?'

'You!' The other defendant pointed at Hanna.

'No, I didn't write it. Does it matter who did?'

A prosecutor suggested that an expert be called to compare the handwriting in the report and the hand-writing of the defendant Schmitz.

'My handwriting? You want my handwriting? . . .'

The judge, the prosecutor, and Hanna's lawyer discussed whether a person's handwriting retains its character over more than fifteen years and can be identified. Hanna listened and tried several times to say or ask something, and was becoming increasingly alarmed. Then she said, 'You don't have to call an expert. I admit I wrote the report.'

CHAPTER TEN

I HAVE NO MEMORY OF THE FRIDAY seminar meetings. Even when I recall the trial, I cannot remember what topics we selected for scholarly discussion. What did we talk about? What did we want to know? What did the professor teach us?

But I remember the Sundays. The days in court gave me a new hunger for the colours and smells of nature. On Fridays and Saturdays I managed to catch up on what I had missed of my studies during the other days of the week, so that I could complete my assignments and pass the course. On Sundays, I took off by myself.

Heiligenberg, St Michael's Basilica, the Bismarck Tower, the Philosophers' Path, the banks of the river – I didn't vary my route much from one Sunday to the next. I found there was enough variety in the greens that became richer and richer from week to week, and in the floodplain of the Rhine, that was sometimes in a heat haze, sometimes hidden behind curtains of rain and sometimes overhung by storm clouds, and in the smells of the berries and wild flowers in the woods when the sun blazed down on them, and of earth and last year's rotting leaves when it rained. Anyway I don't need or seek much variety. Each journey a little further than the last, the next holiday in the new place I discovered during my last holiday and liked . . . For a while I thought I should be more daring, and made myself go to Ceylon, Egypt, and Brazil, before I went back to making familiar regions more familiar. I see more in them.

I have rediscovered the place in the woods where Hanna's secret became clear to me. There is nothing special about it now, nor was there anything special then, no strangely shaped tree or cliff, no unusual view of the city and the plain, nothing that would invite startling associations. In thinking about Hanna, going round and round in the same tracks week after week, one thought had split off, taken another direction, and finally produced its own conclusion. When it did so, it was done – it could have been anywhere, or at least anywhere where the familiarity of the surroundings and the scenery allowed what was truly surprising, what didn't come like a bolt from the blue, but had been growing inside myself, to be recognized and accepted. It happened on a path that climbed steeply up the mountain, crossed the road, passed a spring, and then wound under old, tall, dark trees and out into light underbrush.

Hanna could neither read nor write.

That was why she had had people read to her. That was why she had let me do all the writing and reading on our bicycle trip and why she had lost control that morning in the hotel when she found my note, realized I would assume she knew what it said, and was afraid she'd be exposed. That was why she had avoided being promoted by the tram company; as a conductor she could conceal her weakness, but it would have become obvious when she was being trained to become a driver. That was also why she had refused the promotion at Siemens and become a camp guard. That was why she had admitted to writing the report in order to escape a confrontation with a handwriting expert. Had she talked herself into a corner at the trial for the same reason? Because she couldn't read the daughter's book or the indictment, couldn't see the openings that would allow her to build a defence, and thus could not prepare herself accordingly? Was that why she sent her chosen wards to Auschwitz? To silence them in case they had noticed something? And was that why she always chose the weak ones in the first place?

Was that why? I could understand that she was ashamed at not being able to read or write, and would rather drive me away than expose herself. I was no stranger to shame as the cause of behaviour that was deviant or defensive, secretive or misleading or hurtful. But could Hanna's shame at being illiterate be sufficient reason for her behaviour at the trial or in the camp? To accept exposure as a criminal for fear of being exposed as an illiterate? To commit crimes to avoid the same thing?

How often I have asked myself these same questions, both then and since. If Hanna's motive was fear of exposure – why opt for the horrible exposure as a criminal over the harmless exposure as an illiterate? Or did she believe she could escape exposure altogether? Was she simply stupid? And was she vain enough, and evil enough, to become a criminal simply to avoid exposure?

Both then and since, I have always rejected this. No, Hanna had not decided in favour of crime. She had decided against a promotion at Siemens, and had fallen into a job as a guard. And no, she had not dispatched the delicate and the weak on transports to Auschwitz because they had read to her; she had chosen them to read to her because she wanted to make their last month bearable before their inevitable dispatch to Auschwitz. And no, at the trial Hanna did not weigh exposure as an illiterate against exposure as a criminal. She did not calculate and she did not manoeuvre. She accepted that she would be called to account, and simply did not wish to endure further exposure. She was not pursuing her own interests, but fighting for her own truth, her own justice. Because she always had to dissimulate somewhat, and could never be completely candid, it was a pitiful truth and a pitiful justice, but it was hers, and the struggle for it was her struggle.

She must have been completely exhausted. Her struggle was not limited to the trial. She was struggling, as she always had struggled, not to show what she could do but to hide what she couldn't do. A life made up of advances that were actually frantic retreats and victories that were concealed defeats.

I was oddly moved by the discrepancy between what must have been Hanna's actual concerns when she left my home town and what I had imagined and theorized at the time. I had been sure that I had driven her away because I had betrayed and denied her, when in fact she had simply been running away from being found out by the tram company. However, the fact that I had not driven her away did not change the fact that I had betrayed her. So I was still guilty. And if I was not guilty because one cannot be guilty of betraying a criminal, then I was guilty of having loved a criminal.

CHAPTER ELEVEN

O NCE HANNA ADMITTED HAVING WRITTEN the report, the other defendants had an easy game to play. When Hanna had not been acting alone, they claimed, she had pressured, threatened, and forced the others. She had seized command. She did the talking and the writing. She had made the decisions.

The villagers who testified could neither confirm nor deny this. They had seen that the burning church was guarded by several women who did not unlock it, and they had not dared to unlock it themselves. They had met the women the next morning as they were leaving the village, and recognized them as the defendants. But which of the defendants had been the spokeswoman at the early-morning encounter, or if anyone had played the role of spokeswoman, they could not recall.

'But you cannot rule out that it was this defendant' – the lawyer for one of the other defendants pointed at Hanna – 'who took the decisions?'

They couldn't, how could they even have wanted to, and faced with the other defendants, visibly older, more worn out, more cowardly and bitter, they had no such impulse. In comparison with the other defendants, Hanna was the dominant one. Besides, the existence of a leader exonerated the villagers; having failed to achieve rescue in the face of a fiercely led opposing force looked better than having failed to do anything when confronted by a group of confused women.

Hanna kept struggling. She admitted what was true and disputed what was not. Her arguments became more desperate and more vehement. She didn't raise her voice, but her very intensity alienated the court.

Eventually she gave up. She spoke only when asked a direct question; her answers were short, minimal, sometimes beside the point. As if to make clear that she had given up, she now remained seated when speaking. The presiding judge, who had told her several times at the beginning of the trial that she did not need to stand and could remain seated if she preferred, was put off by this as well. Towards the end of the trial, I sometimes had the sense that the court had had enough, that they wanted to get the whole thing over with, that they were no longer paying attention but were somewhere else, or rather here – back in the present after long weeks in the past.

I had had enough too. But I couldn't put it behind me. For me, the proceedings were not ending, but just beginning. I had been a spectator, and then suddenly a participant, a player, and member of the jury. I had neither sought nor chosen this new role, but it was mine whether I wanted it or not, whether I did anything or just remained completely passive.

'Did anything' – there was only one thing to do. I could go to the judge and tell him that Hanna was illiterate. That she was not the main protagonist and guilty party the way the others made her out to be. That her behaviour at the trial was not proof of singular incorrigibility, lack of remorse, or arrogance, but was born of her incapacity to familiarize herself with the indictment and the manu-script and also probably of her consequent lack of any sense of strategy or tactics. That her defence had been significantly compromised. That she was guilty, but not as guilty as it appeared.

Maybe I would not be able to convince the judge. But I would give him enough to have to think about and inves-tigate further. In the end, it would be proved that I was right, and Hanna would be punished, but less severely. She would have to go to prison, but would be released sooner – wasn't that what she had been fighting for?

Yes, that was what she had been fighting for, but she was not willing to earn victory at the price of exposure as an illiterate. Nor would she want me to barter her self-image for a few years in prison. She could have made that kind of trade herself, and did not, which meant she didn't want it. Her sense of self was worth more than the years in prison to her.

But was it really worth all that? What did she gain from this false self-image which ensnared her and crippled her and paralyzed her? With the energy she put into maintaining the lie, she could have learned to read and write long ago.

I tried to talk about the problem with friends. Imagine someone is racing intentionally towards his own destruction and you can save him – do you go ahead and save him? Imagine there's an operation, and the patient is a drug user and the drugs are incompatible with the anaesthetic, but the patient is ashamed of being an addict and does not want to tell the anaesthetist – do you talk to the anaesthetist? Imagine a trial and a defendant who will be convicted if he doesn't admit to being left-handed – do you tell the judge what's going on? Imagine he's gay, and could not have committed the crime because he's gay, but is ashamed of being gay. It isn't a question of whether the defendant should be ashamed of being left-handed or gay – just imagine that he is.

CHAPTER TWELVE

I DECIDED TO SPEAK TO MY FATHER. Not because we were particularly close. My father was undemonstrative, and could neither share his feelings with his children nor deal with the feelings we had for him. For a long time I believed there must be a wealth of undiscovered treasure behind that uncommunicative manner, but later I wondered if there was anything behind it at all. Perhaps he had been full of emotions as a boy and a young man, and by giving them no outlet had allowed them over the years to wither and die.

But it was because of the distance between us that I

sought him out now. I wanted to talk to the philosopher who had written about Kant and Hegel, and who had, as I knew, occupied himself with moral issues. He should be well positioned to explore my problem in the abstract and, unlike my friends, to avoid getting trapped in the inadequacies of my examples.

When we children wanted to speak to our father, he gave us appointments just like his students. He worked at home and only went to the university to give his lectures and seminars. Colleagues and students who wished to speak to him came to see him at home. I remember queues of students leaning against the wall in the corridor and waiting their turn, some reading, some looking at the views of cities hanging in the corridor, others staring into space, all of them silent except for an embarrassed greeting when we children went down the corridor and said hello. We ourselves didn't have to wait in the hall when our father had made an appointment with us. But we too had to be at his door at the appointed time and knock to be admitted.

I knew two of my father's studies. The windows in the first one, in which Hanna had run her fingers along the books, looked out onto the streets and houses. The windows in the second looked out over the plain along the Rhine. The house we moved to in the early 1960s, and where my parents stayed after we had grown up, was on the big hill above the city. In both places, the windows did not open the room to the world beyond, but framed and hung the world in it like a picture. My father's study was a capsule in which books, papers, thoughts, and pipe and cigar smoke had created their own force field, different from that of the outside world.

My father allowed me to present my problem in its abstract form and with my examples. 'It has to do with the trial, doesn't it?' But he shook his head to show that he didn't expect an answer, or want to press me or hear anything that I wasn't ready to tell him of my own accord. Then he sat, head to one side, hands gripping the arms of his chair, and thought. He didn't look at me. I studied him, his grey hair, his face, carelessly shaven as always, the deep lines between his eyes and from his nostrils to the corners of his mouth. I waited.

When he answered, he went all the way back to first principles. He instructed me about the individual, about freedom and dignity, about the human being as subject and the fact that one may not turn him into an object. 'Don't you remember how furious you would get as a little boy when Mama knew best what was good for you? Even how far one can act like this with children is a real problem. It is a philosophical problem, but philosophy does not concern itself with children. It leaves them to pedagogy, where they're not in very good hands. Philosophy has forgotten about children.' He smiled at me. 'Forgotten them forever, not just sometimes, the way I forget about you.'

'But . . .'

'But with adults I unfortunately see no justification for setting other people's views of what is good for them above their own ideas of what is good for themselves.'

'Not even if they themselves would be happy about it later?'

He shook his head. 'We're not talking about happiness, we're talking about dignity and freedom. Even as a little boy, you knew the difference. It was no comfort to you that your mother was always right.'

Today I like thinking back on that conversation with my father. I had forgotten it until after his death, when I began to search the depths of my memory for happy encounters and shared activities and experiences with him. When I found it, I was both amazed and delighted. At the time I was confused by my father's mixing of abstraction and concreteness. But eventually I sorted out what he had said to mean that I did not have to speak to the judge, that indeed I had no right to speak to him, and was relieved.

My father saw my relief. 'So do you like philosophy?'

'Well, I didn't know if one had to act in the circumstances I described, and I wasn't really happy with the idea that one must, and if one really isn't allowed to do anything at all, I find that . . .' I didn't know what to say. A relief? A comfort? Appealing? That didn't sound like morality and responsibility. 'I think that's good' would have sounded moral and responsible, but I couldn't say I thought it was good, that I thought it was any more than a relief.

'Appealing?' my father suggested.

I nodded and shrugged my shoulders.

'No, your problem has no appealing solution. Of course one must act if the situation as you describe it is one of accrued or inherited responsibility. If one knows what is good for another person who in turn is blind to it, then one must try to open his eyes. One has to leave him the last word, but one must talk to him – to him and not to someone else behind his back.'

Talk to Hanna? What would I say to her? That I had seen through her lifelong lie? That she was in the process of sacrificing her whole life to this silly lie? That the lie wasn't worth the sacrifice? That that was why she should fight not to remain in prison any longer than she had to, because there was so much she could still do with her life afterwards? Could I deprive her of her lifelong lie, without opening some vision of a future to her? I had no idea what that might be, nor did I know how to face her and say that after what she had done it was right that her short- and medium-term future would be in prison. I didn't know how to face her and say anything at all. I didn't know how to face her.

I asked my father: 'And what if you can't talk to him?'

He looked at me doubtfully, and I knew myself that that question was beside the point. There was nothing more to moralize about. I just had to make a decision.

'I haven't been able to help you.' My father stood up and so did I. 'No, you don't have to go, it's just that my back hurts.' He stood bent over, with his hands pressed against his kidneys. 'I can't say that I'm sorry I can't help you. As a philosopher, I mean, which is how you were addressing me. As your father, I find the experience of not being able to help my children almost unbearable.'

I waited, but he didn't say anything else. I thought he was making it easy on himself: I knew when he could have taken care of us more and how he could have helped us more. Then I thought that perhaps he realized this himself and really found it difficult to bear. But either way I had nothing to say to him. I was embarrassed, and had the feeling he was embarrassed too.

'Well then . . .'

'You can come any time.' My father looked at me.

I didn't believe him, and nodded.

CHAPTER THIRTEEN

*I*N JUNE, THE COURT FLEW TO ISRAEL for two weeks. The hearing there took only a few days, but the judge and prosecutors made it a combined judicial and tourist outing, Jerusalem and Tel Aviv, the Negev and the Red Sea. It was undoubtedly all above board as regards rules of conduct, holiday, and expense accounts, but I found it bizarre nonetheless.

I had planned to devote these two weeks to my studies. But it didn't go the way I had imagined and planned. I couldn't concentrate enough to learn anything, either from my teachers or my books. Again and again, my thoughts wandered off and were lost in images.

I saw Hanna by the burning church, hard-faced, in a black uniform, with a riding whip. She drew circles in the snow with her whip, and slapped it against her boots. I saw her being read to. She listened carefully, asked no questions, and made no comments. When the hour was over, she told the reader she would be going on the transport to Auschwitz next morning. The reader, a frail creature with a stubble of black hair and shortsighted eyes, began to cry. Hanna hit the wall with her hand and two women, also prisoners in striped clothing, came in and pulled the reader away. I saw Hanna walking the paths in the camp, going into the prisoners' barracks and overseeing construction work. She did it all with the same hard face, cold eyes, and pursed mouth, and the prisoners ducked, bent over their work, pressed themselves against the wall, into the wall, wanted to disappear into the wall. Sometimes there were many prisoners gathered together or running from one place to the other or standing in line or marching, and Hanna stood among them and screamed orders, her screaming face a mask of ugliness, and helped things along with her whip. I saw the church steeple crashing into the roof and the sparks flying and heard the desperation of the women. I saw the burned-out church next morning.

Alongside these images, I saw the others. Hanna pulling on her stockings in the kitchen, standing by the bath holding the towel, riding her bicycle with skirts flying, standing in my father's study, dancing in front of the mirror, looking at me at the pool, Hanna listening to me, talking to me, laughing at me, loving me. Hanna loving me with cold eyes and pursed mouth, silently listening to me reading, and at the end banging the wall with her hand, talking to me with her face turning into a mask. The worst were the dreams in which a hard, imperious, cruel Hanna aroused me sexually; I woke from them full of longing and shame and rage. And full of fear about who I really was.

I knew that my fantasized images were poor clichés. They were unfair to the Hanna I had known and still knew. But still they were very powerful. They undermined my actual memories of Hanna and merged with the images of the camps that I had in my mind.

When I think today about those years, I realize how little direct observation there actually was, how few photographs that made life and murder in the camps real. We knew the gate of Auschwitz with its inscription, the stacked wooden bunks, the piles of hair and glasses and suitcases; we knew the building that formed the entrance to Birkenau with the tower, the two wings, and the entrance for the trains; and from Bergen-Belsen the mountains of corpses found and photographed by the Allies at the liberation. We were familiar with some of the testimony of prisoners, but many of them were published soon after the war and not reissued until the 1980s, and in the intervening years they were out of print. Today there are so many books and films that the world of the camps is part of our collective imagination and completes our ordinary everyday one. Our imagination knows its way around in it, and since the television series *Holocaust* and movies like *Sophie's Choice* and especially *Schindler's List*, actually moves in it, not just registering, but supplementing and embellishing it. Back then, the imagination was almost static: the shattering fact of the world of the camps seemed properly beyond its operations. The few images derived from Allied photographs and the testimony of survivors flashed on the mind again and again, until they froze into clichés.

CHAPTER FOURTEEN

I DECIDED TO GO AWAY. IF I HAD BEEN able to leave for Auschwitz the next day, I would have gone. But it would have taken weeks to get a visa. So I went to Struthof in Alsace. It was the nearest concentration camp. I had never seen one. I wanted reality to drive out the clichés.

I hitched, and remember a ride in a truck with a driver who downed one bottle of beer after another, and a Mercedes driver who drove wearing white gloves. After Strasbourg I got lucky; the driver was going to Schirmeck, a small town not far from Struthof.

When I told the driver where I was going, he fell

silent. I looked over at him, but couldn't tell why he had suddenly stopped talking in the midst of a lively conversation. He was middle-aged, with a haggard face and a dark red birthmark or scar on his right temple, and his black hair was carefully parted and combed in strands. He stared at the road in concentration.

The hills of the Vosges rolled out ahead of us. We were driving through vineyards into a wide open valley that climbed gently. To the left and right, mixed forests grew up the slopes, and sometimes there was a quarry or a brick-walled factory with a corrugated iron roof, or an old sanatorium, or a large turreted villa among tall trees. A railway line ran alongside us, sometimes to the left and sometimes to the right.

Then he spoke again. He asked me why I was visiting Struthof, and I told him about the trial and my lack of first-hand knowledge.

'Ah, you want to understand why people can do such terrible things.' He sounded as if he was being a little ironic, but maybe it was just the tone of voice and the choice of words. Before I could reply, he went on: 'What is it you want to understand? That people murder out of passion, or love, or hate, or for honour or revenge, that you understand?'

I nodded.

'You also understand that people murder for money or power? That people murder in wars and revolutions?'

I nodded again. 'But . . .'

the people who were murdered in the camps
.n't done anything to the individuals who murdered
them? Is that what you want to say? Do you mean that
there was no reason for hatred, and no war?'

I didn't want to nod again. What he said was true, but
not the way he said it.

'You're right, there was no war, and no reason for
hatred. But executioners don't hate the people they
execute, and they execute them all the same. Because
they're ordered to? You think they do it because they're
ordered to? And you think that I'm talking about orders
and obedience, that the guards in the camps were under
orders and had to obey?' He laughed sarcastically. 'No,
I'm not talking about orders and obedience. An ex-
ecutioner is not under orders. He's doing his work, he
doesn't hate the people he executes, he's not taking
revenge on them, he's not killing them because they're
in his way or threatening him or attacking him. They're
a matter of such indifference to him that he can kill them
as easily as not.'

He looked at me. 'No "buts"? Come on, tell me that
one person cannot be that indifferent to another. Isn't
that what they taught you? Solidarity with everything that
has a human face? Human dignity? Reverence for life?'

I was outraged and helpless. I searched for a word, a
sentence that would erase what he had said and strike him
dumb.

'Once,' he went on, 'I saw a photograph of Jews being

shot in Russia. The Jews were in a long row, naked; some were standing at the edge of a pit and behind them were soldiers with guns, shooting them in the neck. It was in a quarry, and above the Jews and the soldiers there was an officer sitting on a ledge in the rock, swinging his legs and smoking a cigarette. He looked a little morose. Maybe things weren't going fast enough for him. But there was also something satisfied, even cheerful about his expression, perhaps because the day's work was getting done and it was almost time to go home. He didn't hate the Jews. He wasn't . . .'

'Was it you? Were you sitting on the ledge and . . .'

He stopped the car. He was absolutely white, and the mark on his temple glistened. 'Out!'

I got out. He swung the wheel so fast I had to jump aside. I still heard him as he took the next few curves. Then everything was silent.

I walked up the road. No car passed me, none came in the opposite direction. I heard birds, the wind in the trees, and the occasional murmur of a stream. In a quarter of an hour I reached the concentration camp.

CHAPTER FIFTEEN

I WENT BACK THERE NOT LONG AGO. It was winter, a clear, cold day. Beyond Schirmeck the woods were snowy, the trees powdered white and the ground white too. The grounds of the concentration camp, an elongated area on a sloping terrace of mountain with a broad view of the Vosges, lay white in the bright sunshine. The grey-blue painted wood of the two- and three-storey watchtower and the single-storey barracks made a pleasant contrast with the snow. True, there was the entrance festooned with barbed wire and the sign CONCENTRATION CAMP STRUTHOF-NATZWEILER and the double barbed-wire fence that surrounded the camp. But the ground between the remaining barracks, where more barracks had once stood side by side, no longer showed any trace of the camp under its glittering cover of snow. It could have been a sledging slope for children, spending their Christmas holidays in the cheerful barracks with the homely many-paned windows, and about to be called indoors for cake and hot chocolate.

The camp was closed. I tramped around it in the snow, getting my feet wet. I could easily see the whole grounds, and remembered how on my first visit I had gone down the steps that led between the foundations of the former barracks. I also remembered the ovens of the crematorium that were on display in another barracks, and that another barracks had contained cells. I remembered my vain attempts, back then, to imagine in concrete detail a camp filled with prisoners and guards and suffering. I really tried; I looked at a barracks, closed my eyes, and imagined row upon row of barracks. I measured a barracks, calculated its occupants from the information booklet, and imagined how crowded it had been. I found out that the steps between the barracks had also been used for roll call, and as I looked from the bottom of the camp up towards the top, I filled them with rows of backs. But it was all in vain, and I had a feeling of the most dreadful, shameful failure.

On the way back, further down the hill, I found a small house opposite a restaurant that had a sign on it indicating that it had been a gas chamber. It was painted white, had doors and windows framed in sandstone, and could have been a barn or a shed or servants' living quarters. This building, too, was closed and I didn't remember if I had gone inside it on my first visit. I didn't get out of the car. I sat for a while with the motor running, and looked. Then I drove on.

At first I was embarrassed to wander home through the Alsatian villages looking for a restaurant where I could have lunch. But my awkwardness was not the result of real feeling, but of thinking about the way one is supposed to feel after visiting a concentration camp. I noticed this myself, shrugged, and found a restaurant called Au Petit Garçon in a village on a slope of the Vosges. My table looked out over the plain. Hanna had called me Kid.

The previous time I had walked around the concentration camp grounds until they closed. Then I had sat down under the memorial that stood above the camp, and looked down over the grounds. I felt a great emptiness inside, as if I had been searching for some glimpse, not outside but within myself, and had discovered that there was nothing to be found.

Then it got dark. I had to wait an hour until the driver of a small open truck let me climb up and sit on the truck bed and took me to the next village, and I gave up the idea of hitching back that same day. I found a cheap room in a guest house in the village and had a thin steak with chips and peas in the dining room.

Four men were loudly playing cards at the next table. The door opened and a little old man came in without greeting anyone. He wore short trousers and had a wooden leg. He ordered a beer at the bar. He sat facing away from the neighbouring table, so that all they saw was his back and the back of his overly enlarged, bald skull. The card players laid down their cards, reached into the ashtrays, picked up the butts, took aim, and hit him. The man at the bar flapped his hands behind his head as if swatting away flies. The innkeeper set his beer in front of him. No one said a word.

I couldn't stand it. I jumped up and went over to the next table. 'Stop it!' I was shaking with outrage. At that moment, the man half hobbled, half hopped over and began fumbling with his leg; suddenly he was holding the wooden leg in both hands. He brought it crashing down onto the table so that the glasses and ashtrays danced, and fell into an empty chair, laughing a squeaky, toothless laugh as the others laughed in a beery rumble along with him. 'Stop it!' they laughed, pointing at me. 'Stop it!'

During the night the wind howled around the house. I was not cold, and the noise of the wind and the creaking of the tree in front of the house and the occasional banging of a shutter were not enough to have kept me awake. But I became more and more inwardly restless, until my whole body began to shiver. I felt afraid, not in antici-pation that something bad was going to happen, but in a physical way. I lay there, listening to the wind, feeling relieved every time it weakened and died down, but dreading its renewed assaults and not knowing how I would get out of bed next day, hitch back, continue my studies, and one day have a career and a wife and children.

I wanted simultaneously to understand Hanna's crime and to condemn it. But it was too terrible for that. When I tried to understand it, I had the feeling I was failing to condemn it as it must be condemned. When I condemned it as it must be condemned, there was no room for understanding. But even as I wanted to understand Hanna, failing to understand her meant betraying her all over again. I could not resolve this. I wanted to pose myself both tasks — understanding and condemnation. But it was impossible to do both.

The next day was another beautiful summer day. Hitching was easy, and I got back in a few hours. I walked through the city as though I had been away for a long time; the streets and buildings and people looked strange to me. But that didn't mean the other world of the concentration camps felt any closer. My impressions of Struthof joined my few already existing images of Auschwitz and Bergen-Belsen, and froze along with them.

CHAPTER SIXTEEN

I DID GO TO THE PRESIDING JUDGE after all. I couldn't make myself visit Hanna. But neither could I endure doing nothing.

Why didn't I manage to speak to Hanna? She had left me, deceived me, was not the person I had taken her for or imagined her to be. And who had I been for her? The little reader she used, the little bedmate with whom she'd had her fun? Would she have sent me to the gas chamber if she hadn't been able to leave me, but wanted to get rid of me?

Why did I find it unendurable to do nothing? I told myself I had to prevent a miscarriage of justice. I had to make sure justice was done, despite Hanna's lifelong lie, justice both for and against Hanna, so to speak. But I wasn't really concerned with justice. I couldn't leave Hanna the way she was, or wanted to be. I had to meddle with her, have some kind of influence and effect on her, if not directly then indirectly.

The judge knew about our seminar group and was happy to invite me to come and talk after a session in court. I knocked, was invited in, greeted, and offered the chair in front of his desk. He was sitting in his shirtsleeves behind the desk. His robe hung over the back and arms of his chair; he had sat down in the robe and then slipped out of it. He seemed relaxed, a man who had finished his day's work and was content. Without the irritated expression he hid behind during the trial, he had a nice, intelligent, harmless civil servant's face.

He made general easy chitchat, asking me about this and that: what our seminar group thought of the trial, what our professor intended to do with the trial record, which year we were in, which year I was in, why I was studying law and when I planned to take my exams. He told me I must be sure to register for the exams on time.

I answered all his questions. Then I listened while he talked about his studies and his exams. He had done everything the right way. He had taken the right classes and seminars at the right time and with the right degree of success and had passed his final exams. He liked being a lawyer and a judge, and if he had to do it all again he would do it the same way.

The window was open. In the car park, doors were being slammed and engines turned on. I listened to the cars until their noise was swallowed up in the roar of the traffic. Then children came to play and yell in the emptied car park. Sometimes a word came through quite clearly: a name, an insult, a call.

The judge stood up and said goodbye. He told me I could come again if I had any other questions, or if I wanted advice on my studies. And he would like to know our seminar group's evaluation and analysis of the trial.

I walked through the empty car park. One of the bigger boys told me how I could walk to the railway station. Our car pool had driven back right after the session, and I had to take the train. It was a slow rush-hour train that stopped at every station; people got on and off. I sat at the window, surrounded by ever-changing passengers, conversations, smells. Outside, houses passed by, and roads, cars, trees, distant mountains, castles, and quarries. I took it all in and felt nothing. I was no longer upset at having been left, deceived, and used by Hanna. I no longer had to meddle with her. I felt the numbness with which I had followed the horrors of the trial settling over the emotions and thoughts of the past few weeks. It would be too much to say I was happy about this. But I felt it was right. It allowed me to return to and continue to live my everyday life.

CHAPTER SEVENTEEN

*T*HE VERDICT WAS HANDED DOWN AT the end of June. Hanna was sentenced to life. The others received terms in jail.

The courtroom was as full as it had been at the beginning of the trial. People from the justice system, students from my university and the local one, a class of schoolchildren, domestic and foreign journalists, and the people who always find their way into courtrooms. It was loud. At first, no one noticed when the defendants were brought in. But then the spectators fell silent. The first to stop talking were those sitting up front near the defendants. They nudged their neighbours and turned around to those sitting behind them. 'Look,' they whispered, and those who looked fell silent too and nudged their neighbours and turned to those sitting behind them and whispered, 'Look!' Until eventually the whole court-room was silent.

I don't know if Hanna knew how she looked, or maybe she wanted to look like that. She was wearing a black suit and a white blouse, and the cut of the suit and the tie that went with the blouse made her look as if she were in uniform. I have never seen the uniform of the women who worked for the SS. But I believed, and the spectators all believed, that before us we were seeing that uniform, and the woman who had worked for the SS in it, and all the crimes Hanna was accused of doing.

The spectators began to whisper again. Many were audibly outraged. They felt that Hanna was ridiculing the trial, the verdict, and themselves, they who had come to hear the verdict read out. They became more vociferous, and some of them began calling out what they thought of Hanna. But then the court entered the courtroom and after an irritated glance at Hanna, the judge announced the verdict. Hanna listened standing up, straight-backed, and absolutely motionless. She sat down during the reading of the reasons for the verdict. I did not take my eyes off her head and neck.

The entire verdict took several hours to read. When the trial was over and the defendants were being led away, I waited to see whether Hanna would look at me. I was sitting in the same place I always sat. But she looked straight ahead and through everything. A proud, wounded, lost, and infinitely tired look. A look that wished to see nothing and no one.

Part Three

CHAPTER ONE

I SPENT THE SUMMER AFTER THE TRIAL in the reading room of the university library. I arrived as the reading room opened and left when it closed. At the weekends I studied at home. I studied so uninterruptedly, so obsessively, that the feelings and thoughts that had been deadened by the trial remained deadened. I avoided contacts. I moved away from home and rented a room. I brushed off the few acquaintances who spoke to me in the reading room or on my occasional visits to the cinema.

The winter term I was much the same way. Nonetheless, I was asked if I would like to spend the Christmas holidays with a group of students at a ski lodge. Surprised, I accepted.

I wasn't a good skier, but I liked to ski and was fast and kept up with the good ones. Sometimes when I was on slopes that were beyond my ability, I risked falls and broken bones. I did this consciously. The other risk I was taking, and to which I succumbed, was one to which I was oblivious.

I was never cold. While the others skied in sweaters and jackets, I skied in a shirt. The others shook their heads and teased me about it, but I didn't take their worries seriously. I simply didn't feel cold. When I began to cough, I blamed it on the Austrian cigarettes. When I started to feel feverish, I enjoyed it. I felt weak and light-headed at the same time, and all my senses were pleasingly muffled, cottony, padded. I floated.

Then I came down with a high fever and was taken to the hospital. By the time I left, the numbness was gone. All the questions and fears, accusations and self-accusations, all the horror and pain that had erupted during the trial and been immediately deadened were back, and back for good. I don't know what the doctors diagnose when someone isn't freezing even though he should be freezing. My own diagnosis is that the numbness had to overwhelm my body before it would let go of me, before I could let go of it.

When I had finished my degree and began my training, it was the summer of the student upheavals. I was interested in history and sociology, and while clerking with a judge I was still in the university often enough to know what was going on. Knowing what was going on did not mean taking part – university and university reforms were no more interesting to me than the Vietcong and the Americans. As for the third and real theme of the student movement, coming to grips with the Nazi past, I felt so removed from the other students that I had no desire to agitate and demonstrate with them.

Sometimes I think that dealing with the Nazi past was not the reason for the generational conflict that drove the student movement, but merely the form it took. Parental expectations, from which every generation must free itself, were nullified by the fact that these parents had failed to measure up during the Third Reich, or after it ended. How could those who had committed Nazi crimes or watched them happen or looked away while they were happening or tolerated the criminals among them after 1945 or even accepted them – how could they have anything to say to their children? But on the other hand, the Nazi past was an issue even for children who couldn't accuse their parents of anything, or didn't want to. For them, coming to grips with the Nazi past was not merely the form taken by a generational conflict, it was the issue itself.

Whatever validity the concept of collective guilt may or may not have, morally and legally – for my generation of students it was a lived reality. It did not just apply to what had happened in the Third Reich. The fact that Jewish gravestones were being defaced with swastikas, that so many old Nazis had made careers in the courts, the administration, and the universities, that the Federal Republic had not recognized the State of Israel, that emigration and resistance were handed down as traditions less often than a life of conformity – all this filled us with shame, even when we could point at the guilty parties. Pointing at the guilty parties did not free us from shame, but at least it overcame the suffering we went through on account of it. It converted the passive suffering of shame into energy, activity, aggression. And coming to grips with our parents' guilt took a great deal of energy.

I had no one to point at. Certainly not my parents, because I had nothing to accuse them of. The zeal for letting in the daylight, with which, as a member of the concentration camps seminar, I had condemned my father to shame, had passed, and it embarrassed me. But what other people in my social environment had done, and that guilt, were in any case a lot less bad than what Hanna had done. I had to point at Hanna. But the finger I pointed at her turned back to me. I had loved her. Not only had I loved her, I had chosen her. I tried to tell myself that I had known nothing of what she had done when I chose her. I tried to talk myself into the state of innocence in which children love their parents. But love of our parents is the only love for which we are not responsible.

And perhaps we are responsible even for the love we

feel for our parents. I envied other students back then who had dissociated themselves from their parents and thus from the entire generation of perpetrators, voyeurs, and the wilfully blind, accommodators and accepters, thereby overcoming perhaps not their shame, but at least their suffering because of the shame. But what gave rise to the swaggering self-righteousness I so often encountered among these students? How could one feel guilt and shame, and at the same time parade one's self-righteousness? Was their dissociation of themselves from their parents mere rhetoric: sounds and noise that were supposed to drown out the fact that their love for their parents made them irrevocably complicit in their crimes?

These thoughts did not come until later, and even later they brought no comfort. How could it be a comfort that the pain I went through because of my love for Hanna was, in a way, the fate of my generation, a German fate, and that it was only more difficult for me to evade, more difficult for me to manage than for others? All the same, it would have been good for me back then to be able to feel I was part of my generation.

CHAPTER TWO

I MARRIED WHILE I WAS STILL CLERK-
ing. Gertrud and I had met at the ski
lodge, and when the others left at the end of the
holiday, she stayed behind until I was released from the
hospital and she could take me home. She was also studying law; we studied together, passed our exams together,
and began our clerking together. We got married when
Gertrud got pregnant.

I did not tell her about Hanna. Who, I thought, wants
to know about the other's earlier relationships, if he or
she is not the fulfilment of their promise? Gertrud was
smart, efficient, and loyal, and if our life had involved

running a farm with lots of farmhands and farmgirls, lots of children, lots of work, and no time for each other, it would have been fulfilling and happy. But our life was a three-room flat in a modern building on the edge of the city, our daughter Julia and Gertrud's and my work as legal clerks. I could never stop comparing the way it was with Gertrud and the way it had been with Hanna; again and again, Gertrud and I would hold each other, and I would feel that something was wrong, that she was wrong, that she moved wrong and felt wrong, smelled wrong and tasted wrong. I thought I would get over it. I hoped it would go away. I wanted to be free of Hanna. But I never got over the feeling that something was wrong.

We got divorced when Julia was five. Neither of us could keep things going; we parted without bitterness and retained our loyalty to each other. It tormented me that we were denying Julia the sense of security she obviously craved. When Gertrud and I were open and warm with each other, Julia swam in it like a fish in water. She was in her element. When she sensed tension between us, she ran from one to the other to assure us that we were good and she loved us. She longed for a little brother and probably would have been happy with siblings. For a long time, she didn't understand what divorce meant; when I came to visit, she wanted me to stay, and when she came to visit me, she wanted Gertrud to come too. When it was time to go, and she watched me from the window, and I had to get into the car under her sad gaze, it broke my heart. And I had the feeling that what we were denying her was not only her wish, but her right. We had cheated her of her rights by getting divorced, and the fact that we did it together didn't halve the guilt.

I tried to approach my later relationships better, and to get into them more deeply. I admitted to myself that a woman had to move and feel a bit like Hanna, smell and taste a bit like her for things to be good between us. I told them about Hanna. And I told them more about myself than I had told Gertrud; they had to be able to make sense of whatever they might find disconcerting in my behaviour and moods. But the women didn't want to hear that much. I remember Helen, an American literary critic who stroked my back silently and soothingly as I talked, and continued to stroke me just as silently and soothingly after I'd stopped speaking. Gesina, a psycho-analyst, thought I needed to work through my relationship with my mother. Did it not strike me that my mother hardly appeared in my story at all? Hilke, a dentist, kept asking about the time before we met, but immediately forgot whatever I told her. So I stopped talking about it. There's no need to talk, because the truth of what one says lies in what one does.

CHAPTER THREE

S I WAS TAKING MY SECOND STATE
exam, the professor who had given the
concentration camps seminar died. Gertrud
came across the obituary in the newspaper. The funeral
was at the mountain cemetery. Did I want to go?

I didn't. The burial was on a Thursday afternoon, and
on both Thursday and Friday morning I had exams. Also,
the professor and I had never been particularly close. And
I didn't like funerals. And I didn't want to be reminded
of the trial.

But it was already too late. The memory had been
awakened, and when I came out of the exam on Thursday,

it was as if I had an appointment with the past that I couldn't miss. I did something I never did otherwise: I took the tram. This in itself was an encounter with the past, like returning to a place that once was familiar but has changed its appearance. When Hanna worked for the tram company, there were long trams made up of two or three carriages, platforms at the front and back, running boards along the platforms that you could jump onto when the tram had pulled away from the stop, and a cord running through the carriages that the conductor rang to signal departure. In summer there were trams with open platforms. The conductor sold, punched, and inspected tickets, called out the stations, signalled departures, kept an eye on the children who pushed their way onto the platforms, fought with passengers who jumped off and on, and denied further entry if the tram was full. There were cheerful, witty, serious, grouchy, and coarse conductors, and the temperament or mood of the conductor often defined the atmosphere in the tram. How idiotic of me that after the failed surprise on the ride to Schwetzingen, I had been afraid to waylay Hanna and see what she was like as a conductor.

I got onto the conductor-less tram and rode to the mountain cemetery. It was a cold autumn day with a cloudless, hazy sky and a yellow sun that no longer gave off any heat, the kind you can look at directly without hurting your eyes. I had to search awhile before finding the grave where the funeral ceremony was being held. I walked beneath tall, bare trees, between old gravestones. Occasionally I met a cemetery gardener or an old woman with a watering can and gardening shears. It was absolutely still, and from a distance I could hear the hymn being sung at the professor's grave.

I stopped a little way off and studied the small group of mourners. Some of them were clearly eccentrics and misfits. In the eulogies for the professor, there were hints that he himself had withdrawn from the pressures of society and thus lost contact with it, remaining a loner and thereby becoming something of an oddball himself.

I recognized a former member of the concentration camps seminar. He had taken his exams before me, had become a lawyer, and then opened a pub; he was dressed in a long red coat. He came to speak to me when everything was over and I was making my way to the cemetery gate. 'We were in the same seminar – don't you remember?'

'I do.' We shook hands.

'I was always at the trial on Wednesdays, and sometimes I gave you a lift.' He laughed. 'You were there every day, every day and every week. Can you say why, now?' He looked at me, good-natured and ready to pounce, and I remembered that I had noticed this look even in the seminar.

'I was very interested in the trial.'

'You were very interested in the trial?' He laughed again. 'The trial, or the defendant you were always staring at? The only one who was quite good-looking. We all used to wonder what was going on between you and her, but none of us dared ask. We were so terribly sensitive and considerate back then. Do you remember . . .' He recalled another member of the seminar, who stuttered or lisped and held forth incessantly, most of it nonsense, and to whom we listened as though his words were gold. He went on to talk about other members of the seminar, what they were like back then and what they were doing now. He talked and talked. But I knew he would get back to me eventually and ask: 'So — what was going on between you and the defendant?' And I didn't know what to answer, how to betray, confess, parry.

Then we were at the entrance to the cemetery, and he asked. A tram was just pulling away from the stop and I called out, 'Bye,' and ran off as though I could jump onto the running board, ran alongside the tram beating the flat of my hand against the door, and something happened that I wouldn't have believed possible, hadn't even hoped for. The tram stopped, the door opened, and I got on.

CHAPTER FOUR

FTER MY STATE EXAM, I HAD TO decide on a profession within the law. I gave myself a little time; Gertrud, who immediately began working in the judiciary, had her hands full, and we were happy that I could remain at home and take care of Julia. Once Gertrud had got over all the difficulties of getting started and Julia was in kindergarten, I had to make a decision.

I had a hard time of it. I didn't see myself in any of the roles I had seen lawyers play at Hanna's trial. Prosecution seemed to me as grotesque a simplification as defence, and judging was the most grotesque oversimplification of all. Nor could I see myself as an administrative official; I had worked at a local government office during my training, and found its rooms, corridors, smells, and employees grey, sterile, and dreary.

That did not leave many legal careers, and I don't know what I would have done if a professor of legal history had not offered me a research job. Gertrud said it was an evasion, an escape from the challenges and responsibilities of life, and she was right. I escaped and was relieved that I could do so. After all, it wasn't forever, I told both her and myself; I was young enough to enter any solid branch of the legal profession after a few years of legal history. But it was forever; the first escape was followed by a second, when I moved from the university to a research institution, seeking and finding a niche in which I could pursue my interest in legal history, in which I needed no one and disturbed no one.

Now escape involves not just running away, but arriving somewhere. And the past I arrived in as a legal historian was no less alive than the present. It is also not true, as outsiders might assume, that one can merely observe the richness of life in the past, whereas one can participate in the present. Doing history means building bridges between the past and the present, observing both banks of the river, taking an active part on both sides. One of my areas of research was law in the Third Reich, and here it is particularly obvious how the past and present come together in a single reality. Here, escape is not a preoccupation with the past, but a determined focus on the present and the future that is blind to the legacy of the past which brands us and with which we must live.

In saying this, I do not mean to conceal how gratifying it was to plunge into different stretches of the past that were not so urgently connected to the present. I felt it for the first time when I was working on the legal codes and drafts of the Enlightenment. They were based on the belief that a good order is intrinsic to the world, and that therefore the world can be brought into good order. To see how legal provisions were created paragraph by paragraph out of this belief as solemn guardians of this good order, and worked into laws that strove for beauty and by their very beauty for truth, made me happy. For a long time I believed that there was progress in the history of law, a development towards greater beauty and truth, rationality and humanity, despite terrible setbacks and retreats. Once it became clear to me that this belief was a chimera, I began playing with a different image of the course of legal history. In this one it still has a purpose, but the goal it finally attains, after countless disruptions, confusions, and delusions, is the beginning, its own original starting point, which once reached must be set off from again.

I reread the *Odyssey* at that time, which I had first read in school and remembered as the story of a homecoming. But it is not the story of a homecoming. How could the Greeks, who knew that one never enters the same river twice, believe in homecoming? Odysseus does not return home to stay, but to set off again. The *Odyssey* is the story of motion both purposeful and purposeless, successful and futile. What else is the history of law?

CHAPTER FIVE

I BEGAN WITH THE *ODYSSEY*. I READ it after Gertrud and I had separated. There were many nights when I couldn't sleep for more than a few hours; I would lie awake, and when I switched on the light and picked up a book, my eyes closed, and when I put the book down and turned off the light, I was wide awake again. So I read aloud, and my eyes didn't close. And because in all my confused half-waking thoughts that swirled in tormenting circles of memories and dreams around my marriage and my daughter and my life, it was always Hanna who predominated, I read to Hanna. I read to Hanna on tape.

It was several months before I sent off the tapes. At first I didn't want to send just bits of it, so I waited until I had recorded all of the *Odyssey*. Then I began to wonder if Hanna would find the *Odyssey* sufficiently interesting, so I recorded what I read next after the *Odyssey*, stories by Schnitzler and Chekhov. Then I put off calling the court that had convicted Hanna to find out where she was serving her sentence. Finally I had everything together, Hanna's address in a prison near the city where she had been tried and convicted, a cassette player, and the cassettes, numbered from Chekhov to Schnitzler to Homer. And so finally I sent off the package with the machine and the tapes.

Recently I found the notebook in which I entered what I recorded for Hanna over the years. The first twelve titles were obviously all entered at the same time; at first I probably just read, and then realized that if I didn't keep notes I would not remember what I had already recorded. Next to the subsequent titles there is sometimes a date, sometimes none, but even without dates I know that I sent Hanna the first package in the eighth year of her imprisonment, and the last in the eighteenth. In the eighteenth, her plea for clemency was granted.

In general I read to Hanna the things I wanted to read myself at any given moment. With the *Odyssey*, I found at first that it was hard to take in as much when I read aloud as when I read silently to myself. But that changed. The disadvantage of reading aloud remained the fact that it took longer. But books read aloud also stayed long in my memory. Even today, I can remember things in them absolutely clearly.

But I also read books I already knew and loved. So Hanna got to hear a great deal of Keller and Fontane, Heine and Mörike. For a long time I didn't dare to read poetry, but eventually I really enjoyed it, and I learned many of the poems I read by heart. I can still recite them today.

Taken together, the titles in the notebook testify to a great and fundamental confidence in bourgeois culture. I do not ever remember asking myself whether I should go beyond Kafka, Frisch, Johnson, Bachmann, and Lenz, and read experimental literature, literature in which I did not recognize the story or like any of the characters. To me it was obvious that experimental literature was experimenting with the reader, and Hanna didn't need that and neither did I.

When I began writing myself, I read these pieces aloud to her as well. I waited until I had dictated my handwritten text, and revised the typewritten version, and had the feeling that now it was finished. When I read it aloud, I could tell if the feeling was right or not. And if not, I could revise it and record a new version over the old. But I didn't like doing that. Hanna became the court before which once again I concentrated all my energies, all my creativity, all my critical imagination. After that, I could send the manuscript to the publisher.

I never made a personal remark on the tapes, never asked after Hanna, never told her anything about myself. I read out the title, the name of the author, and the text. When the text was finished, I waited a moment, closed the book, and pressed the Stop button.

CHAPTER SIX

*I*N THE FOURTH YEAR OF OUR word-driven, wordless contact, a note arrived. 'Kid, the last story was especially nice. Thank you. Hanna.'

It was lined paper, torn out of a notebook, and cut smooth. The message was right up at the top, and filled three lines. It was written in blue smudged ballpoint pen. Hanna had been pressing hard on the pen; the letters went through to the other side. She had also written the address with a great deal of pressure; the imprint was legible on the bottom and top halves of the paper, which was folded in the middle.

At first glance, one might have taken it for a child's handwriting. But what is clumsy and awkward in children's handwriting was forceful here. You could see the resistance Hanna had had to overcome to make the lines into letters and the letters into words. A child's hand will wander off this way and that, and has to be kept on track. Hanna's hand didn't want to go anywhere and had to be forced. The lines that formed the letters started again each time on the upstroke, the downstroke, and before the curves and loops. And each letter was a victory over a fresh struggle, and had a new slant or slope, and often the wrong height or width.

I read the note and was filled with joy and jubilation. 'She can write, she can write!' In these years I had read everything I could lay my hands on to do with illiteracy. I knew about the helplessness in everyday activities, finding one's way or finding an address or choosing a meal in a restaurant, about how illiterates anxiously stick to prescribed patterns and familiar routines, about how much energy it takes to conceal one's inability to read and write, energy lost to actual living. Illiteracy is dependence. By finding the courage to learn to read and write, Hanna had advanced from dependence to independence, a step towards liberation.

Then I looked at Hanna's handwriting and saw how much energy and struggle the writing had cost her. I was proud of her. At the same time, I was sorry for her, sorry for her delayed and failed life, sorry for the delays and failures of life in general. I thought that if the right time gets missed, if one has refused or been refused something for too long, it's too late, even if it is finally tackled with energy and received with joy. Or is there no such thing as 'too late'? Is there only 'late', and is 'late' always better than 'never'? I don't know.

After the first note came a steady stream of others. They were always only a few lines, a thank you, a wish to hear more of a particular author or to hear no more, a comment on an author or a poem or a story or a character in a novel, an observation about prison. 'The forsythia is already in flower in the yard' or 'I like the fact that there have been so many storms this summer' or 'From my window I can see the birds flocking to fly south' – often it was Hanna's note that first made me pay attention to the forsythia, the summer storms, or the flocks of birds. Her remarks about literature were often right on the mark. 'Schnitzler barks, Stefan Zweig is a dead dog' or 'Keller needs a woman' or 'Goethe's poems are like tiny paintings in beautiful frames' or 'Lenz must write on a typewriter.' Because she knew nothing about the authors, she assumed they were contemporaries, unless something indicated this was obviously impossible. I was astonished at how much older literature can actually be read as if it were contemporary; to anyone ignorant of history, it would be easy to see ways of life in earlier times simply as ways of life in foreign countries.

I never wrote to Hanna. But I kept reading to her.

When I spent a year in America, I sent cassettes from there. When I was on holiday or was particularly busy, it might take longer for me to finish the next cassette; I never established a definite rhythm, but sent cassettes sometimes every week or two weeks, and sometimes only every three or four weeks. I didn't worry that Hanna might not need my cassettes now that she had learned to read by herself. She could read as well. Reading aloud was my way of speaking to her, with her.

I kept all her notes. The handwriting changed. At first she forced the letters into the same slant and the right height and width. Once she had managed that, she became lighter and more confident. Her handwriting never became fluid, but it acquired something of the severe beauty that characterizes the writing of old people who have written little in their lives.

CHAPTER SEVEN

T THE TIME I NEVER THOUGHT ABOUT the fact that Hanna would be released one day. The exchange of notes and cassettes was so normal and familiar, and Hanna was both close and removed in such an easy way, that I could have continued the situation indefinitely. That was comfortable and selfish, I know.

Then came the letter from the prison governor.

For years you and Frau Schmitz have corresponded with each other. This is the only contact Frau Schmitz has with the outside world, and so I am turning to you, although I do not know how close your relationship is, nor whether you are a relative or a friend.

Next year Frau Schmitz will again make an appeal for clemency, and I expect the parole board to grant the appeal. She will then be released quite shortly — after eighteen years in prison. Of course we can find or try to find her a flat and a job; a job will be difficult at her age, even though she is in excellent health and has shown great skill in our sewing shop. But rather than us taking care of her, it would be better for relatives or friends to do so, to have the released prisoner live nearby, and keep her company and give her support. You cannot imagine how lonely and helpless one can be on the outside after eighteen years in prison.

Frau Schmitz can take care of herself quite well, and manages on her own. It would be enough if you could find her a small flat and a job, visit her, and invite her to your house occasionally during the first weeks and months and make sure she knows about the programmes offered by the local congregation, adult education, family support groups, and so on.

It is not easy, after eighteen years, to go into the city for the first time, go shopping, deal with the authorities, go to a restaurant. Doing it with someone else helps.

I have noticed that you do not visit Frau Schmitz. If you did, I would not have written to you, but would have asked to talk to you during one of your visits. Now it seems as if you will have to visit her before she is released. Please come and see me at that opportunity.

The letter closed with sincere greetings, which I did not think referred to me but to the fact that the governor was sincere about the issue. I had heard of her; her institution was considered extraordinary, and her opinion on questions of penal reform carried weight. I liked her letter.

But I did not like what was coming my way. Of course I would have to see about a job and a flat, and I did. Friends who neither used nor rented out the flat attached to their house agreed to let it to Hanna at a low rent. The Greek tailor who occasionally altered my clothes was willing to employ Hanna; his sister, who ran the tailoring business with him, wanted to return to Greece. And long before Hanna could have used them, I looked into the social services and educational programmes run by churches and secular organizations. But I put off the visit to Hanna.

Precisely because she was both close and removed in such an easy way, I didn't want to visit her. I had the feeling she could only be what she was to me at an actual distance. I was afraid that the small, light, safe world of notes and cassettes was too artificial and too vulnerable to withstand actual closeness. How could we meet face to face without everything that had happened between us coming to the surface?

So the year passed without me going to the prison. For a long time I heard nothing from the governor; a letter in which I described the housing and job situation for Hanna went unanswered. She was probably expecting to talk to me when I visited Hanna. She had no way to know that I was not only putting off this visit, but avoiding it. Finally, however, the decision came down to pardon and release Hanna, and the governor called me. Could I come now? Hanna was getting out in a week.

CHAPTER EIGHT

I WENT THE NEXT SUNDAY. IT WAS MY first visit to a prison. I was searched at the entrance, and a number of doors were unlocked and locked along the way. But the building was new and bright, and in the inner area the doors were open, allowing the women to move about freely. At the end of a corridor a door opened to the outside, onto a little lawn with lots of people and trees and benches. I looked around, searching. The guard who had brought me pointed to a nearby bench in the shade of a chestnut tree.

Hanna? The woman on the bench was Hanna? Grey hair, a face with deep furrows on brow and cheeks and around the mouth, and a heavy body. She was wearing a light blue dress that was too tight and stretched across her breasts, stomach, and thighs. Her hands lay in her lap holding a book. She wasn't reading it. Over the top of her half-glasses, she was watching a woman throwing breadcrumbs to a couple of sparrows. Then she realized that she was being watched, and turned her face to me.

I saw the expectation in her face, saw it light up with joy when she recognized me, watched her eyes scan my face as I approached, saw them seek, inquire, then look uncertain and hurt, and saw the light go out of her face. When I reached her, she smiled a friendly, weary smile. 'You've grown up, kid.' I sat down beside her and she took my hand.

In the past, I had particularly loved her smell. She always smelled fresh, freshly washed or of fresh laundry or fresh sweat or freshly loved. Sometimes she used perfume. I don't know which one, and its smell, too, was more fresh than anything else. Under these fresh smells was another, heavy, dark, sharp smell. Often I would sniff at her like a curious animal, starting with her throat and shoulders, which smelled freshly washed, soaking up the fresh smell of sweat between her breasts mixed in her armpits with the other smell, then finding this heavy dark smell almost pure around her waist and stomach and between her legs with a fruity tinge that excited me; I would also sniff at her legs and feet – her thighs, where the heavy smell disappeared, the hollows of her knees again with that light, fresh smell of sweat, and her feet, which smelled of soap or leather or tiredness. Her back and arms had no special smell; they smelled of nothing and yet they smelled of her, and the palms of her hands smelled of the day and of work – the ink of the tickets, the metal of the ticket puncher, onions or fish or frying fat, soapsuds or the heat of the iron. When they are freshly washed, hands betray none of this. But soap only covers the smells, and after a time they return, faint, blending into a single scent of the day and work, a scent of work and day's end, of evening, of coming home and being at home.

I sat next to Hanna and smelled an old woman. I don't know what makes up this smell, which I recognize from grandmothers and elderly aunts, and which hangs in the rooms and halls of old-people's homes like a curse. Hanna was too young for it.

I moved closer. I had seen that I had disappointed her before, and I wanted to do better, make up for it.

'I'm glad you're getting out.'

'You are?'

'Yes, and I'm glad you'll be nearby.' I told her about the flat and the job I had found for her, about the cultural and social programmes available in that part of the city, about the public library. 'Do you read a lot?'

'A little. Being read to is nicer.' She looked at me. 'That's over now, isn't it?'

'Why should it be over?' But I couldn't see myself

talking into cassettes for her or meeting her to read aloud. 'I was so glad and so proud of you when you learned to read. And what nice letters you wrote me!' That was true; I had admired her and been glad, because she was reading and she wrote to me. But I could feel how little my admiration and happiness were worth compared to what learning to read and write must have cost Hanna, how meagre they must have been if they could not even get me to answer her, visit her, talk to her. I had granted Hanna a small niche, certainly an important niche, one from which I gained something and for which I did something, but not a place in my life.

But why should I have given her a place in my life? I reacted indignantly against my own bad conscience at the thought that I had reduced her to a niche. 'Didn't you ever think about the things that were discussed at the trial, before the trial? I mean, didn't you ever think about them when we were together, when I was reading to you?'

'Does that bother you very much?' But she didn't wait for an answer. 'I always had the feeling that no one understood me anyway, that no one knew who I was and what made me do this or that. And you know, when no one understands you, then no one can call you to account. Not even the court could call me to account. But the dead can. They understand. They don't even have to have been there, but if they were, they understand even better. Here in prison they were with me a lot. They came every night, whether I wanted them or not. Before the trial I could still chase them away when they wanted to come.'

She waited to see if I had anything to say, but I couldn't think of anything. At first, I wanted to say that I wasn't able to chase anything away. But it wasn't true. You can chase someone away by setting them in a niche.

'Are you married?'

'I was. Gertrud and I have been divorced for many years and our daughter is at boarding school; I hope she won't stay there for the last years of school, and will move in with me.' Now I waited to see if she would say or ask anything. But she was silent. 'I'll pick you up next week, all right?'

'All right.'

'Quietly, or can there be a little noise and hoopla?'

'Quietly.'

'Okay, I'll pick you up quietly, with no music or champagne.'

I stood up, and she stood up. We looked at each other. The bell had rung twice, and the other women had already gone inside. Once again her eyes scanned my face. I took her in my arms, but she didn't feel right.

'Take care, kid.'

'You too.'

So we said goodbye, even before we had to separate inside.

CHAPTER NINE

THE FOLLOWING WEEK WAS PAR-
ticularly busy. I don't remember whether
I was under actual pressure to finish the lecture
I was working on, or only under self-inflicted pressure to
work and succeed.

The idea I had had when I began working on the lecture
was no good. When I began to revise it, where I expected
to find meaning and consistency, I encountered one *non
sequitur* after another. Instead of accepting this, I kept
searching, harassed, obsessed, anxious, as though reality
itself could fail along with my concept of it, and I was
ready to twist or exaggerate or play down my own find-

ings. I got into a state of strange disquiet; I could go to sleep if I went to bed late, but a few hours later I would be wide awake, until I decided to get up and continue reading or writing.

I also did what needed to be done to prepare for Hanna's release. I furnished her apartment with furniture from IKEA and some old pieces, advised the Greek tailor that Hanna would be coming in, and brought my information about social services and educational programmes up to date. I bought groceries, put books on the bookshelves, and hung pictures. I had a gardener come to tidy up the little garden surrounding the terrace outside the living room. I did all this with unnatural haste and doggedness; it was all too much for me.

But it was just enough to prevent me from thinking about my visit to Hanna. Only occasionally, when I was driving my car, or when I was in Hanna's flat, did thoughts of it get the upper hand and trigger memories. I saw her on the bench, her eyes fixed on me, saw her at the swimming pool, her face turned to me, and again had the feeling that I had betrayed her and owed her something. And again I rebelled against this feeling; I accused her, and found it both shabby and too easy, the way she had wriggled out of her guilt. Allowing no one but the dead to demand an accounting, reducing guilt and atonement to insomnia and bad feelings – where did that leave the living? But what I meant was not the living, it was me.

Did I not have my own accounting to demand of her? What about me?

On the afternoon before I was due to pick her up, I called the prison. First I spoke to the governor.

'I'm a bit nervous. You know, normally people aren't released after such long sentences before spending a few hours or days outside. Frau Schmitz refused this. It won't be easy for her.'

Then I spoke to Hanna.

'Think about what we should do tomorrow. Whether you want to go straight home, or whether we might go to the woods or the river.'

'I'll think about it. You're still a big planner, aren't you?'

That annoyed me. It annoyed me the way it did when girlfriends told me I wasn't spontaneous enough, that I operated too much through my head and not enough through my heart.

She could tell by my silence that I was annoyed, and laughed. 'Don't be cross, kid. I didn't mean anything by it.'

I had met Hanna again on the benches as an old woman. She had looked like an old woman and smelled like an old woman. I hadn't noticed her voice at all. Her voice had stayed young.

CHAPTER TEN

*N*EXT MORNING, HANNA WAS DEAD. She had hanged herself at dawn.

When I arrived, I was taken to the governor. I saw her for the first time — a small, thin woman with dark blonde hair and glasses. She seemed insignificant until she began to speak, with force and warmth and a severe gaze and energetic use of both hands and arms. She asked me about my telephone conversation of the night before and the meeting the previous week. Had I picked up any signals, had it made me fear for her? I said no. Indeed, I had had no suspicions or fears that I had ignored.

'How did you get to know each other?'

'We lived in the same neighbourhood.'

She looked at me searchingly, and I saw that I would have to say more.

'We lived in the same neighbourhood and we got to know each other and became friends. When I was a young student, I was at the trial that convicted her.'

'Why did you send Frau Schmitz cassettes?'

I was silent.

'You knew that she was illiterate, didn't you? How did you know?'

I shrugged my shoulders. I didn't see what business the story of Hanna and me was of hers. Tears were filling my chest and throat, and I was afraid I wouldn't be able to speak. I didn't want to cry in front of her.

She must have seen how I was feeling. 'Come with me, I'll show you Frau Schmitz's cell.' She went ahead, but kept turning around to tell me things or explain them to me. Here is where there had been a terrorist attack, here was the sewing shop where Hanna had worked, this is where Hanna once held a sit-down strike until cuts in library funding were revoked, this was the way to the library. She stopped in front of the cell. 'Frau Schmitz didn't pack. You'll see her cell the way she lived in it.'

Bed, closet, table, chair, a shelf on the wall over the table, a sink and toilet in the corner behind the door. Glass bricks instead of window glass. The table was bare. The shelf held books, an alarm clock, a stuffed bear, two mugs, instant coffee, tea caddies, the cassette machine, and on two lower shelves, the cassettes I had made.

'They aren't all here.'

The warden had followed my glance. 'Frau Schmitz always lent some tapes to the aid society for blind prisoners.'

I went over the bookshelf. Primo Levi, Elie Wiesel, Tadeusz Borowski, Jean Améry – the literature of the victims, next to the autobiography of Rudolf Hess, Hannah Arendt's report on Eichmann in Jerusalem, and scholarly literature on the camps.

'Did Hanna read these?'

'Well, she at least ordered them with care. Several years ago I had to get her a general concentration-camp bibliography, and then one or two years ago she asked me to suggest some books on women in the camps, both prisoners and guards; I wrote to the Institute for Contemporary History, and they sent a specialized bibliography. As soon as Frau Schmitz learned to read, she began to read about the concentration camps.'

Above the bed hung many small pictures and slips of paper. I knelt on the bed and read. There were quotations, poems, little articles, even recipes that Hanna had written down or cut out like pictures from newspapers and magazines. 'Spring lets its blue banner flutter through the air again,' 'Cloud shadows fly across the fields' – the poems were all full of delight in nature, and yearning for it, and the pictures showed woods bright with spring, meadows splattered with flowers, autumn foliage and single trees, a pasture by a stream, a cherry tree with ripe red cherries, and autumnal chestnut flamed in yellow and orange. A newspaper photograph showed an older man and a younger man, both in dark suits, shaking hands. In the young one, bowing to the older one, I recognized myself. I was graduating from school, and was getting a prize from the headmaster at the ceremony. That was a long time after Hanna had left the city. Had Hanna, who could not read, subscribed to the local paper in which my photo appeared? In any case she must have gone to some trouble to find out about the photo and get a copy. And had she had it with her during the trial? I felt the tears again in my chest and throat.

'She learned to read with you. She borrowed the books you read on tape out of the library, and followed what she heard, word by word and sentence by sentence. The tape machine couldn't handle all that constant switching on and off, and rewinding and fast-forwarding. It kept breaking down and having to be repaired, and because that required permission, I finally found out what Frau Schmitz was doing. She didn't want to tell me at first; when she also began to write, and asked me for a writing manual, she didn't try to hide it any longer. She was also just proud that she had succeeded, and wanted to share her happiness.'

As she spoke, I had continued to kneel, my eyes on the pictures and notes, fighting back tears. When I turned around and sat down on the bed, she said, 'She so hoped you would write. You were the only one she got mail from, and when the mail was distributed and she said "No letter for me?" she wasn't talking about the packages the tapes came in. Why did you never write?'

I still said nothing. I could not have spoken; all I could have done was to stammer and weep.

She went to the shelf, picked up a tea caddy, sat down next to me, and took a folded sheet of paper from her suit pocket. 'She left a letter for me, a sort of will. I'll read the part that concerns you.' She unfolded the sheet of paper. 'There is still money in the lavender tea caddy. Give it to Michael Berg; he should send it, along with the 7,000 marks in the bank, to the daughter who survived the fire in the church with her mother. She should decide what to do with it. And tell him I said hello.'

So she had not left any message for me. Did she intend to hurt me? Or punish me? Or was her soul so tired that she could only do and write what was absolutely necessary? 'What was she like all those years?' I waited until I could go on. 'And how was she these last few days?'

'For years and years she lived here the way you would live in a convent. As if she had moved here of her own accord and voluntarily subjected herself to our system, as if the rather monotonous work was a sort of meditation. She was greatly respected by the other women, to whom she was friendly but reserved. More than that, she had authority, she was asked for her advice when there were problems, and if she intervened in an argument, her decision was accepted. Then a few years ago she gave up. She had always taken care of herself personally, she was slender despite her strong build, and meticulously clean. But now she began to eat a lot and seldom washed; she got fat and smelled. She didn't seem unhappy or dissatisfied. In fact it was as though the retreat to the convent was no longer enough, as though life in the convent was still too sociable and talkative, and she had to retreat even further, into a lonely cell safe from all eyes, where looks, clothing, and smell meant nothing. No, it would be wrong to say that she had given up. She redefined her place in a way that was right for her, but no longer impressed the other women.'

'And the last days?'

'She was the way she always was.'

'Can I see her?'

She nodded, but remained seated. 'Can the world become so unbearable to someone after years of lone-liness? Is it better to kill yourself than to return to the world from the convent, from the hermitage?' She turned to me. 'Frau Schmitz didn't write anything about why she was going to kill herself. And you won't say what there was between you that might have led to Frau Schmitz's killing herself at the end of the night before you were due to pick her up.' She folded the piece of paper, put it away, stood up, and smoothed her skirt. 'Her death is a blow to me, you see, and at the moment I'm very angry, with Frau Schmitz, and with you. But let's go.'

She led the way again, this time silently. Hanna lay in the infirmary in a small cubicle. We could just fit between the wall and the stretcher. The warden pulled back the sheet.

A cloth had been tied around Hanna's head to hold up her chin until the onset of rigor mortis. Her face was neither particularly peaceful nor particularly agonized. It looked rigid and dead. As I looked and looked, the living face became visible in the dead, the young in the old. This is what must happen to old married couples, I thought: the young man is preserved in the old one for her, the beauty and grace of the young woman stay fresh in the old one for him. Why had I not seen this reflection a week ago?

I must not cry. After a time, when the governor looked at me questioningly, I nodded, and she spread the sheet over Hanna's face again.

CHAPTER ELEVEN

*I*T WAS AUTUMN BEFORE I COULD carry out Hanna's instructions. The daughter lived in New York, and I used a meeting in Boston as the occasion to bring her the money: a bank cheque plus the tea caddy with the cash. I had written to her, introduced myself as a legal historian, and mentioned the trial. I told her I would be grateful for a chance to talk to her. She invited me to tea.

I took the train from Boston to New York. The woods were a triumphal parade of brown, yellow, orange, tawny red, and chestnut, and the flaming glowing scarlet of the maples. It made me think of the autumn pictures in

Hanna's cell. When the rhythm of the wheels and the rocking of the car tired me, I dreamed of Hanna and myself in a house in the autumn-blazed hills that were lining our route. Hanna was older than when I had met her and younger than when I had met her again, older than me, more attractive than in earlier years, more relaxed in her movements with age, more at home in her own body. I saw her getting out of the car and picking up shopping bags, saw her going through the garden into the house, saw her set down the bags and go upstairs ahead of me. My longing for Hanna became so strong that it hurt. I struggled against the longing, argued that it went against Hanna's and my reality, the reality of our ages, the reality of our circumstances. How could Hanna, who spoke no English, live in America? And she couldn't drive a car either.

I woke up and knew that Hanna was dead. I also knew that my desire had fixed on her without her being its object. It was the desire to come home.

The daughter lived in New York on a street near Central Park. The street was lined on both sides with old row houses of dark sandstone, with front steps of the same sandstone leading up to the door on the first floor. This created an effect of severity — house after house with almost identical façades, front steps after front steps, trees only recently planted at regular intervals along the pavement, with a few yellowing leaves on thin twigs.

The daughter served tea by large windows looking

out on the pocket-sized back gardens, some green and colourful and some merely collections of rubbish. As soon as we had sat down, the tea had been poured, and the sugar added and stirred, she switched from the English in which she had welcomed me, to German. 'What brings you here?' The question was neither friendly nor unfriendly; her tone was absolutely matter-of-fact. Everything about her was matter-of-fact: her manner, her gestures, her dress. Her face was oddly ageless, the way faces look after being lifted. But perhaps it had set because of her early sufferings; I tried and failed to remember her face as it had been during the trial.

I told her about Hanna's death and her last wishes.

'Why me?'

'I suppose because you are the only survivor.'

'And how am I supposed to deal with it?'

'However you think fit.'

'And grant Frau Schmitz her absolution?'

At first I wanted to protest, but Hanna was indeed asking a great deal. Her years of imprisonment were not merely to be the required atonement: Hanna wanted to give them her own meaning, and she wanted this giving of meaning to be recognized. I said as much.

She shook her head. I didn't know if this meant she was refusing to accept my interpretation or refusing to grant Hanna the recognition.

'Could you not recognize it without granting her absolution?'

She laughed. 'You like her, don't you? What was your relationship?'

I hesitated a moment. 'I read aloud to her. It started when I was fifteen and continued while she was in prison.'

'How did you . . .'

'I sent her tapes. Frau Schmitz was illiterate almost all her life; she only learned to read and write in prison.'

'Why did you do all this?'

'When I was fifteen, we had a relationship.'

'You mean you slept together?'

'Yes.'

'That woman was truly brutal . . . what kind of a jolt did it give you, that you were only fifteen when she . . . No, you said yourself that you began reading to her again when she was in prison. Did you ever get married?'

I nodded.

'And the marriage was short and unhappy, and you never married again, and the child, if there is one, is at boarding school.'

'That's true of thousands of people, it doesn't take a Frau Schmitz.'

'Did you ever feel, when you had contact with her in those last years, that she knew what she had done to you?'

I shrugged my shoulders. 'In any case, she knew what she had done to people in the camp and on the march. She didn't just tell me that, she dealt with it intensively during her last years in prison.' I told her what the warden had said.

She stood up and took long strides up and down the room. 'How much money is it?'

I went to the coat cupboard, where I had left my bag, and returned with the cheque and the tea caddy. 'Here.'

She looked at the cheque and put it on the table. She opened the caddy, emptied it, closed it again, and held it in her hand, her eyes riveted on it. 'When I was a little girl, I had a tea caddy for my treasures. Not like this, although these sorts of tea caddies already existed, but one with Cyrillic letters, not one with a top you push in, but one you snap shut. I brought it with me to the camp, but then one day it was stolen from me.'

'What was in it?'

'What you'd expect. A piece of hair from our poodle. Tickets to the operas my father took me to, a ring I won somewhere or found in a package – the caddy wasn't stolen for what was in it. The caddy itself, and what could be done with it, were worth a lot in the camp.' She put the caddy down on top of the cheque. 'Do you have a suggestion for what to do with the money? Using it for something to do with the Holocaust would really seem like an absolution to me, and that is something I neither wish nor care to grant.'

'For illiterates who want to learn to read and write. There must be non-profit organizations, foundations, societies you could give the money to.'

'I'm sure there are.' She thought about it.

'Are there corresponding Jewish organizations?'

'You can depend on it, if there are organizations for something, then there are Jewish organizations for it. Illiteracy, it has to be admitted, is hardly a Jewish problem.' She pushed the cheque and the money back to me. 'Let's do it this way. You find out what kind of relevant Jewish organizations there are, here or in Germany, and you pay the money to the account of the organization that seems most plausible to you.' She laughed. 'If the recognition is so important, you can do it in the name of Hanna Schmitz.' She picked up the caddy again. 'I'll keep the caddy.'

CHAPTER TWELVE

ALL THIS HAPPENED TEN YEARS AGO. In the first few years after Hanna's death, I was tormented by the old questions of whether I had denied and betrayed her, whether I owed her something, whether I was guilty for having loved her. Sometimes I asked myself if I was responsible for her death. And sometimes I was in a rage at her and at what she had done to me. Until finally the rage faded and the questions ceased to matter. Whatever I had done or not done, whatever she had done or not to me — it was the path my life had taken.

Soon after her death, I decided to write the story of

me and Hanna. Since then I've done it many times in my head, each time a little differently, each time with new images, and new strands of action and thought. Thus there are many different stories in addition to the one I have written. The guarantee that the written one is the right one lies in the fact that I wrote it and not the other versions. The written version wanted to be written, the many others did not.

At first I wanted to write our story in order to be free of it. But the memories wouldn't come back for that. Then I realized our story was slipping away from me and I wanted to recapture it by writing, but that didn't coax up the memories either. For the last few years I've left our story alone. I've made peace with it. And it came back, detail by detail and in such a fully rounded fashion, with its own direction and its own sense of completion, that it no longer makes me sad. What a sad story, I thought for so long. Not that I now think it was happy. But I think it is true, and thus the question of whether it is sad or happy has no meaning whatever.

At any rate, that's what I think when I just happen to think about it. But if something hurts me, the hurts I suffered back then come back to me, and when I feel guilty, the feelings of guilt return; if I yearn for something today, or feel homesick, I feel the yearnings and home-sickness from back then. The geological layers of our lives rest so tightly one on top of the other that we always come up against earlier events in later ones, not as matter

that has been fully formed and pushed aside, but absolutely present and alive. I understand this. Nevertheless,
I sometimes find it hard to bear. Maybe I did write our
story to be free of it, even if I never can be.

As soon as I returned from New York, I donated
Hanna's money in her name to the Jewish League Against
Illiteracy. I received a short, computer-generated letter
in which the Jewish League thanked Ms Hanna Schmitz
for her donation. With the letter in my pocket, I drove
to the cemetery, to Hanna's grave. It was the first and
only time I stood there.

The Reader

READING GROUP NOTES

IN BRIEF

*S*et in post-war Germany, *The Reader* begins as an erotic love story but later becomes a philosophical enquiry into the effects of the Holocaust on a generation whose parents are perceived as at best complicit, at worst perpetrators. Central to the novel is the question: what is to be done with the knowledge and the guilt of the Holocaust?

When Michael Berg is taken ill on his way home from school a stranger helps him out. After a winter spent sick with hepatitis, Michael's mother sends him to thank the stranger. Finding his way into Hanna's house, he surprises her when she arrives home. While she changes out of her work clothes, Michael watches through the crack of the door, running away when she catches his eye. He returns and their affair begins.

When Hanna asks Michael to read to her it soon becomes an essential part of their routine. Then one day Hanna disappears.

When Michael next sees her, he is a law student and she is on trial for her part in a war crime. During a bombing raid, while guarding a group of women in transit between camps, Hanna and her fellow SS guards locked the women inside a church. All but two were burnt to death. The author of the report describing this terrible event is considered the most culpable defendant. Hanna refuses to deny that she wrote it despite the fact that, as Michael has finally realised, she is illiterate.

Michael is faced with a dilemma: if he convinces the judge of Hanna's illiteracy she will be given a lighter sentence, but given that she is too proud to confess it herself, would she want it exposed? He seeks advice but eventually lets it go and when Hanna is sentenced to life he is haunted by guilt. His marriage fails after five years and he struggles to find some sort of meaning in his work. Eventually, he begins to record his favourite books for Hanna. When the prison governor writes to tell him that Hanna will soon be leaving prison, he visits her for the first, and last, time.

ABOUT THE AUTHOR

*B*ernhard Schlink was born in Germany in 1944. A professor of law at the University of Berlin and former judge, he is the author of the major international bestseller *Flights of Love*, and several prize-winning crime novels. His latest novel, *Homecoming*, is also available from Orion. He lives in Berlin.

FOR DISCUSSION

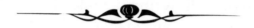

• Who do you think 'the reader' of the title is, or can it be applied to more than one character? At what point was it apparent to you that Hanna was illiterate? What is the importance of literacy in the book?

• How would you describe the tone and style of Bernhard Schlink's writing in part one of the book? How does it differ from the second and third parts? What effect does this difference achieve?

• The relationship between Hanna and Michael begins with an act of kindness on her part but we later learn of her involvement in the concentration camps. Does Hanna engage your sympathy at any point after you found out that she was a camp guard? On pages 131–132, Michael suggests reasons why Hanna became a guard and for her selection of girls to read to her. How convincing are his arguments? How can we explain why ordinary people commit atrocities without resorting to calling them monsters?

• Why does Michael find it so difficult to make his relationship with women work? How does the affair with Hanna affect him as an adolescent?

• On page 133, Michael says, 'And if I was not guilty because one cannot be guilty of betraying a criminal, then I was guilty of having loved a criminal'. Michael did not know of Hanna's crime during their affair so why does he feel guilty? How do other characters of his generation appear to feel about the Holocaust? What about his father's generation?

• On page 146–147, Michael refers to the many images that have been produced of the camps, particularly in films. Is there a danger that the continued exposure of Holocaust images lessens their impact until they become frozen into clichés, as Michael suggests? How do you feel about the images of war which are recorded in the newspapers and on television?

• Is Hanna a scapegoat just for her co-defendants or in a more general way? When she turns to the judge and asks him what he would have done in her position (page 110), what does his answer imply? Could the judge be considered as guilty as Hanna if he knew about the camps but did nothing?

• Why do you think Hanna does what she does at the end of the novel? How do you think learning to read might have changed her view of what she had done in the camps?

• Does the novel answer the question posed on page 102: 'What should our second generation have done, what should it do with the knowledge of the horrors of the extermination of the Jews?' What do you think the answer might be or is it an unanswerable question?

• Does the novel give any grounds for hopes of forgiveness, and if so what are they?

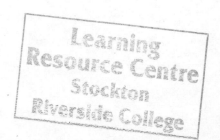

SUGGESTED FURTHER READING

NOVELS

Crime and Punishment by Fyodor Dostoevsky
War Story by Gwen Edelman
The Tin Drum by Gunter Grass
Stones from the River by Ursula Hegi
Schindler's List by Thomas Keneally
The Twins by Tessa de Loo
Fugitive Pieces by Anne Michaels
The Dark Room by Rachel Seiffert
Sophie's Choice by William Styron
Everything is Illuminated by Jonathan Safran Foer

NON-FICTION

Eichmann in Jerusalem by Hannah Arendt
    (History)

If This is a Man / The Truce by Primo Levi
    (Autobiography)

The Holocaust and Collective Memory by
    Peter Novick (History)

Night by Elie Weisel (Autobiography)

OTHER BOOKS BY BERNHARD SCHLINK

Flights of Love

Self's Punishment (writing as Thomas Richter)

All Orion/Phoenix titles are available at your local bookshop or from the following address:

> Mail Order Department
> Littlehampton Book Services
> FREEPOST BR535
> Worthing, West Sussex, BN13 3BR
> *telephone* 01903 828503, *facsimile* 01903 828802
> *e-mail* MailOrders@lbsltd.co.uk
> (Please ensure that you include full postal address details)

Payment can be made either by credit/debit card (Visa, Mastercard, Access and Switch accepted) or by sending a £ Sterling cheque or postal order made payable to *Littlehampton Book Services*.
DO NOT SEND CASH OR CURRENCY.

Please add the following to cover postage and packing

UK and BFPO:
£1.50 for the first book, and 50p for each additional book to a maximum of £3.50

Overseas and Eire:
£2.50 for the first book plus £1.00 for the second book and 50p for each additional book ordered

---

BLOCK CAPITALS PLEASE

name of cardholder ....

address of cardholder ....

delivery address
(if different from cardholder)

....

....

postcode ....

postcode ....

☐ I enclose my remittance for £...........................

☐ please debit my Mastercard/Visa/Access/Switch (delete as appropriate)

card number ☐☐☐☐ ☐☐☐☐ ☐☐☐☐ ☐☐☐☐

expiry date ☐☐☐☐   Switch issue no. ☐☐